UNLOCKING
MEDICAL LAW
AND ETHICS

Claudia Carr

UNLOCKING THE LAW

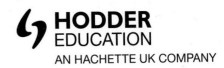

HODDER
EDUCATION
AN HACHETTE UK COMPANY

Orders: please contact Bookpoint Ltd, 130 Milton Park, Abingdon, Oxon OX14 4SB.
Telephone: (44) 01235 827720. Fax: (44) 01235 400454. Lines are open from 9.00 - 5.00,
Monday to Saturday, with a 24 hour message answering service. You can also order through
our website www.hoddereducation.co.uk

If you have any comments to make about this, or any of our other titles, please send them to
educationenquiries@hodder.co.uk

British Library Cataloguing in Publication Data
A catalogue record for this title is available from the British Library

ISBN: 978 1 444 12095 0

First Edition Published 2012
Impression number   10 9 8 7 6 5 4 3 2 1
Year   2015 2014 2013 2012

Copyright © 2012 Claudia Carr

Hachette Livre UK's policy is to use papers that are natural, renewable and
recyclable products and made from wood grown in sustainable forests.
The logging and manufacturing processes are expected to conform to the
environmental regulations of the country of origin.

Cover photo © Thomas Perkins/iStockphoto.com
Typeset by Datapage India Pvt Ltd
Printed in Italy for Hodder Education, an Hachette UK Company,
338 Euston Road, London NW1 3BH

Contents

3   MENTAL HEALTH LAW   81

Dedication

This book is dedicated to the memory of my brother Lloyd Carr (Aviv Carmel) and with love and thanks to my husband John Rose and children Ella and Hannah for their unconditional and never ending love and support.

Guide to the book

In the Unlocking the Law books all the essential elements that make up the law are clearly defined to bring the law alive and make it memorable. In addition, the books are enhanced with learning features to reinforce learning and test your knowledge as you study. Follow this guide to make sure you get the most from reading this book.

AIMS AND OBJECTIVES

Defines what you will learn in each chapter.

definition
Find key legal terminology at-a-glance.

SECTION

Highlights sections from Acts.

ARTICLE

Defines Articles of the EC Treaty or of the European Convention on Human Rights or other Treaty.

CLAUSE

Shows a Bill going through Parliament or a draft Bill proposed by the Law Commission.

CASE EXAMPLE

 Illustrates the law in action.

JUDGMENT

Provides extracts from judgments on cases.

Indicates that you will be able to test yourself further on this topic using the Key Questions and Answers section of this book on www. unlockingthelaw. co.uk.

QUOTATION

Encourages you to engage with primary sources.

ACTIVITY

Enables you to test yourself as you progress through the chapter.

SAMPLE ESSAY QUESTIONS

Provide you with real-life sample essays and show you the best way to plan your answer.

SUMMARY

Concludes each chapter to reinforce learning.

Preface

The 'Unlocking' series is designed to make learning each subject area more accessible by focusing on learning needs, and by providing a range of different supporting materials and features.

All topic areas are broken up into 'bite size' sections with a logical progression and extensive use of headings and numerous sub-headings. Each book in the series also contains a variety of charts, diagrams and key fact summaries to reinforce the information in the body of the text. Diagrams and flow charts are particularly useful because they can provide a quick and easy understanding of the key points, especially when revising for examinations. Key facts charts not only provide a quick visual guide through the subject but are useful for revision purposes also.

The books have a number of common features in the layout. Important cases are separated out for easy access and have full citation in the text as well as the table of cases for ease of reference. The emphasis of the series is on depth of understanding much more than breadth. For this reason each text also includes key extracts from judgments where appropriate. Extracts from academic comment from journal articles and leading texts are also included to give some insight into the debates on complex or controversial areas. In both cases these are indented to make them clear from the body of the text.

Finally, the books also include much formative 'self-testing', with a variety of activities including subject specific comprehension and application of the law amongst others to help the student gain a good idea of his or her progress in the course.

Medical law and ethics is a relatively new area of law that is growing in complexity by the day. Controversial and contemporary, medical law and ethics often acts as a reflection of our own society, as it is hoped does the material in the book. Throughout the book, the medical professional is referred to as 'he' and the patient as 'she'. Whilst the stereotypical nature of the analogy is regretted, the descriptions are accepted and commonplace.

The first part of the book considers the law. The book begins with an introduction to Medical Negligence before moving onto the issue of Consent in Chapter 2. Mental Health Law is considered in Chapter 3, where it is recognised that a book of this depth cannot do true justice to such a complex area. From there we concentrate on Resource Allocation or rationing of NHS resources, where there is a consideration of the controversial Health and Social Care Bill 2011. After Confidentiality, the book then moves on to consider medical ethics and begins with a discussion of the prevailing medical theories and illustrates their application with issues considered throughout the book, in order that the role of ethical theories can be appreciated in isolation. We move from birth to death throughout this part of the book and in Assisted Conception discuss cloning, Pre-implantation Genetic Diagnosis (PGD), sex selection, 'saviour siblings' and surrogacy. These issues are contemporary, ongoing and steeped in ethical argument. After Abortion we explore Organ Transplantation, an area brought to life by the question of whether it is ethically acceptable to sell a kidney. End of life decisions and assisted suicide are never far from the gaze of the press and Assisted Suicide discusses the current law and ethics in as much depth as the book allows. The recent case of *W (by her litigation friend, B) v M (by her litigation friend, the Official Solicitor) and S and A NHS Primary Care Trust)* [2011] EWHC 2443 is included in order to chart the development of the law in relation to withholding and withdrawing medical treatment from an incompetent patient. It is hoped that the reader will find this area of the law fascinating and the book truly engaging.

The law is stated as we believe it to be on 1st December 2011.

Claudia Carr

Table of Cases

Table of Statutes and other Legislation

1

Medical negligence

After reading this chapter you should be able to:

- Understand how and when a duty of care is established
- Understand and appreciate what amounts to the legal standard of care
- Understand and appreciate the common law test for breach of duty of care
- Understand and appreciate subsequent decisions and how they have been subsequently applied (appreciate the effect of the case of *Bolitho* on the *Bolam* test)
- Appreciate the complexity of the common law in the area of causation and understand the difficulties that arise in this area in medical negligence claims
- Be able to apply duty of care and breach of duty of care together with causation to a hypothetical situation

1.1 Part 1: Introduction to medical negligence

The study of medical negligence is about the legal consequences where a medical professional negligently treats a patient. Here, we are concerned with the civil law, although there can be criminal consequences, albeit rarely. The prevailing issue is whether the claimant will be able to recover damages or compensation for the negligent act caused to them. In order to establish this, we must consider duty of care, breach of duty of care, causation and remoteness.

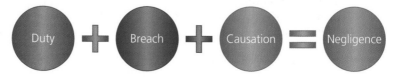

Figure 1.1 The acts which result in negligence

---

claimant

the aggrieved patient himself/herself, or a person claiming on their behalf

---

defendant

the person against whom the claim is brought

For a **claimant** (either the aggrieved patient himself/herself, or a person claiming on their behalf) to be able to succeed in an action for negligence, the claimant must be able to establish three elements:

- that she is owed a *duty of care* by the defendant (this will be the team of medical professionals treating the patient)
- that the defendant failed to use reasonable care and skill in treating the claimant and therefore *breached* his duty
- that the **defendant**'s breach *caused* the claimant's injuries and that the injuries sustained are not too *remote*.

Firstly, we will consider the duty of care.

1.2 Duty of care

1.2.1 The principle

You may remember the case of *Caparo Industries plc v Dickman* [1990] 2 AC 605 from your studies of the law of tort. In that case the House of Lords set out the three essential elements to establish whether a defendant owes a claimant a duty of care. The *Caparo* criteria are as follows:

- Was the damage caused to the claimant by the defendant *reasonably foreseeable*?
- Was the relationship between the defendant and the claimant reasonably *proximate*?
- Is it *fair, just and reasonable* to impose a duty of care on the defendant?

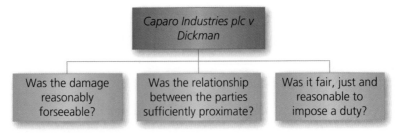

Figure 1.2 The *Caparo* test

The *Caparo* test *only* needs to be applied in a novel duty situation; that is, in cases where the facts are such that they have not fallen for consideration by the courts before. In the case of negligence claims involving medical professionals, it has long been established that they owe their patients a duty of care.

The historical reasoning for why a duty of care is owed by a medical professional to his or her patient is based largely on the approach taken by Lord Atkin in the seminal tort case of *Donoghue v Stevenson* [1932] AC 562.

Lord Atkin held that a person owes a duty of care to another where injury to that person is reasonably foreseeable. But how do we define what amounts to reasonably foreseeable?

Lord Atkin explained that one must take care not to injure one's 'neighbour', that is, one who is 'so closely and directly affected by my actions that I ought reasonably to have them in contemplation as being so affected when I am directing my mind to the acts or omissions that are called into question'.

The basic approach is that since any patient is clearly 'closely and directly affected' by their doctor's act, it follows that any doctor 'ought reasonably to have (his patient) within his contemplation' as someone who would be closely and directly affected by their actions. Consequently, any injury caused by a doctor is reasonably foreseeable. Thus, it follows that hospital doctors, nurses and any other staff employed by the Health Authority or Trust owe their patients a duty of care.

It is usually extremely straightforward to establish that a doctor owes a duty of care to his/her patients. He owes a duty of care to *you*, his patient, simply because he is *your* doctor. It can be compared to train drivers or pilots owing a duty of care to their passengers.

We can see the principle in action in the following cases.

CASE EXAMPLE

Pippin v Sheppard (1822) 11 Price 400

The plaintiff's wife sustained injuries that were treated by the defendant. The injuries became inflamed and painful, and further treatment was required.

The defendant surgeon was liable for the worsening injuries caused simply because he had treated her. The court said 'an undertaking to do a thing, even without consideration, creates a liability for negligence and want of due care'. No other reason was required. The treating surgeon lacked the necessary 'due care'.

While we are largely unconcerned with discussing the criminal liability of medical practitioners (which will only be an issue in the rarest of cases), the principle above is supported by the dictum in the criminal gross negligence manslaughter case of *R v Bateman* (1925) 19 Cr App R 18. Lord Hewart CJ famously stated:

JUDGMENT

'If a doctor holds himself out as possessing special skill and knowledge, and he is consulted as possessing such skill and knowledge, by or on behalf of the patient, he owes a duty to the patient to use caution in the undertaking the treatment.'

In contrast, the modern day *Caparo* test will be used in situations where it is more difficult to determine whether a duty of care arises between the claimant and the defendant.

CASE EXAMPLE

Kent v Griffiths [2001] QB 36

A pregnant woman suffered an asthma attack. The emergency services were called and the message was relayed to the ambulance centre. The ambulance took 36 minutes to arrive, even though the journey was only 6.5 miles. The patient lost her baby and suffered brain damage as a result. She sued the ambulance service in negligence.

It was held that the ambulance service owed a duty of care to those who dialled 999. If due to carelessness they fail to reach the caller within a reasonable amount of time and further loss is suffered as a result, the ambulance service will be liable in negligence.

The court's decision to impose liability on the defendant in this case can be easily explained in light of the *Caparo* test discussed above.

Lord Woolf MR explained:

JUDGMENT

'the fact that it was a person who foreseeably would suffer further injuries by a delay in providing an ambulance ... is important in establishing the necessary proximity and thus duty of care in this case ... as there are no circumstances which made it unfair or unreasonable or unjust that liability should exist, there is no reason why there should not be liability if the arrival of the ambulance is delayed for no good reason.'

If we apply the *Caparo* test we can see that a duty was owed to the patient for whom the 999 call was made. The necessary proximity was established as the ambulance was responding to a call to this particular patient, and the courts decided there was no state of affairs that made it unfair, unjust or unreasonable to impose a duty. Therefore, the three elements were satisfied.

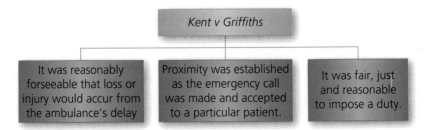

Figure 1.3 The *Caparo* test in action

A distinction was made between the ambulance service and the fire service, as seen in *Capital and Counties v Hants CC* [1996] 1 WLR 1553. A duty of care was owed in *Kent v Griffiths* because the ambulance service had accepted the call to the individual patient whose call they were responding to, whereas in *Capital and Counties v Hants CC* they were responding to the public's need at large.

Any study of the cases governing the courts' approach to determining the existence, or otherwise, of a duty of care will reveal that the courts are keen to keep a realistic check on the scope of an individual's duty of care. The courts state that an individual simply cannot be held to owe a duty of care to the world at large.

Discussion point

It is worth considering whether there are any limitations on the duty of care. Hospital authorities have finite resources (as we will see when we discuss the case of *Bull v Devon Health Authority* [1993] 4 Med LR 117 below), and there may sometimes be difficult decisions to be made about how those limited resources should be allocated between those with competing interests in accessing them. In *Bull v Devon Health Authority* the obstetrician was split over two hospital sites. The result of the Health Authority's decision to allocate their resources in this way resulted in a tragic outcome. In *Kent v Griffiths* (2001) discussed above, Lord Woolf MR indicated that the situation could arise where there could be conflicting interests and if there was a 'conflict in priorities' or an 'allocation of resources' question, different considerations may apply. The suggestion is that a duty may not be breached if an ambulance takes longer than the ideal time to arrive if it is required elsewhere as a priority, or if there are limited available ambulances.

1.2.2 The duty of care owed to a stranger

It is worth pausing to consider what duty a doctor owes a complete stranger, for example a person who may have collapsed in the street or where a person on an aeroplane needs urgent medical attention. English law does not impose a duty upon a person to act as a Good Samaritan. A doctor is not required to respond to a call for help, but if he does so, a duty of care arises.

This ethical limitation on the doctor's duty to act is highlighted in the case of *F v West Berkshire Health Authority* [1990] 2 AC 1, which will be discussed in more detail in Chapter 2, Consent. For current purposes, the key point comes from Lord Goff's judgment where he said:

JUDGMENT

'the doctor in the house who volunteers to assist a lady in the audience who, overcome by the drama or by the heat in the theatre, has fainted away is impelled to act by no greater duty than that imposed by his own Hippocratic Oath'.

Stuart-Smith LJ expressed a similar view in *Capital and Counties v Hants CC* (1996) (albeit the comment was made *obiter*) that a doctor is under no legal obligation to treat a stranger; however, if he chooses to do so and '... volunteers his assistance, his only duty as a matter of law is not to make the victim's condition worse'.

1.2.3 The relationship between GP and patient

While it may be easy to establish that a medical professional owes a duty of care to the patient, we need to explore *when* that duty begins.

You know that your General Practitioner (GP) owes you a duty of care, but when is that duty created? This is quite straightforward: you become the GP's patient as soon as you become registered on the GP list by virtue of the NHS (Choice of Medical Practitioner) Regulations 1998 (amended 1999). However, the duty of care does not arise until the GP becomes aware of your need for medical attention. Therefore when you, as a patient, request the services of a GP, the duty of care comes into existence.

Certain statutory requirements are imposed upon a GP by virtue of the National Health Service (General Medical Services) Regulations 1992 SI 1992/635. Schedule 2, para 4(1)(h) states that a GP is obliged to treat a person if requested to in the event of an accident or other emergency in the area of his practice. This applies if the GP is available to provide such treatment and there is no other doctor available. This however will not apply if the GP, being elderly or infirm or for any other reason, has been relieved of liability to provide treatment.

1.2.4 The relationship between hospital professional and the patient

The essential difference here is that while the doctor/patient relationship discussed above comes into being when the doctor has undertaken to provide the medical services, the case of *Barnett v Chelsea and Kensington Management Committee* (1969) establishes the principle that a duty of care can arise when a patient presents himself at the Accident and Emergency Department, even though that patient may not see a doctor. It was also relevant in this case, that the Casualty Department was open; if it had been closed, then no duty of care would have arisen.

CASE EXAMPLE

Barnett v Chelsea and Kensington Hospital Management Committee [1969] 1 QB 428

Three night watchmen drank tea which contained arsenic. They began to vomit and attended the local Accident and Emergency Department. They were seen by a triage nurse who telephoned the on-call doctor. The doctor did not see them but told them to return home and see their own doctors. One of the men died and his widow brought an action for negligence.

While the action failed for reasons concerning causation that will be discussed later in this chapter, it was held that even though the doctor had not seen the men he still owed them a duty of care.

Nield J stated that:

JUDGMENT

'there was here such a close and direct relationship between the hospital and the watchmen that there was imposed upon the hospital a duty of care which they owed to the watchmen'.

Furthermore, Nield J referred to the earlier case of *Cassidy v Minister of Health* [1951] 1 ALL ER 574 where Denning LJ emphasised that hospital authorities owe the same duty to patients as any doctor. Therefore:

JUDGMENT

'authorities who run a hospital, be they local authorities, government boards or any other corporation, are in law under the self-same duty as the humblest doctor; whenever they accept a patient for treatment they must still use reasonable care and skill to cure him of an ailment.'

Key facts on duty of care

Case or statute	Principle or provision
Donoghue v Stevenson (1932)	Establishes a duty of care between parties: neighbour principle *per* Lord Atkin.
Pippin v Sheppard (1822)	Illustrates one of the earliest cases of a medical professional owing a patient a duty of care.
Caparo Industries plc v Dickman (1990)	Only to be applied in a novel situation (e.g. *Kent v Griffiths* (2001)) but the damage caused must be reasonably foreseeable; the relationship between the parties must be sufficiently proximate; and it must be fair, just and reasonable to impose a duty.
NHS (Choice of Medical Practitioner) Regulations 1998 (amended 1999)	Procedure and provisions relating to patient choice of GP.
National Health Service (General Medical Services) Regulations 1992 SI 1992/635, Schedule 2, para 4(1)(h)	Obligation imposed upon GPs to treat.
F v West Berkshire Health Authority (1990) *Capital and Counties v Hants CC* (1996)	Illustrates limited duty imposed upon a doctor to assist a stranger.
Barnett v Chelsea and Kensington Hospital Management Committee (1969)	A duty of care was owed by the hospital doctor to the patient who presented himself at Accident and Emergency Department.
Cassidy v Minister of Health (1951)	The same duty is owed by hospital doctors as any other doctor.

1.2.5 The relationship between doctors and third parties

So far, there has been little difficulty is establishing when a duty of care exists, even if it has not always been obvious at first! One of the key problem areas which remains in medical negligence claims (in the context of issues relating to duties of care at least) is the question of whether a medical professional owes a duty of care to those harmed by the actions of their patients.

These claims seem to fall into three key categories:

- claims for wrongful conception
- claims for failure to warn of possible harms, and
- claims for psychiatric injury.

The essence in each of these claims is that the third party has suffered some form of harm which they allege was caused by the negligent way in which the medical professional handled their patient. As will be seen, the success of such claims, or otherwise, seems to hinge entirely upon whether the court takes the view that there was sufficient proximity between the claimant and the defendant medical professional.

Claims for wrongful conception

The need for proximity in such claims is neatly illustrated by comparing the decisions in *Thake v Maurice* (1986) and *Goodwill v British Pregnancy Advisory Service* (1996).

CASE EXAMPLE

Thake v Maurice [1986] QB 644

The plaintiff underwent a **vasectomy**. The defendant failed to warn either the husband (patient) or his wife of the risk of spontaneous reversal of the vasectomy. The couple stopped using contraception but the wife became pregnant. The wife tried to claim damages on the basis that she was owed a duty of care.

The Court of Appeal held that a duty of care existed between the parties because it was reasonably foreseeable that the wife could become pregnant if the vasectomy failed to be effective. As such, there was sufficient proximity and a duty of care was owed.

Whether there is a sufficient relationship of proximity between the defendant and the claimant can depend on the facts of the case. The more direct the relationship is between the parties, the more likely it is that a duty of care will be inferred.

CASE EXAMPLE

Goodwill v British Pregnancy Advisory Service [1996] 2 ALL ER 161

A man underwent a vasectomy performed by the defendant. He was advised that the operation was successful and it was unnecessary to use contraception. He met the claimant some three years after his operation. They had sexual intercourse without any contraception and the claimant became pregnant. The claimant alleged that the defendant had been negligent in failing to advise her partner of the risk that the vasectomy might reverse itself and that he may become fertile once more. The question was whether there was a sufficiently proximate relationship between the claimant and the defendants to establish a duty of care.

The court held the defendant did not owe the claimant a duty of care. The claimant was not in a relationship with the patient at the time of the operation. The British Pregnancy Advisory Service (BPAS) owed a duty of care to the patient who underwent the operation and any partner whom he was with at the time of the operation. The defendant did not owe a duty of care to any partner whom the claimant subsequently had a relationship with as it would not have been foreseeable to the defendant that the claimant might suffer harm if they were negligent in the treatment of their patient. There was insufficient proximity between the claimant and the defendant.

The court will only impose a duty of care in those circumstances where it was foreseeable that the claimant might suffer harm as a result of the defendant's actions, because it is only in such situations that the defendants will be in a position to take steps to protect the claimant from possible harm.

Claims for failure to warn of possible harm

CASE EXAMPLE

Palmer v Tees Health Authority [1999] EWCA Civ 1533

A man with extensive psychiatric problems abducted, sexually abused and killed the claimant's young daughter. Prior to his release the patient had warned that he would harm a child. The claimant argued that the defendants had failed to identify the extent of the risk which the man posed to her daughter, and therefore the defendant should be held liable in negligence for the child's death.

While the injuries caused to a child might have been reasonably foreseeable, there was a lack of proximity between the health authority and the claimant's daughter. The category of potential victims in this case was large and there was no evidence which would have identified Mrs Palmer's daughter as being at particular risk of harm. It would have placed an excessive burden on the defendants to try and protect all the children in the area potentially at risk. On this basis the court decided that it was not fair, just or reasonable to impose a duty of care on the defendants.

vasectomy

a surgical procedure for male sterilisation

Claims for psychiatric injury

The courts have been reluctant to impose liability on defendants where psychiatric damage has been caused to a third party as a result of the defendant's negligence. This will usually be as a result of witnessing the negligent treatment of a patient or of witnessing its immediate consequences. The problem in such cases, however, is that it is often difficult to determine whether there is sufficient proximity between the defendant and the person who suffers the injury, and whether it might be considered fair, just and reasonable to impose such a duty.

CASE EXAMPLE

JD (FC) v East Berkshire Community Health NHS Trust [2005] UKHL 23

Parents had been accused by healthcare professionals of abusing or harming their children. The allegations were based on negligent diagnosis of injuries sustained by the children. It was suggested that the injuries were intentionally inflicted. The negligent diagnosis had resulted in psychiatric injury caused to the parents. It was argued that the Trust owed a duty of care not only to the child but to the parents as well.

While the Trust owed a duty of care to the child, the duty did not extend to the parents. The decision turned on the application of *Caparo* and the House of Lords held that it was not fair, just and reasonable to impose a policy, as healthcare professionals should not be under a conflict of duties when determining whether a child had been abused.

A series of attempts to recover damages for psychiatric injury followed the tragic events at the Hillsborough football stadium in 1989, in which 96 football fans died. The cases which followed led to the development of limited principles which would govern claims for recovery of damages for psychiatric illness allegedly caused by a defendant's negligence.

The seminal tortious case of *Alcock v Chief Constable of South Yorkshire* [1992] 4 ALL ER 907 (see Turner, C. and Hodge, S. (2010) *Unlocking Torts*, third edition. London: Hodder Education, page 124 for a more detailed discussion) set down three elements that had to be satisfied in order to establish whether the injury sustained was foreseeable.

1. There has to be sufficient proximity in the relationship between the victim and the claimant; that is, there needed to be a close tie of love and affection between the victim and the claimant.
2. There has to be sufficient proximity in time and space between the claimant and the event which caused the psychiatric harm suffered by the claimant; that is, the claimant must have seen or heard the event or its immediate aftermath.
3. The psychiatric harm was caused by seeing or hearing the event or its immediate aftermath; there needed to be a causal link between witnessing the event and the harm suffered.

Subsequent cases have also suggested that the claimant will only be able to recover damages where:

1. It was reasonably foreseeable that a person of normal fortitude in the claimant's position might suffer psychiatric harm, and
2. The damage was caused as the result of a sudden, shocking event.

Claimants in early cases, such as *Sion v Hampstead Health Authority* (1994) and *Taylor v Somerset Health Authority* (1993), failed on the grounds that the courts were not satisfied that the *Alcock* criteria were fulfilled.

CASE EXAMPLES

Sion v Hampstead Health Authority [1994] 5 Med LR 170

The courts were unwilling to allow a claim where the father's psychiatric illness was brought on as a result of watching his son die over a two-week period. While the claimant could clearly establish a close relationship, the action failed as the harm had not been caused by a sudden, shocking event. The court felt that, sadly, the child's death was an expected event.

CASE EXAMPLE

Taylor v Somerset Health Authority [1993] 4 Med LR 34

The deceased died from a heart attack as a result of the defendant's negligence. The defendants had been treating the victim for some years, but had negligently failed to diagnose his heart condition. His widow was told he had died and it was necessary for her to identify her husband's body. She went on to develop a psychiatric illness for which she claimed damages. The court dismissed the claim on the grounds that Mrs Taylor could not satisfy the requirement for the claimant to have witnessed the death itself or its immediate aftermath. According to Auld J there were two factors necessary if a claimant was to succeed in fulfilling this element of the test, namely:

1. An external, traumatic event caused by the defendant's breach of duty which immediately causes some personal injury or death; and
2. A perception by the claimant of the event as it happens, normally by his presence at the scene, or exposure to the scene and/or to the primary victim so shortly afterwards that the shock of the event as well as of its consequences is brought home to him.

Mrs Taylor's claim could not satisfy these requirements. Mr Taylor died at work and was subsequently transferred to the hospital. Once there, it was a full hour before Mrs Taylor was informed of her husband's death. Furthermore, Mrs Taylor already knew that her husband was dead by the time she saw his body in the mortuary. When considered together, the events show that there was not the immediacy between the traumatic event and the discovery of death needed to give rise to a claim for nervous shock.

In contrast, in the case of *Tredget & Tredget v Bexley Health Authority* (1994) the Courts sought not to draw a distinction between the trauma of the horrifying event and the subsequent death.

CASE EXAMPLE

Tredget & Tredget v Bexley Health Authority [1994] 5 Med LR 178

The defendant delivered Mrs Tredget's baby in such a way that he was severely deprived of oxygen and died two days later. The delivery of baby Callum was steeped in 'chaos' and 'pandemonium'. Both Mr and Mrs Tredget were able to recover damages for psychiatric illness. The Court opined that the circumstances of the baby's birth, the recognition of his condition, followed by his subsequent death were part of the same event, even though they lasted for some 48 hours. It was unrealistic to separate and distinguish one traumatic event from the other.

CASE EXAMPLE

Froggatt v Chesterfield and North Derbyshire Royal Hospital NHS Trust [2002] All ER 218

mastectomy
a surgical procedure for the removal of one or both of a woman's breasts

Mrs Froggatt, a young mother, had been misdiagnosed breast cancer when an overworked pathologist mixed up tissue samples. She underwent an unnecessary **mastectomy**, suffering pain and distress as a result.

Her husband was able to recover damages for the psychiatric illness he suffered as a result of seeing his wife undressed for the first time. Her son, who was ten years old, was also able to recover damages for being told the news that his mother had been diagnosed with breast cancer and was likely to die as a result.

The case of *Froggatt v Chesterfield and North Derbyshire Royal Hospital NHS Trust* (2002) demonstrates the courts' increased willingness to allow a claim for damages for psychiatric illness or nervous shock. It has been labelled a claimant-friendly decision on the basis that the judge appears to have adopted a very generous interpretation of the requirement from *Alcock*.

The court also allowed the claimant in *North Glamorgan NHS Trust v Walters* (2002) to recover damages for psychiatric illness.

CASE EXAMPLE

North Glamorgan NHS Trust v Walters [2002] EWCA Civ 1792

This catalogue of events began when the claimant, a mother who was in hospital with her baby, woke to find the baby was suffering a fit. The fit was caused by the defendant's negligent treatment. The baby suffered brain damage as a direct result of that negligence and died in the claimant's arms within 36 hours.

The potential difficulty for the claimant in this claim was that there was a delay of 36 hours between the negligent act which caused the baby's brain damage, and the baby's eventual death which caused the claimant to suffer a pathological grief reaction.

Nevertheless the court held that in spite of the delay between the two events, the claimant's psychiatric injury could still be said to have been the result of a sudden, shocking event. According to the Court of Appeal the 36-hour period from the child's seizure to his death could be viewed as a seamless ongoing experience.

However, despite the above cases which illustrate the courts' willingness to allow claims for psychiatric illness where the defendants have acted negligently, the courts will ensure that the *Alcock* criteria is satisfied before a claim can be allowed and damages recovered.

KEY FACTS

Key facts on relationship between doctors and third parties

Case	Principle
Thake v Maurice (1986)	Sufficient proximity between the wife of the patient and the defendant for a duty of care to arise.
Goodwill v British Pregnancy Advisory Service (1996)	Insufficient proximity between the claimant and the defendant to establish a duty of care.
Palmer v Tees Health Authority (1999)	A lack of proximity between the victim and the defendant meant it was not fair, just or reasonable to impose a duty of care.
Sion v Hampstead Health Authority (1994)	Damages for psychiatric illness could not be recovered as the damage was not caused by a sudden shocking event.
Taylor v Somerset Health Authority (1993)	Damages for psychiatric illness could not be recovered as the claimant had not witnessed the death itself or the immediate aftermath.
Tredget and Tredget v Bexley Health Authority (1994)	Damages for psychiatric illness could be recovered as the baby's birth and death were treated as one continuing event.
Froggatt v Chesterfield and North Derbyshire Royal Hospital NHS Trust (2002)	Damages for psychiatric illness could be recovered.
North Glamorgan NHS Trust v Walters (2003)	Damages for psychiatric illness could be recovered despite a delay between the baby's birth and death.

1.2.6 Who can a potential claimant sue?

Assuming that the claimant has a case which has a reasonable chance of success, the question still remains, 'who to sue?' There appear to be three possible defendants:

- The medical professional treating the claimant may be sued **directly**.
- Under the doctrine of vicarious liability, the claimant may sue the treating medical professional's **employer**.
- The claimant may sue the **provider** of the medical services directly.

Suing the individual medical practitioner directly

It has been suggested that 'a lawyer will usually advise against suing individuals working for NHS bodies directly' (Pattinson, 2006, page 63) largely because that individual is unlikely to have the means available to pay the level of damages which the claimant is likely to be seeking. There is, however, nothing to prevent the claimant pursuing an individual if they wish.

If such an individual is found to be liable, is required to pay compensation to the claimant and is employed by the NHS, then that individual may be indemnified for their losses by the NHS because of the provisions of the NHS indemnity arrangements (Department of Health (1996) *NHS Indemnity: Arrangements for Clinical Negligence Claims in the NHS*, Catalogue number 96 HR 0024).

The position is different however if the defendant is a GP, as they are personally responsible for meeting the costs of litigation and are insured accordingly to meet this risk.

Suing the individual medical professional's employer

Vicarious liability is a legal concept whereby an employer can be held liable for the torts of his employees, providing the torts are committed in the course of their employment (see Turner, C. and Hodge, S. (2010) *Unlocking Torts*, third edition. London: Hodder Education, page 400). There are two requirements that must be satisfied in order for an employer to be held vicariously liable.

- The tort must have been committed by an employee.
- The employee must have committed the tort in the course of their employment.

CASE EXAMPLE

Cassidy v Ministry of Health [1951] 2 KB 343

The defendant hospital was held liable for the negligence of a house surgeon employed as part of the permanent staff. Denning LJ provides the most useful judgment in this case:

JUDGMENT

'In my opinion authorities who run a hospital ... are in law under the self-same duty as the humblest doctor; whenever they accept a patient for treatment, they must use reasonable care and skill to cure him of his ailment. The hospital authorities cannot, of course, do it by themselves: they have no ears to listen through the stethoscope, and no hands to hold the surgeon's knife. They must do it by the staff which they employ; and if their staff are negligent in giving the treatment, they are just as liable for the negligence as anyone else who employs others to do his duties for him ... It is no answer for them to say that their staff are professional men and women who do not tolerate any interference by their lay masters in the way they do their work.'

Lord Justice Denning continues:

JUDGMENT

'I think it depends on this: who employs the doctor or surgeon – is it the patient or the hospital authorities? If the patient himself selects and employs a doctor or surgeon, as in *Hillyer*'s case, the hospital authorities are of course not liable for his negligence, because he is not employed by them. But where the doctor or surgeon, be he a consultant or not, is employed and paid, not by the patient but by the hospital authorities, I am of the opinion that the hospital authorities are liable for his negligence in treating the patient. It does not depend on whether the contract under which he was employed was a contract of service or a contract for services. That is a fine distinction which is sometimes of importance; but not in cases such as the present, where the hospital authorities are themselves under a duty to use care in treating the patient.'

In short, what Lord Justice Denning does in that section of his judgment is make it clear that were the patient to have been injured as the result of a medical practitioner's negligence, and that medical practitioner was employed by a hospital, it is open for that employer to be held vicariously liable for the negligent actions of its employees.

Suing the healthcare provider directly

On occasions, the NHS Trust or other public unit provider may also be held liable for breach of its primary duty; for example, if there has been a failure to provide staff who possess a reasonable level of skill and care (see *Wilsher v Essex Area Health Authority* [1987] 1 QB 730) or if there has been a failure to ensure that staff are kept up to date with medical developments.

A key case dealing with direct liability is *Bull v Devon Area Health Authority* (1993).

CASE EXAMPLE

Bull v Devon Area Health Authority [1993] 4 Med LR 117

The plaintiff was in labour giving birth to twins. After the first twin was born, the junior doctor called for urgent assistance from a more senior colleague. Due to the hospital's design, the other doctor was on another site which was over a mile away. It took him over an hour to attend the call. The second twin was born with severe brain damage as a result of the delay. The health authority argued that since the hospital was situated on two sites, there would inevitably be the occasional delay in attending a call.

While Mrs Bull was not entitled to expect that an obstetrician would be available immediately, the delay of over an hour was unreasonable.

Slade LJ said

JUDGMENT

'The duty of a hospital is to provide a woman admitted in labour with a reasonable standard of skilled obstetric and paediatric care ...'

Concurring with Slade LJ, Dillon LJ said:

JUDGMENT

'In my judgment, the plaintiff has succeeded in proving, by the ordinary civil standards of proof, that the failure to provide for Mrs Bull the prompt attendance she needed was attributable to the negligence of the defendants in implementing an unreliable and essentially unsatisfactory system for calling the registrar.'

The case underlines the difficult balance between the issue of unit providers allocating their own resources and accountability where the courts may decide that a safe system of care has not been provided. The key point to take from *Bull v Devon* however is that the defendant healthcare provider cannot simply use an alleged lack of resources as the Ace of Spades with which to defeat any claim which alleges primary liability.

The subsequent case of *Garcia v St Mary's NHS Trust* (2006) was similar to *Bull* on its facts, but no reference was made to the decision in that case.

CASE EXAMPLE

Garcia v St Mary's NHS Trust [2006] EWHC 2314 (QB)

The claimant underwent coronary artery bypass surgery. The operation appeared to be a success and Mr Garcia was returned to the ward to recover. Later that evening, however, the claimant's condition deteriorated rapidly. It transpired that a clip that had been used during surgery had slipped, causing a severe bleed which required emergency surgery. The on-call surgeon was called at home and arrived at the hospital some 27 minutes later. The bleeding was stopped a further 15 minutes later. As a result of the substantial bleed Mr Garcia suffered brain damage.

The claimant framed his claim in two ways. Firstly he argued that the clip had slipped as a result of it being applied in a negligent manner. Secondly, Mr Garcia argued that the defendant had failed to take reasonable care to ensure that their staff were adequately available so that his post-operative bleed could have been stopped before he suffered brain damage. The claimant failed in his action. On the first ground, on hearing expert evidence, the court found that the treatment was not negligent. On the second ground, the court found that the Trust had not been negligent in the delay in attending the patient. The court accepted that even if there had been a specialist on site at the time Mr Garcia's bleed began, the delay experienced by the patient was not unreasonable and it would have been likely that Mr Garcia would have suffered severe brain damage in any event.

Interestingly, it is worthwhile noting that it is not just the unit provider that can be sued directly. The case of *Re HIV Haemophiliac Litigation* (1990) 140 NLJ illustrates the situation where the Secretary of State was sued in negligence for a failure to treat blood products from the USA adequately, and for a failure to warn patients of any potential risks. The case was settled before trial; therefore there was no determination of this particular issue, but the case of *Danns v Department of Health* [1997] EWCA Civ 1168 demonstrates the difficulties in attempting to impose a duty of care, where it was alleged that the Department of Health had failed to advise patients of the risk of spontaneous reversal of vasectomies.

KEY FACTS

Key facts on who may be sued

Case	Principle
Cassidy v Ministry of Health (1951)	Defendant health authority liable for negligence of its surgeon.
Bull v Devon Area Health Authority (1993)	Defendant liable in negligence for an unavailable surgeon.
Garcia v St Mary's NHS Trust (2006)	Trust liable for unavailability of on-call surgeon.

ACTIVITY

Self-test questions for duty of care

Ensure that all your answers are supported by case law.

- What authorities can be relied upon to support a common law duty between doctor and patient?
- What principle of law does the case of *Kent v Griffiths* (2001) demonstrate?
- Which case supports the principle that a hospital doctor owes the same duty of care as a general practitioner?
- In order to be successful in a wrongful conception claim, what would a claimant have to establish? Which case is a good example?
- What principle does *Cassidy v Ministry of Health* (1951) illustrate? See Lord Denning's judgment.
- Which case illustrates that a hospital can be sued directly for breach of its primary duty? Why was the hospital liable?

1.3 Part 2: Breach of duty of care

We have looked at when a duty is owed and by whom. Once the claimant has established this element, it is then necessary for the claimant to demonstrate that the owed duty was breached.

We need to consider whether the standard of care that was owed was breached.

1.3.1 The standard of care

CASE EXAMPLE

Bolam v Friern Hospital Management Committee [1957] 1 WLR 582

The plaintiff was suffering with a mental illness and was being treated with electroconvulsive therapy (ECT). The treatment was known to induce convulsions or fits. The hospital failed to warn the patient of the risk of bone fracture associated with the treatment, and did not provide the patient with a muscle relaxant or other form of restraint to minimise the risk of harm during the treatment. This was the hospital's normal practice and the plaintiff was treated in much the same way as any other patient. However, he suffered fractures to his hip, and alleged negligence for the failure to provide relaxants and the failure to advise of the risks of fracture. The plaintiff was unable to prove his case.

McNair J stated that a doctor will *not* be negligent if 'he has acted in accordance with a practice acceptable as proper by a responsible body of medical men skilled in that particular art'.

```
            Bolam v Friern Hospital Management
                   Committee (1957)
                     per McNair J
```

'A doctor is not guilty of negligence if he has acted in accordance with a practice accepted as proper by a responsible body of medical men skilled in that particular art'.

'A man is not negligent, if he is acting in accordance with such a practice, merely because there is a body of opinion that takes a contrary view'.

Figure 1.4 McNair J's test in *Bolam*

In simple terms, a defendant could avoid liability by establishing that there existed a responsible body of medical men practising in the same field of medicine who agreed that the defendant's actions were appropriate in the circumstances.

The more controversial part of the test is shown on the right hand side of the diagram. McNair J stated in *Bolam* that 'a doctor is not negligent if acting in accordance with a practice accepted as proper by a responsible body of medical opinion merely because there is a body of opinion that takes a contrary view.' The practical effect of this was that when the court applied the *Bolam* test in situations where there were conflicting views, the courts effectively paid no attention to those views which did not support the defendant's conduct, and thus reached the conclusion that the defendant was not liable.

1.3.2 Interpretation of the *Bolam* test

It appears that cases of medical negligence are treated differently from most other negligence claims when they come before the courts. In other areas of the law, the standard of care is set by the courts by applying an objective standard, that is, the test of the reasonable man. However, where defendants are medical professionals, the reasonable man test seems to be inappropriate because:

'where you get a situation which involves the use of some special skill or competence, then the test whether there has been negligence or not is not the test of the man [*in the street*], because he has not got this special skill.' (*per* McNair J)

1.3.3 Application of the *Bolam* test

The reasonable man test is an objective test; the court will seek to determine what a reasonable man would have done (or would not have done) in the circumstances if they had been faced with the same circumstances as the defendant. Under the second limb of the *Bolam* test however, all the defendant has to do to successfully defend a claim in negligence is to demonstrate that there exists a responsible body of medical opinion which accepts his conduct as reasonable. This has led to the suggestion that this leaves the medical profession (rather than the courts) free to set the standard of care required of medical practitioners.

Although *Bolam* was a first instance case, its impact and application has been extensive and was applied by the House of Lords in both *Whitehouse v Jordan* (1981) and *Maynard v West Midlands Regional Health Authority* (1985), cases which involved treatment and diagnosis respectively. In both cases however, the *Bolam* test was applied in a way which effectively suggested that it would be virtually impossible to demonstrate that a defendant medical professional was liable in negligence.

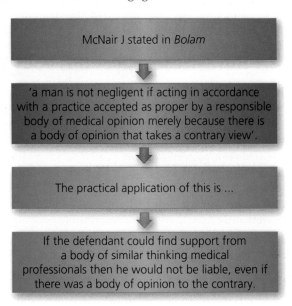

Figure 1.5 *Bolam's* controversial limb

CASE EXAMPLE

Maynard v West Midlands Regional Health Authority [1985] 1 All ER 635

The plaintiff was suffering from one of two possible conditions and was advised to undergo a diagnostic procedure to help determine which of the two conditions she was suffering from. During the procedure a nerve was damaged which affected her vocal cord. She alleged negligence in the diagnosis as she maintained that one condition was so certain that it was negligent to undertake the procedure at all. There was a conflict of opinion as to whether it was negligent to carry out that procedure in the circumstances.

In the High Court the trial judge, confronted with conflicting views on what an appropriate course of action would have been in the circumstances, concluded that the approach advocated by the claimant's expert witness was preferable to that supported by the defendant's witness. On that basis, the trial judge had concluded that the defendant had not met the standard of care required of him.

The House of Lords, however, criticised the approach taken in the High Court and declared that negligence is not to be established by simply 'preferring one respectable opinion over another'.

Lord Scarman stated that where treatment and diagnosis is concerned, there will inevitably be differences in opinion and a doctor is *not* negligent just because his opinion is different from another. He referred to the dictum of Lord President Clyde in *Hunter v Hanley* (1955) SLT 213 with approval: 'the true test ... is whether he has proved to be guilty of such failure as no doctor of ordinary skill would be guilty of if acting with ordinary care.'

This suggests that the defendant will only be liable in negligence if he can find *no* other similar-minded professional who would have taken the same action.

CASE EXAMPLE

Whitehouse v Jordan [1981] 1 All ER 26

The plaintiff was born by Caesarean section, but it was apparent that the baby had suffered severe brain damage as a result of alleged negligence sustained during a protracted and failed delivery using forceps.

In approving the *Bolam* test to treatment specifically, the court held that even if the defendant had caused the brain damage by the way the forceps delivery was carried out, this was not negligence in itself, simply an error of clinical judgment for which the defendant was not liable.

These cases illustrate that provided the defendant can show a body of opinion that supports the defendant's act, the defendant will not be negligent.

1.3.4 How sizeable does this body of opinion need to be?

The *Bolam* test requires the defendant in a medical negligence claim to show that their conduct is supported by a 'body of medical men skilled in that particular art'. *Bolam* is silent however on the issue of just how many professionals would have to agree that the defendant's course of action was acceptable in the circumstances before they could be classified as 'a body of opinion'.

In *Defreitas v O'Brien* [1995] 6 Med LR 108, a case which involved orthopedics and neurosurgery, only a small minority of similarly qualified professionals would have acted as the defendant did. The size of the supporting body of medical opinion was not relevant, only that 'there was a responsible body' (*per* Otton LJ).

1.3.5 A changing tide?

Despite the seemingly impregnable position that the decision in *Bolam* put defendants in medical negligence claims, there was some limited evidence that the courts would be willing to challenge expert opinion. One such example is *Hucks v Cole*, a case that was decided in 1968 but was not reported until 1993.

CASE EXAMPLE

Hucks v Cole [1993] 4 Med LR 393

A doctor failed to treat a pregnant patient with penicillin. He was aware that a failure to treat septic areas of her skin could lead to puerperal fever. There were however a number of doctors who supported the defendant's judgment not to treat her in this situation.

The Court of Appeal, clearly rejecting the *Bolam*-style approach, stated that if the opinion not to provide the patient with antibiotics was unreasonable then it did not automatically follow that the court should find that the defendant had met the standard of care, even if a body of expert opinion considered the conduct to be acceptable.

Sachs LJ stated:

JUDGMENT

'the fact that other practitioners would have done the same thing as the defendant practitioner is a very weighty matter to be put on the scales on his behalf; but is not conclusive.'

This move towards adopting a more critical approach to expert opinion in medical negligence claims reached recognition in the seminal case of *Bolitho v Hackney Health Authority* (1997). The case of *Bolitho* is widely recognised as a robust attempt by the courts to control the expansion of the *Bolam* test as the application of the test had clearly pervaded areas of medical negligence, which would have been neither intended nor anticipated by McNair J when he first devised the test.

CASE EXAMPLE

Bolitho v Hackney Health Authority [1997] 4 All ER 771

The plaintiff in this case was a two-year-old boy, Patrick, who was admitted to hospital suffering from a common childhood respiratory infection called croup. He was admitted, treated and discharged home. There is no allegation of negligence or complaint during this period.

The following day, his parents became concerned about his condition. He had been restless and was having difficulty in breathing. He was admitted to hospital, seen by a doctor and was admitted for observation. There was no suggestion there was anything improper about the defendant's conduct at this point.

There came a point when the nurse became concerned about Patrick's condition and called Dr Horn, the senior pediatric registrar, directly as she considered his condition was so severe. Dr Horn failed to attend and neither did her senior house officer but, as it was, his condition appeared to have improved a little. This episode repeated itself again and once more Dr Horn did not attend. It appeared that the boy's condition was fluctuating significantly.

Eventually Patrick's respiratory system became entirely blocked and he was unable to breathe. He suffered cardiac arrest. Although he was revived, Patrick was left with severe brain damage.

It was accepted by the defendants that the duty of care was breached as Dr Horn failed to attend Patrick when she was asked to do so. She also failed to send a junior doctor in her place. It was the defendant's case however that even if she had attended, she would not have intubated Patrick in any event. The claim failed on the question of causation, which we will consider in more detail a little later.

For our present purposes, we need to consider the judgment of Lord Browne-Wilkinson who discussed the situation of whether the courts would determine there had been negligence despite the defendant's case being supported by expert evidence.

The judgment of Lord Browne-Wilkinson took a robust approach. He began by critcising the simplistic application of the *Bolam* test evidenced in cases such as *Maynard*:

JUDGMENT

'... in my view, the court is not bound to hold that a defendant doctor escapes liability for negligent treatment or diagnosis just because he leads evidence from a number of medical experts who are genuinely of the opinion that the defendant's treatment or diagnosis accorded with sound medical practice.'

Lord Browne-Wilkinson then notes McNair J's reference in *Bolam* to a 'responsible body of medical men' and a 'reasonable body of opinion'. Furthermore he comments that Lord Scarman (presumably in *Sidaway* (1985), see Chapter 2 for full citation and examination) talks about 'a respectable body of medical opinion' and concludes:

JUDGMENT

'The use of these adjectives – responsible, reasonable and respectable – all show that the court has to be satisfied that the exponents of the body of opinion relied upon can demonstrate that such opinion has a logical basis.'

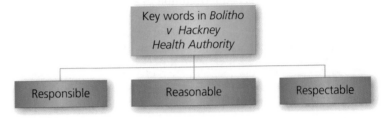

Figure 1.6 Key words in *Bolitho* (1997)

So, how can it be determined whether the opinion is capable of withstanding logical analysis or not? Lord Browne-Wilkinson explained thus:

JUDGMENT

'… the judge before accepting a body of opinion as being responsible, reasonable or respectable, will need to be satisfied that, in forming their views, the experts have directed their minds to the question of comparative risks and benefits and have reached a defensible conclusion on the matter.'

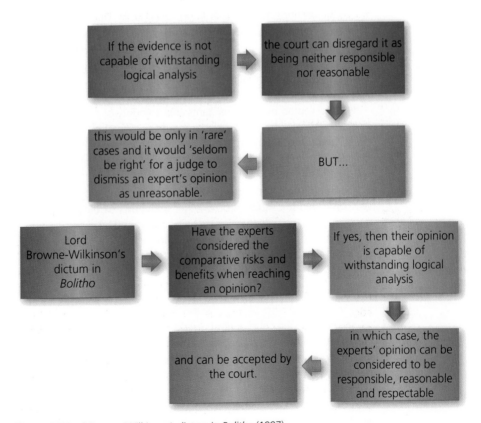

Figure 1.7 Lord Browne-Wilkinson's dictum in *Bolitho* (1997)

However, although Lord Browne-Wilkinson encouraged the courts to adopt a more robust position in relation to expert evidence, there are aspects of his judgment in which he seems to remain rather deferential to the medical profession.

He comments that 'if, in a rare case, it can be demonstrated that the professional opinion is not capable of withstanding logical analysis, the judge is entitled to hold that the body of opinion is not reasonable or responsible'. However, this is tempered with, 'it will very seldom be right for a judge to reach the conclusion that views genuinely held by a competent medical expert are unreasonable.'

1.3.6 The impact of *Bolitho* (1997) on subsequent case law

The case of *Wisniewski v Central Manchester Health Authority* (1998) gave the courts an opportunity to consider the effect of *Bolitho*.

CASE EXAMPLE

Wisniewski v Central Manchester Health Authority [1998] Lloyd's Rep Med 223 CA

The claimant alleged that her labour had been negligently managed. She contended that a failure to intervene at a sufficiently early stage and deliver baby Philip by Caesarean section led to the baby being born with irreversible brain damage. This had shown up in the form of abnormalities in the foetal heartbeat which had been picked up by the monitors.

The claimant argued that these abnormalities should have prompted further investigations, which would have revealed the need to carry out delivery by way of a Caesarean section.

The defendant presented expert evidence to support their claims that there was a responsible body of medical opinion that would not have carried out further investigations in the circumstances.

The trial judge dismissed the defendant's evidence, choosing instead to decide himself what should have been done in the circumstances. However, in the Court of Appeal, the court reflected on *Bolitho* and applied Lord Browne-Wilkinson's judgment, stating that it would only be in the rarest of situations that the views of eminent experts would not withstand logical analysis.

JUDGMENT

'It is quite impossible for a court to hold that the views sincerely held by doctors of such eminence cannot be logically supported at all.' (*per* Brook LJ)

Wisniewski can be contrasted with the case below, where the court *was* willing to find that the body of opinion put forward in support of the defendant's conduct was illogical.

CASE EXAMPLE

Marriott v West Midlands Health Authority [1999] Ll Med Rep 23

Mr Marriot had been involved in a fall which left him unconscious. During the week following his fall, he displayed symptoms such as lethargy and a general feeling of being unwell. He sought his GP's advice who prescribed painkillers, and advised Mr Marriott's wife to monitor her husband's condition and call the doctor if there was any further deterioration in his condition. The GP failed, however, to give him a full neurological examination despite his case history. A short period of time later, Mr Marriott collapsed and had to undergo surgery to relieve a haematoma. His condition left him permanently disabled.

There was disagreement at the trial between Mr Marriott's expert witness and the defendant's expert witness. The claimant's expert said the symptoms shown by Mr Marriott should have led to the GP sending him to the hospital. The defendant's expert said that the risk of a clot on the brain was so small that it was reasonable to send him home with instructions to review his condition.

> Beldam LJ observed that although the risk of harm materialising was small, it was clear that if such a risk *did* materialise, the outcome for the patient would be catastrophic. Consequently, the only reasonably prudent course of action in those circumstances would have been to send Mr Marriott back to hospital for further tests.

The *Bolitho* approach indicates the court's willingness to reject expert evidence if they consider it to be indefensible. In cases such as *Marriott*, one can see less deference being paid to the medical profession with the courts demonstrating a greater willingness to take responsibility for setting the standard of care in negligence claims away from the medical profession.

However, the courts have tempered the *Bolitho* judgment in different ways:

- In *Glicksman v Redbridge NHS Trust* [2001] EWCA Civ 1097 the judge had preferred to follow one expert's opinion above another, but failed to give any reasons for rejecting the alternative point of view. As such, it was not possible to determine whether the judge's opinion was 'reasonable and capable of being supported'.
- A similar point was made in *Smith v Southampton University Hospital NHS Trust* [2007] EWCA Civ 387 where the Court of Appeal stated that if a judge is to prefer one expert's opinion over another, then the judge must explain the reasoning behind that decision.
- In *M (a Child by his Mother) v Blackpool Victoria Hospital NHS Trust* [2003] EWHC 1744 it was observed *per* Silber LJ that it would 'very seldom be right' for the court to reject a medical expert's views on the grounds that the court considered it unreasonable.
- In *Burne v A* [2006] EWCA Civ 24 Ward LJ said that he was 'not convinced that we are entitled to rely on what seems common sense to judges, and consequently dismiss the views of experts as illogical … at least not until experts are given an opportunity to explain and justify their practice.'
- In the more recent case of *Birch v University College London Hospital* [2008] EWHC 2237 (QB) the High Court interpreted the decision in *Bolitho* in a rather restrictive way. Cranston J opined that a body of medical opinion advanced in support of the defendant's conduct would only be 'incapable of withstanding logical analysis' where it 'cannot be logically supported at all'. Cranston J then continued by saying that it would be 'folly' if judges who had no medical training were to decide whether one body of professional opinion was to be 'preferred over another when both are professionally sanctioned and both withstand logical analysis'. The opinion suggests that the judiciary are not in a position to adjudicate on medical negligence cases without accepting medical expert opinion.

1.3.7 What effect has *Bolitho* really had?

It would appear from the case law above that the courts remain unwilling to disregard expert opinion altogether, and if the court is to choose between two conflicting expert opinions then a reasoned explanation must justify the decision. This would suggest that *Bolitho* actually had little to no impact on how the courts subsequently set the standard of clinical negligence claims. This suggestion also appears to be supported by the following authors.

- Herring correctly observes that since cases subsequent to *Bolitho* cite *Bolam* in reference and not *Bolitho*, it could be argued that 'the courts do not regard Bolitho as having made a change of any great significance' (2010, page 108).
- Brazier and Miola described the failure of *Bolitho* to totally overthrow the *Bolam* test in poetic terms: 'the revolution, if it can be so styled, will be a velvet revolution, not a bloodbath' (2000).
- Mason and Laurie comment that while *Bolitho* 'undoubtedly devalues the trump card which *Bolam* presented to the medical profession', it only does so in limited circumstances (2010, page 139).

Key facts on a breach of care

Case	Principle
Hunter v Hanley (1955)	The defendant will be negligent if no doctor of ordinary skill would have acted the same way.
Bolam v Friern Hospital Management Committee (1957)	**Two-part test established. A doctor will not be negligent if he has acted in accordance with a practice acceptable as proper by a responsible body of medical men skilled in that particular art, even if there is a contrary body of opinion.**
Whitehouse v Jordan (1981)	A supporting body of opinion will exonerate the defendant of liability.
Hucks v Cole (1968) reported 1993	If the defendant had not met the standard of care, the defendant was liable even if there was a supporting body of opinion.
Maynard v West Midlands Regional Health Authority (1985)	House of Lords – negligence is not established by preferring one respectable opinion over another. Defendant is not negligent just because there is an opposing view.
DeFreitas v O'Brien (1995)	The size of the supporting body of opinion can be small.
Bolitho v Hackney Health Authority (1997)	**Expert medical opinion needed to be responsible, reasonable and respectable for it to be accepted by the court.**
Wisniewski v Central Manchester Health Authority (1998)	Only in the rarest of situations would experts not withstand logical analysis.
Marriott v West Midlands Health Authority (1999)	Rejected expert evidence as indefensible.
Glicksman v Redbridge NHS Trust (2001)	Judge failed to give reasons why one expert's opinion was preferred over another and therefore not clear if the judge's opinion was reasonable.
M (a child by his Mother) v Blackpool Victoria Hospital NHS Trust (2003)	Very seldom would it be acceptable to reject an expert's opinion as unacceptable.
Burne v A (2006)	Experts must be able to justify their practice before they are dismissed as illogical.
Smith v Southampton University Hospital NHS Trust (2007)	Judge must explain why one expert's opinion was preferred over another.
Birch v University College London Hospital (2008)	Restrictive interpretation of *Bolitho*. Defendant expert's opinion will only be rejected if it cannot withstand logical analysis.

21

BREACH OF DUTY OF CARE

1.3.8 Is the standard of care fixed or flexible?

The courts are reluctant to make allowances for a person who is less experienced than another. This is not a concept unique to medical law as we can see in the tort case of *Nettleship v Weston* [1971] 3 All ER 581. Here, the court held that a learner driver is deemed in law to have the same skills as an experienced driver, and no recognition could be made of the fact that she was a learner driver.

Similarly, in *Wilsher v Essex AHA* (1987) the Court of Appeal had to consider the liability of junior staff in a hospital. The courts had to consider the defendants' argument that the staff were inexperienced and did the best they could in the circumstances.

Glidewell LJ held that 'the law requires the trainee or learner to be judged by the same standard as his more experienced colleagues'.

Is this not unduly harsh on the young junior doctor who has only been working in the hospital for only a week? That may be, but a junior doctor has more experienced staff to call upon for advice and assistance. Only by applying a consistent standard owed regardless of experience can the law be evenly and equally applied. Glidewell LJ explained that if inexperience was taken into account then it would often be used as a defence in litigation.

Nevertheless, Mustill LJ did indicate that account could be taken of 'battle conditions'; for example, where a doctor attends the scene of a road accident or train crash, suggesting that when he needs to do many tasks at once in situations that are far from ideal, 'the fact that he does one of them incorrectly should not lightly be taken as negligence.'

1.3.9 Other factors

Other factors besides the relative experience of the defendant are relevant when setting the standard of care expected of the defendant. As we know, some cases can take several years to come to trial, and in this situation we need to consider whether the standard of care will be judged at the time that the alleged negligence took place or at the time of trial.

CASE EXAMPLE

Roe v Minister of Health [1954] 2 QB 66

In this unusual case, anaesthetic that was being given to the plaintiff had been stored in glass vials. The vials had been placed into a phenol solution. The phenol had seeped through minute cracks in the glass contaminating the anaesthetic. The defendant's use of this contaminated anaesthetic left the plaintiff permanently paralysed.

The incident took place in 1947. The risk of phenol seeping through cracks in the glass vials and contaminating anaesthetic did not come to light however until four years later. The defendants were not held liable as, while we all may appreciate the benefit of hindsight, Lord Denning stated that one cannot look 'at the 1947 accident with 1954 spectacles'.

Before we conclude our study of breach of duty of care it is useful to consider one last point: how up to date must the defendant keep their knowledge before it can be established that a duty of care is breached?

The case of *Crawford v Board of Governors of Charing Cross Hospital* (1953), *The Times*, 8 December 1953 draws the distinction between isolated articles in medical journals and material that is 'so well accepted that it should be adopted'. Lord Denning in exonerating the defendant stated that it would place 'too high a burden on a medical man to say that he has to read every article appearing in the current medical press.'

1.3.10 Criticisms of the *Bolam* test

- The interpretation of McNair J's words led to difficulties. Undue deference by the courts to the medical profession resulted in the medical profession setting their own standard of care.
- As Brazier and Miola state, 'Bolam ran out of control. The test became no more than a requirement to find some other expert(s) who would declare that they would have done as the defendant did.' (2000)
- It follows that the claimant faces significant difficulties when trying to establish breach of duty of care.

1.3.11 Approval of the *Bolam* test

◼ Those involved with the profession are best placed to determine medical negligence. Since the court has no medical expertise, the court cannot adjudicate matters involving the medical profession.

◼ If the *Bolam* test was not applied, then the floodgates could open and claims involving alleged medical negligence could increase significantly. This would in turn place an undue burden on the NHS's already over-stretched purse.

ACTIVITY

Self-test questions on breach of duty of care

Ensure that all your answers are supported by case law.

- How is the standard of care determined in medical negligence cases?
- Is the same standard applied in other professional cases?
- What impact has *Bolam* had on cases involving treatment and diagnosis?
- Critically evaluate the *Bolam* test.
- What is your understanding of the judgment of *Bolitho*?
- Through a close consideration of the above judgment, consider the impact which you believe the judgment of *Bolitho* has had.
- What standard of care is required of a newly qualified doctor?
- Can any adjustments be made to this standard?

ACTIVITY

Applying the law

Test your understanding of the legal principles you have just read about by reading the following scenario and advising A.

A is in the late stages of pregnancy, and having felt the baby kicking regularly is rather alarmed one day when she feels the baby is a little less active. On advice from her midwife, she attends hospital and is seen by Dr Y. He admits her and she is taken to the labour ward for observations. She is attached to a **CTG** which records the foetal heartbeat.

Two hours later, Nurse X notices a sudden deceleration in the foetal heart rate which causes her concern. She bleeps Dr Y who says he will attend shortly. He fails to arrive and Nurse X bleeps him again. He admits that he forgot. He is a little embarrassed and tells Nurse X that the deceleration is not a problem. Twenty minutes later it occurs again and Nurse X tries once again to bleep Dr Y. Her attempts prove unsuccessful and so she bleeps Mr Z, the obstetric consultant. He arrives, looks at the CTG trace and is extremely alarmed. He insists on an emergency Caesarean section and baby B is born 15 minutes later. The baby fails to breathe spontaneously and once resuscitated, it becomes apparent that he will be severely brain damaged.

A believes that if baby B was born by Caesarean section when the CTG first began to record decelerations in the foetal heart rate, he would not have suffered brain damage.

Points to consider in your answer:

- Your starting point should be a discussion of whether there is a duty of care. However, taking into account what you have previously learnt, it would be appropriate to begin by simply explaining that a duty of care exists between A and the hospital. Illustrate with reference to case law how that arises.
- Once the duty has been established, consider the area of breach.
- You will probably have already established in your mind that although the hospital will be liable for the acts or omissions committed by its employees (vicarious liability), we are really looking at the acts of Dr Y. Has he breached his duty of care by not acting upon the decreased foetal heart rate?

CTG
cardiotocography is the technology which records the foetal heartbeat

- Firstly, you will need to establish what the standard of care is. You will need to apply the *Bolam* test.
- Ensure that your answer provides an accurate account of McNair's test.
- It is advisable to apply the law to the question throughout, so state that Dr Y will need to be able to demonstrate a body of opinion that would have done as he did.
- Use case examples throughout: you should probably consider *Maynard* and also *Whitehouse v Jordan* as illustrations of where the *Bolam* test has been applied in the areas of treatment and diagnosis.
- Consider also the case of *Defreitas* and the size of the body of opinion that is needed to support his opinion. This case shows that the size of opinion can be quite small.
- Move on now to *Bolitho*: this case is particularly pertinent because it concerns an omission, a failure to act. This is the same in the scenario above; Dr Y failed to attend the patient. Had he attended, would he have arranged an emergency Caesarean section?
- So as a result of *Bolitho*, even if Dr Y supports his position with a body of similar minded professionals, Lord Browne-Wilkinson stated that the opinion needs to be 'respectable, responsible and reasonable' so the courts will now look beyond just the credibility of a witness.
- You need to explain that even if Dr Y could find a body of professional opinion to support what he did, it is open to the court to reject it. It may be that, given that his failure to act is so significant, the courts may consider that this may be one of the rare occasions in which expert opinion could be rejected.
- The problem is, of course, that even in the period post-*Bolitho* the courts have largely continued to set the standard of care in clinical negligence cases in a way that is closer to a straightforward application of the *Bolam* test. Reference to the decision in *Wisniewski v Central Manchester Health Authority* would be appropriate at this point (it is also highly pertinent as the facts of *Wisniewski* closely mirror those of the problem scenario).
- Ensure that you conclude clearly – in this case it is possible that the courts will conclude, much like in *Bolitho*, that the defendant breached his duty of care. Whether the claimant is ultimately successful depends largely on causation.

1.4 Part 3: Causation

We have considered how a duty of care might arise in a healthcare setting, and also how and why that duty of care can be breached. We continue by considering the next element that must be established in order to succeed in a claim for negligence: causation.

Once the claimant has proved a breach of duty of care, it is still necessary to prove that the defendant caused the injuries of which the claimant complains. The claimant must be able to prove the existence of the causal link on a balance of probabilities; that is, a likelihood of 50 per cent or more.

The claimant must be able to show that the defendant's negligence was the cause of the injury they suffered, and that the injury was a foreseeable consequence of the defendant's negligence.

In your study of tort you learnt the application of the 'but for' test. As a reminder, it can be expressed as follows: 'but for' the defendant's negligence, would the claimant have suffered those injuries?

One can also ask: how far can the injuries from which the claimant now suffers be attributable to the defendant's negligence? This particular question raises other issues, because it is sometimes necessary to distinguish the injuries which the claimant alleges stem from the defendant's negligence, from any pre-existing injuries the claimant may have suffered from.

We start by looking at the 'but for' test.

causation

Causation is the term where the treating doctor/ medical practitioner will be responsible if his negligent act or his omission to act results in the claimant's injuries.

1.4.1 *'But for'* test

CASE EXAMPLE

Barnett v Chelsea and Kensington Hospital Management Committee [1969] QB 428

Three nightwatchmen drank some tea which contained arsenic. The men presented themselves at the defendant's casualty department complaining of symptoms which included vomiting. The triage nurse called the on-call doctor but he refused to see them, saying that they should go home and call their own doctors if they still felt ill later on. Five hours later, one of the men died from arsenic poisoning ingested from the tea. An action in negligence was brought by the deceased's widow.

While it was clear that there was a breach of duty of care as the doctor was negligent in refusing to see the men, it was not clear that the negligence caused the man's death. 'But for' the defendant's negligence, would the claimant have died?

The court held that even if the doctor had admitted the man, he would still have died. Therefore, causation was *not* satisfied as the defendant's negligent act did not cause the plaintiff's death, and the claim failed.

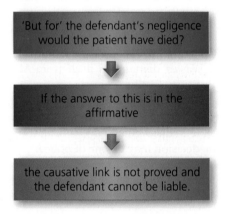

Figure 1.8 'But for' – an explanation

1.4.2 Multiple causes

The 'but for' test is relatively straightforward to apply in cases such as *Barnett* where there is only *one* possible cause of the claimant's injury, but it becomes more complicated where there is *more than one* potential cause, and it is not clear whether the injury was caused by the defendant or by one of the other causes.

CASE EXAMPLE

Wilsher v Essex Area Health Authority [1988] AC 1074

In this case, a baby was born three months prematurely. He suffered from a number of disabling conditions. As he had breathing difficulties he required additional oxygen. He was negligently given excess oxygen on two occasions. He developed retrolental fibroplasia which resulted in near blindness. The plaintiff sued the health authority on the grounds that the negligent use of excess oxygen was the cause of the blindness.

It was apparent that any one of six possible causes could have caused **retrolental fibroplasia** but only one of which was due to the defendant's negligent actions. At trial the medical evidence was inconclusive as to whether the excess of oxygen caused or materially contributed to the baby's condition. The House of Lords held that it was necessary for the claimant to be able to establish (on the balance of probabilities) that the defendant caused the claimant's injuries. As the claimant was unable to do this, causation failed.

retrolental fibroplasia

an eye disease detected in babies born prematurely

The case of *Wilsher* was distinguished from the (non-medical) House of Lords case of *McGhee v National Coal Board* (1973). It is worth noting, however, that although the decision in *McGhee* was not followed in *Wilsher*, it has since been applied in the more recent case of *Fairchild v Glenhaven* [2002] UKHL 22.

CASE EXAMPLE

McGhee v National Coal Board [1973] 1 All ER 871

The claimant in *McGhee* was exposed to brick dust as a result of his job working in a brick kiln. The defendants had negligently failed to supply adequate washing facilities. Mr McGhee developed dermatitis and sought to claim damages.

While the defendants accepted that exposure to brick dust had caused his skin condition, he would only be able to succeed in his claim if he could show that the defendant's negligence was *the* cause of that injury.

On a straightforward application of the 'but for' test, Mr McGhee's claim should have failed.

The court however altered their approach to causation in this case and held that causation could be established if Mr McGhee could prove that the defendant's negligence had 'materially increased the risk' of him developing dermatitis (which was a much easier test to satisfy). The court accepted that this requirement had been fulfilled because the defendant's negligent failure to provide adequate washing facilities (unnecessarily) prolonged Mr McGhee's exposure to brick dust, thereby increasing the chances of him developing dermatitis.

Discussion point

Why did *Wilsher* distinguish itself from *McGhee*? There are a number of possibilities for this decision. Firstly, there was a division of medical opinion in *Wilsher*, a complex medical case which was simply not evident in *McGhee*. Secondly, Lord Bridge's opinion was that *McGhee* 'laid down no new principle of law whatsoever' and so it was therefore possible to distinguish *Wilsher* from the case of *McGhee* and not be bound by it, and finally, the decision may be one of policy.

In medical, potentially high value cases, the courts are often keen to place a narrow interpretation on principles of law for fear of placing an unduly high financial burden on the NHS. While the burden on the claimant is often more difficult to prove, the reasoning is clearly expressed by Lord Hoffman as he distinguishes 'the political and economic arguments involved in the massive increase in the liability of the National Health Service' which would have followed if the principle in *Wilsher* had been applied from 'imposing liability upon an employer who has failed to take simple precautions.'

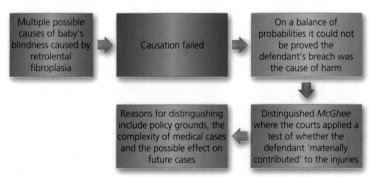

Figure 1.9 Judgment in *Wilsher v Essex Area Health Authority* (1988)

1.4.3 A more 'flexible' approach to establishing causation?

No discussion of the rules governing factual causation in clinical negligence claims would be complete without a discussion of the key cases of *Chester v Afshar* (2004) and *Bailey v Ministry of Defence* (2008).

CASE EXAMPLE

Chester v Afshar [2004] UKHL 41

The claimant, Mrs Chester, suffered from severe back pain and sought the advice of the defendant, a neurosurgeon. He recommended surgery but failed to warn Mrs Chester of the one to two per cent risk of significant nerve damage that could occur. Mrs Chester consented to the surgery and while the surgery was carried out correctly, the one to two per cent risk materialised and she was left partially paralysed. Mrs Chester maintained that had she been advised of the risk, she would not have undergone the operation that day but would have sought a second opinion. She accepted, however, that she probably would still have undergone the surgery with Mr Afshar, albeit on a different day.

The court had to consider whether there was causal link between a breach of duty of care caused by the failure to inform and the claimant's injuries.

In a majority opinion, the House of Lords held that where a patient has not been advised of the risks of surgery *and* as a result of injury undergoes an operation where the risk of which she was unaware materialises *and* is a situation where the claimant says that she would not have undergone the operation at that time if she had been advised of the risks, the claimant can claim damages.

The decision was complicated by the fact that the claimant accepted that she would have probably been operated on by the defendant once she had sought a second opinion. Therefore, she would have been in exactly the same position, facing exactly the same risks to the operation which she underwent.

The House of Lords' focus appeared to be on delivering a just and fair result to Mrs Chester rather than applying the more conventional 'but for' test. In what has been described as a 'very pro-claimant, patient-centred decision' (Pattinson, (2006), page 130), their Lordships differed considerably in their reasoning.

However, the majority of the House of Lords considered that it was necessary to find in favour of the claimant as she had not been fully informed. Had she been, on her evidence, she would have taken a second opinion. Therefore, her right to autonomy and self-determination had been denied. She had a right to be informed of the risks; the neurosurgeon had breached the duty and she had suffered injury as a result.

The majority's reasons for finding in favour of Mrs Chester in this case are evident in the views of Lord Hope and Lord Steyn:

JUDGMENT

'The function of the law is to enable rights to be vindicated and to provide remedies when duties have been breached. Unless this is done the duty is a hollow one, stripped of all practical force and devoid of all content. It will have lost its ability to protect the patient and thus to fulfil the only purpose which brought it into existence. On policy grounds therefore I would hold that the test of causation is satisfied in this case. The injury was intimately involved with the duty to warn. The duty was owed by the doctor who performed the surgery that Miss Chester consented to. It was the product of the very risk that she should have been warned about when she gave her consent. So I would hold that it can be regarded as having been caused, in the legal sense, by the breach of that duty.' (Lord Hope)

'... it is a distinctive feature of the present case that but for the surgeon's negligent failure to warn the claimant of the small risk of serious injury the actual injury would not have occurred when it did and the chance of it occurring on a subsequent occasion was very small. It could therefore be said that the breach by the surgeon resulted in the very injury about which the claimant was entitled to be warned.' (Lord Steyn)

The majority in the House of Lords seem to have been inspired by the suggestion in *Fairchild* (2002) that the courts should adopt a flexible approach to causation on policy grounds where justice demanded it. As such, the court delivered a judgment which provides a just and fair result to Mrs Chester rather than worrying about ensuring strict compliance with the basic requirements of the 'but for' test.

This more recent case of *Bailey v Ministry of Defence* [2008] EWCA Civ 883 demonstrates an interesting development in the rules of causation in the context of clinical negligence claims.

CASE EXAMPLE

Bailey v Ministry of Defence [2008] EWCA Civ 883

The claimant returned from holiday with suspected gallstones. She was admitted to hospital where she had the gallstones removed. However, during that night she bled a considerable amount and was extremely unwell in the morning. Unrelated to the treatment for the gallstones she developed pancreatitis. She spent time in ICU and after several days was transferred back to the ward. There, she drank some lemonade but as she was so weak, choked on her own vomit and suffered brain damage before she could be resuscitated.

Had the Ministry of Defence hospital caused her brain damage? Could it be said that 'but for' the defendant's acts, the claimant's injuries would not have occurred?

If we look at the facts, her weakness that led to the choking was not necessarily the hospital's fault. Clearly, some of her weakness was caused by the pancreatitis, which was also not the fault of the hospital. Nevertheless, the claimants argued that the lack of care materially increased the risk of harm. It was not possible to argue that 'but for' the lack of care, the harm would not have been caused as it was in part caused by the pancreatitis.

The Court of Appeal took a creative approach and held that the material increase of risk which emanated from the defendant's hospital amounted to a sufficient causal link.

Perhaps the key part of the judgment can be found in the words of Waller LJ. Having dismissed the contention that clinical negligence claims should be treated any differently from any other negligence claim where the harm in question is the result of cumulative causes (as was the case in *McGhee*), Waller LJ stated:

JUDGMENT

'If the evidence demonstrates on a balance of probabilities that the injury would have occurred as a result of the non-tortious cause or causes in any event, the Claimant would have failed to establish that the tortious cause contributed … If the evidence demonstrates that "but for" the contribution of the tortious cause the injury would probably not have occurred, the Claimant will (obviously) have discharged the burden. In a case where medical science cannot establish the probability that "but for" an act of negligence the injury would not have happened but can establish that the contribution of the negligent cause was more than negligible, the "but for" test is modified, and the claimant will succeed.'

In short this meant that in cases where there was a lack of medical certainty so that one could not say on the balance of probabilities that 'but for' the defendant's negligence the injuries would not have occurred, it would be open to the court to draw a conclusion that the defendant had caused the harm suffered, on the basis that 'the contribution of the negligent cause [*to the harm suffered by the claimant*] was more than negligible'. The claimant in *Bailey* was, therefore, able to recover damages.

So, after *Bailey* we can say as follows:

If negligence is more than a negligible contribution to the claimant's injuries, it is a material cause. Causation need not be satisfied by a 'but for' test.

1.4.4 Criticism of *Bailey* (2008)

The decision in *Bailey* has received a mixed judicial response, and has been distinguished by the Court of Appeal.

CASE EXAMPLE

Ministry of Defence v AB and others [2010] EWCA Civ 1317

This case involved a claim by war veterans who were attempting to argue, among other things, that they had suffered injury as a result of exposure to radiation during nuclear testing carried out by the British Government in the Pacific during the 1950s.

The Court of Appeal held that in this case the issue of causation was to be resolved in line with the approach taken in *Wilsher v Essex Area Health Authority* (1987). The decisions in *McGhee* and *Bailey* were distinguished on the basis that the 'material contribution to risk' principle derived from those cases should only apply 'where the disease or condition is divisible so that an increased dose of the harmful agent worsens the disease' (*per* Lady Justice Smith).

Nevertheless the decision in *Bailey* was applied in the High Court cases of *Canning-Kishver v Sandwell and West Birmingham Hospitals NHS Trust* [2008] EWHC 2384 and followed in the case of *Ingram v Williams* [2010] EWHC 758 (QB).

CASE EXAMPLE

Canning-Kishver v Sandwell and West Birmingham Hospitals NHS Trust [2008] EWHC 2384 (QB)

In the case of *Canning-Kishver* the defendant NHS Trust was held liable for the cerebral atrophy suffered by a premature baby who had been in the care of the defendant's neonatal intensive care unit. The cerebral atrophy was the result of a cardiac collapse. The claimant argued that the harm suffered had been the result of the failure of the nursing staff to respond adequately to falls in the baby's heart and respiratory rate. It was suggested that if these rates had been monitored appropriately, the cardiac collapse could have been avoided.

The court applied Waller LJ's judgment in *Bailey* and went on to use that test and to find in favour of the claimant. He stated:

JUDGMENT

'... I am entitled to find – and I do find – that on balance of probabilities the contribution of the collapse occasioned by the breach of duty constituted a contribution to the atrophy of the cerebellum that was more than negligible so that the claim succeeds.

On a balance of probabilities, the 'but for' test could not be satisfied. Nevertheless, the court concluded that the cardiac collapse (which was the result of the defendant's negligence) made more than a negligible contribution to the resulting cerebral atrophy. This was enough, according to the rule set out in *Bailey*, to allow the court to conclude that there was a causal link between the defendant's negligence and the harm suffered by the baby.

Given that, in the cases of *Canning-Kishver* and *Ingram* the decision in *Bailey* has allowed the courts to take an approach which seemingly goes against the decision in *Wilsher*, it is understandable that the decision in *Bailey* has been criticised. It is indeed possible that its life is limited.

The practical effect of *Bailey* is that it allows claimants to successfully claim against health providers where they suffer harm, but that harm was inextricably linked to their poor physical health. Arguably this vastly increases the potential scope of the NHS's liability.

There are clear policy reasons which support not widening the scope of claims against health providers.

Medical negligence cases can and should be distinguished from industrial disease cases. In the latter, while there may be more than one possible cause of the claimant's injury, they still all invariably derive from the workplace. The defendant guards against such a risk by insurance.

Conversely, in medical negligence cases, if the claimant is successful in cases where the causative link is not clearly established with blurred parameters, the effect is simply a negative impact on resources for other patients' clinical care.

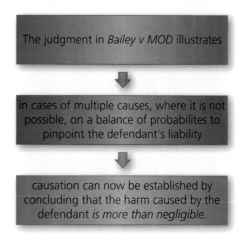

Figure 1.10 The judgment in *Bailey v MOD* (2008)

1.4.5 A failure or an omission to act

We have looked at the difficulties which the courts have in determining whether the defendant's act has caused the claimant's injuries. Further problems are caused where a claimant alleges that the defendant has been negligent in failing or omitting to act. Our consideration concerns the difficulty of causation where the defendant has failed to act rather than has acted.

CASE EXAMPLE

CJL (A Child) v West Midlands Strategic Health Authority [2009] EWHC 259 (QB)

The claimant was in labour. The midwives who were caring for her grew concerned about the foetus and called the obstetrician. The obstetrician had however failed to arrive within a reasonable time which put him in breach of his duty of care to the patient. Expert evidence determined that had the baby been delivered earlier, he would have suffered either no brain damage or minor brain damage.

The defendants were held vicariously liable for the obstetrician's failure to deliver the baby quickly enough after it was discovered that a baby's condition was deteriorating.

Things become more complicated however where the failure in question is not a failure to act quickly enough (as in *CJL (A Child)*), but rather it is a failure to act at all.

CASE EXAMPLE

Bolitho v Hackney Health Authority [1997] 4 All ER 771

This case was also examined on page 17. A doctor failed to attend to a two-year-old boy who had been admitted to hospital with respiratory difficulties. She had been asked by the nurse to attend the child on two occasions but had negligently failed to do so. The child subsequently suffered cardiac arrest and died. The doctor alleged that her failure to attend did not cause the child's death as even if she had attended, she would not have intubated the child (as the claimant alleged she should) and there was a body of professional opinion that supported her decision. Therefore, the defendant alleged that the child would have died in any event.

Although the defendants admitted a breach of their duty of care, they denied that the failure to act had caused Patrick's injuries. The claimant argued that the doctor should have attended Patrick when she was called and, if she had, she could have prevented the injuries he suffered by intubating him. The doctor claimed, however, that even if she had not been negligent and had attended Patrick when she was called, she would not have intubated the child in any event.

The House of Lords held that on the evidence the claimant could not establish causation. The court accepted the defendant's evidence that there were inherent risks with intubating a young child and therefore even if she had attended the child, she would not have intubated him and it was not negligent not to do so. Hence, we can see that the *Bolam* test applies to causation.

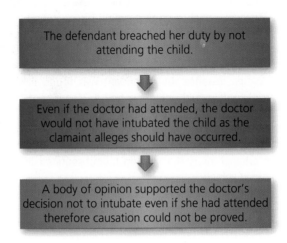

Figure 1.11 Causation in *Bolitho*

A more recent case which builds upon this aspect of the decision in *Bolitho* is the Court of Appeal case of *Gouldsmith v Mid Staffordshire General Hospitals NHS Trust* (2007).

CASE EXAMPLE

Gouldsmith v Mid Staffordshire General Hospitals NHS Trust [2007] EWCA Civ 397

The claimant suffered from lesions on her left hand. The defendants treated her but it was necessary to amputate her left index finger. She was later re-admitted and due to further deterioration, it became necessary to amputate her other fingers. The claimant alleged that if she had been referred to a specialist hospital then they would have operated earlier which would have avoided subsequent amputation.

The court therefore had to consider, as in *Bolitho*, what the claimant's position would have been had she been referred to the specialist.

The Trust had breached its duty as it failed to refer the claimant to a specialist hospital. The court needed to consider what would have happened if the claimant had been referred, and whether on a balance of probabilities the hospital would have operated on the lesion.

In applying the *Bolitho* test, the court held that the claimant should have been referred to the specialist hospital and, had she been referred, she would on a balance of probabilities been operated upon, which would have avoided the subsequent amputation to her fingers.

1.4.6 Loss of chance

This complicated area of law arises where the doctor breaches his duty to his patient and the breach deprives the patient of the chance to make a full recovery from their condition.

CASE EXAMPLE

Hotson v East Berkshire Area Health Authority [1987] AC 750

A 13-year-old boy injured his hip as a result of falling from a tree at home. He was taken to hospital and sent home without his injury being correctly diagnosed. After five days, he returned to hospital still in pain. There, his condition was correctly diagnosed and he received appropriate treatment. He was, however, left permanently disabled. The plaintiff alleged that, had he been correctly diagnosed when he first attended the hospital, he would have been treated accordingly at the time and he would have had a 25 per cent chance of recovery. He sued the defendant on these grounds.

The evidence showed that even if his injury had been correctly diagnosed/treated during his first hospital visit, he could have been one of those patients who still go on to develop that disability in 75 per cent of cases. His claim was therefore for the loss of a 25 per cent chance to make a full recovery from his condition due to the negligent misdiagnosis.

At first instance the defendant was found liable; however, in light of the fact that the plaintiff would only have had a 25 per cent chance of making a full recovery even if the defendant had not been negligent, Hotson was awarded damages equivalent to 25 per cent of the full value of the claim. This approach was supported by the Court of Appeal. However, the House of Lords took a different approach and concluded that it was the original injury that caused his subsequent disability. The defendant health authority avoided liability.

Lord Bridge stated in that case:

JUDGMENT

'... unless the plaintiff could prove on a balance of probabilities that the delayed treatment was at least a material contributory cause ... he failed on the issue of causation and no quantification could arise.'

The problem this creates for a claimant who tries to base their claim on an alleged 'loss of a chance' to make a full recovery should be clear. The court's reasoning in such cases is very simplistic. When the courts are trying to decide whether, by their negligence, the defendant caused the claimant's loss of a chance to make a full recovery from their condition, they apply the 'but for' test as follows:

- If the court concludes that there was a greater than 50 per cent chance that an event might happen, the court will conclude that the event was definitely going to happen.
- If the court concludes that there was a lower than 50 per cent chance that an event might happen, the court will conclude that the event was definitely *not* going to happen.

This approach is neatly summarised in the words of Lord Nicholls in the case of *Gregg v Scott* (2005) below:

JUDGMENT

'The present state of the law is crude to an extent bordering on arbitrariness. It means that a patient with a 60 per cent chance of recovery reduced to a 40 per cent prospect by medical negligence can obtain compensation. But he can obtain nothing if his prospects were reduced from 40 per cent to nil.'

CASE EXAMPLE

Gregg v Scott [2005] UKHL 2

The claimant, Mr Gregg, attended his GP, Dr Scott, as he was concerned about a lump under his arm. The doctor failed to refer him to hospital and negligently diagnosed the lump as benign. Nine months later Mr Gregg returned to see another GP who referred him to hospital. Mr Gregg was subsequently diagnosed with cancer of the lymph glands but by the time it was detected, the cancer had spread.

Statistics showed that had Mr Gregg been treated promptly, his chances of surviving for a further 10 years stood at 42 per cent. Following Mr Gregg's second relapse, however, his chances of surviving a further ten years had dropped to 25 per cent. The claimant argued that the defendant GP's failure to refer him on to hospital had cost him a 17 per cent chance of being 'cured'. In this context the term 'cure' meant surviving for a period of ten years.

It was accepted that the examination carried out by the claimant's original general practitioner was negligent. The key question therefore was whether it could be said, on the balance of probabilities, that this negligent examination had caused the harm suffered by Mr Gregg (that is, the 17 per cent drop in his chances of being 'cured').

In order to succeed in his claim, Mr Gregg had to prove that, on the balance of probabilities, he would have survived for a further ten years if the GP had not negligently failed to refer him to a specialist. Statistics showed however that even if the doctor *had* referred him to a specialist, he only stood a 42 per cent chance of reaching the ten-year mark; that is to say, according to the balance of probabilities test it was unlikely he would have survived that long even if the original examination had not been carried out negligently and he had been referred to hospital at that point.

The way the courts work the 'balance of probabilities' test means that, in the eyes of court, if there is a less than 50 per cent chance that something would have occurred then it is deemed legally certain that it would not have happened. Since Mr Gregg only had a 42 per cent chance of surviving prior to the defendant's negligence, legally speaking it was a certainty that he would not have been 'cured' even if the defendant had not been negligent. As such it is unsurprising that the court could not hold that the defendant's negligence had caused Mr Gregg's injury (that is, the loss of a chance to survive ten years). Mr Gregg's claim was dismissed.

The House of Lords in *Gregg v Scott* was divided 3:2 in favour of denying Mr Gregg a chance to recover damages. The dissenting judgments in that case were delivered by Lord Nicholls and by Lord Hope.

Lord Nicholls was highly critical of the 'all-or-nothing balance of probabilities approach' adopted by the House of Lords in *Hotson*. He states:

JUDGMENT

'The loss of a 45 per cent prospect of recovery is just as much a real loss for a patient as the loss of a 55 per cent prospect of recovery. In both cases the doctor was in breach of his duty to the patient. In both cases the patient was worse off. He lost something of importance and value. But, it is said, in one case the patient has a remedy, in the other he does not.'

For Lord Nicholls therefore, a loss of a percentage chance to make a full recovery from illness/injury was a real and actionable loss, deserving of compensation regardless of what the claimant's prospects of making a full recovery were at the time of the negligent act. Any approach which took a different view was in Lord Nicholls' view 'irrational and indefensible'. This approach was supported by Lord Hope. Like Lord Nicholls, Lord Hope agreed that the loss of a prospect of making a recovery as a result of the defendant's negligence was a loss for which Mr Gregg deserved to be compensated. Furthermore, Lord Hope agreed that the correct way to compensate such individuals would be to calculate damages in accordance with the approach of the lower courts in *Hotson*.

KEY FACTS

Key facts on loss of chance cases

	Hotson v East Berkshire Health Authority (1987)	*Chester v Afshar* (2004)	*Gregg v Scott* (2005)
Facts	13-year-old boy fell out of a tree. Delayed diagnosis and treatment for 5 days.	Defendant failed to warn the patient of 1–2% risk of nerve damage during surgery. The risk materialised.	Delayed diagnosis of cancer of the lymph gland.
House of Lords	Unanimous judgment	Majority judgment	Majority judgment
Judgment	Claimant needed to prove on a balance of probabilities that the delayed treatment was at least a material contribution of the cause. The claimant failed on causation.	The claimant had not been properly and fully informed. The defendant had violated the claimant's autonomy. She underwent the operation which she probably would have had at a later stage but she suffered injury as a result of this operation. The claimant was successful in her claim.	It could not be proved that the delayed diagnosis and delay had caused the claimant's loss. The claimant failed in his claim.

ACTIVITY

Self-test questions on causation

Ensure that all your answers are supported by case law.

- Clearly express the 'but for' test.
- What is the difficulty of multiple causes in medical cases, and what approach do the courts take?
- Distinguish the case you used to answer the above question with non-medical cases. How does the approach differ?
- Consider two cases that are relevant to an omission or a failure to act. Ensure that you can clearly express the principles in both cases.
- Why did the courts find for the defendant in *Hotson*?
- As far as you are able, compare and contrast the judgments of *Chester v Afshar* and *Gregg v Scott*.

We now revisit the Applying the Law activity on page 23, and consider the problems of causation that may arise. The facts have been altered slightly. Invariably, if you are faced with a question on breach, causation will also be relevant.

SAMPLE ESSAY QUESTION

Test your understanding of the legal principles you have just read about by reading and discussing the following scenario:

A is in the late stages of pregnancy, and having felt the baby kicking regularly is rather alarmed one day when she feels the baby is a little less active. On advice from her midwife, she attends a hospital run by West County NHS Trust and is seen by Dr Y. He admits her and she is taken to the labour ward for observations. She is attached to a CTG which records the foetal heartbeat. Two hours later, Nurse X notices a sudden deceleration which causes her concern. She bleeps Dr Y who says he will attend shortly. He fails to arrive and Nurse X bleeps him again. He admits that he forgot. He is a little embarrassed and tells Nurse X that the deceleration is not a problem. Twenty minutes later it occurs again and Nurse X, being unable to bleep Dr Y bleeps Mr Z, the obstetric consultant. He arrives, looks at the CTG trace and is extremely alarmed. He insists on an emergency Caesarean section and baby B is born 15 minutes later. The baby fails to breathe spontaneously and, once resuscitated, it becomes apparent that he will be severely brain damaged. However, later blood tests reveal that the brain damage caused could have been as a result of A contracting rubella during pregnancy, a known cause of brain damage in babies.

- We have already considered the duty of care and breach of duty elements of this claim, and these will not be discussed further. It will be assumed for present purposes that Dr Y has breached the duty of care expected of him and thus he is negligent.
- It will also be assumed for present purposes that the requisite tests have been satisfied and West County NHS Trust is vicariously liable for the negligence of their employee, Dr Y.
- Even though Dr Y is negligent, West County NHS Trust will not be liable to pay any damages unless the court is satisfied that, on the balance of probabilities, Dr Y's negligent failure to attend caused the brain damage suffered by baby B.

- Your starting point should be a discussion of the decision in *Bolitho*, as the facts are very similar. As in *Bolitho*, this claim involves a negligent failure to act. This means you are faced with a two-stage test you need to apply (see Figure 1.12 below for a visual guide to how this section of the answer works).
- Ask yourself what the defendant would have done if he had attended when he was first summonsed. Would Dr Y have recommended a Caesarean section at that point? If the answer to that question is 'Yes, if Dr Y had attended he would have made such a recommendation', then you would be one step closer to establishing causation (though such a finding would not be the end of the matter). If, on the other hand, the answer is 'No, even if Dr Y had attended he would not have called for a Caesarean section' then you would need to consider the next step in the *Bolitho* test.

- The second step of the *Bolitho* test requires you to ask yourself whether Dr Y's decision not to recommend a Caesarean section in that hypothetical scenario would have been negligent. This will require you to apply the *Bolam* test. If you conclude that Dr Y's decision not to recommend a Caesarean section in that hypothetical situation *would not* have been negligent, then that brings the claim to a close and West County NHS Trust will not be liable to pay out damages to baby B.
- If, on the other hand, you conclude that Dr Y's decision not to recommend a Caesarean section in that situation *would* have been negligent then you need to move on to consider the next issue.

- The next issue is the question of whether Dr Y's negligence was the cause of baby B's brain damage. This brings us to the factual causation element of a negligence claim. This requires you to look at the 'but for' test from the case of *Barnett v Chelsea and Kensington Hospital Management Committee* (1969).
- You should ask yourself whether, on a balance of probabilities, baby B would have suffered brain damage 'but for' Dr Y's negligence.
- You should also realise that the scenario contains a major problem. On the facts there are two potential causes of baby B's injury. As we know, the 'but for' test is not suited to those cases where there is more than one possible cause of the injury in question. As such, reference will need to be made to those cases which consider the issue of multiple causes.

- It would appear that the case of *Wilsher* is applicable here. There are multiple potential causes of baby B's injury and so reference to the decisions in *McGhee* and *Fairchild* would not be appropriate. Of course, the decision in *Wilsher* would pose a major obstacle to any claim in negligence based on these facts. The House of Lords in that case states that the defendant had to prove, on the balance of probabilities, that the defendant's negligence was *the* cause of the claimant's injury. We may not be able to do that here.
- However, discussion of the more recent case of *Bailey* (2008) highlighted the Court of Appeal's creative approach to cases where there are multiple potential causes of the injury. The Court of Appeal said in *Bailey* that where there was a lack of medical certainty so that one cannot say 'but for' the defendant's negligence the injuries would not have occurred, factual causation could be established if it could be shown that the defendant's negligence had made a 'more than negligible' contribution to the likelihood that the claimant would go on to suffer the injury in question.

- How to conclude? If you have highlighted the relevant issues, discussed the relevant law and applied the law throughout your answer to the facts of the question, all you need to do is offer your opinion whether, on the basis of your discussion, you believe West County NHS Trust will be required to pay damages. The answer you reach will, most likely, be dependent upon whether you believe *Wilsher* or *Bailey* should apply here.

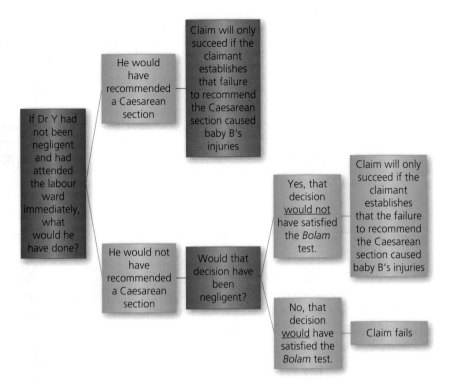

Figure 1.12 Applying the law

1.4.7 Remoteness

The last element that a claimant is required to prove after establishing causation is that the damage claimed for is not too remote. Remoteness tends not to be an issue in cases of medical negligence, but the seminal case in tort, *The Wagon Mound* [1961] AC 388 reminds us that the type of damage needs to be foreseeable although the extent of it does not.

CASE EXAMPLE

R v Croydon Health Authority [1998] PIQR Q26

The claimant underwent a chest x-ray which was required for employment purposes. The defendant failed to warn her of an abnormality. She subsequently became pregnant and argued that had she been aware of the abnormality she would not have become pregnant.

It was too remote to hold the defendant health authority liable for the failure to warn of abnormalities which may affect her personal life. The defendant was only responsible to the extent that it was required to undertake the chest x-ray initially.

1.4.8 Defences

It is worth exploring this area, even though in reality, its use in medical negligence litigation is likely to be limited.

There are three defences that could be raised:

- *Volenti non fit injuria*
- *Ex turpi causa*
- Contributory negligence.

The first defence, *volenti non fit injuria* (translated as 'to a willing person, no injury is done') is unlikely ever to be applied to medical negligence cases as it means that the claimant would be voluntarily assuming the risk of being injured.

The second defence, *ex turpi causa* (no action may be founded on illegal or immoral conduct) is only slightly more likely and means that an action cannot arise from the claimant's illegal act. This may be difficult to understand without the benefit of one of the few medical cases on the subject.

CASE EXAMPLE

Clunis v Camden and Islington Health Authority [1998] QB 978

In this highly publicised case, the claimant who had mental health problems stabbed a tube passenger (Jonathan Zito) to death. He sued the health authority, alleging that they breached their duty of care in treating him and had they acted properly, he would not have been released to kill.

In refusing his claim, the Court of Appeal emphasised that as a matter of public policy it would be wrong to allow a claim that arose only because of the commission of a criminal offence.

The last defence is also unlikely to arise. The only way in which one could visualise a patient having been contributory negligent would be where a patient has acted directly against medical advice in such a way that it has an immediate effect on her wellbeing. In these circumstances, s 1, Law Reform (Contributory Negligence) Act 1945 will reduce the amount of damages awarded to the claimant reflecting her percentage contribution to the negligence alleged.

SUMMARY

■ A duty of care exists in the doctor–patient relationship, and it is generally straightforward to establish such a duty. There are however examples in common law where the courts have held there is insufficient proximity between the parties for a duty to exist.

■ Occasionally there are novel situations where a duty of care has been determined by the courts, although these are increasingly infrequent.

■ Whether a breach of duty of care has occurred will be determined by applying the *Bolam* test, which has been controversial in its application but is applied nonetheless.

■ The case of *Bolitho* attempted to limit its boundaries and application to cases of medical and clinical negligence but, while sometimes relevant, it is the *Bolam* test that pervades medical law.

■ In order to establish negligence, causation must also be tested and is often satisfied by the traditional 'but for' test. In cases of multiple causes, which is often the case where medical negligence is alleged, the test is simply not suitable.

■ Causation must then be proved on a balance of probabilities, but creative interpretation by the courts has often led to perceived injustice although there is also evidence of more patient-centred cases decided.

Further reading

Students must ensure that they read the judgments of the most significant cases, such as *Bolam*, *Bolitho*, *Wilsher* and *Bailey*.

Bailey, S. H. (2010) 'Causation in negligence: what is a material contribution?' *Legal Studies*, Vol. 30. No. 2, pages 167–85.

Brazier, M. and Miola, J. (2000) 'Bye-bye Bolam: A Medical Litigation Revolution', *Medical Law Review* 8, 85.

Herring, J. (2010) *Medical Law and Ethics*, third edition. Oxford: OUP.

Mason, J. K. and Laurie, G. T. (2010) *Mason and McCall Smith's Law and Medical Ethics*, eighth edition. Oxford: OUP.

Pattinson, S. D. (2006) *Medical Law and Ethics*, London: Sweet & Maxwell.

Woolf, Lord, (2001) 'Are the Courts Excessively Deferential To The Medical Profession?' *Medical Law Review* 9, 1.

2

Consent

This chapter considers the issue of consent in a number of various forms. For the sake of clarity, it will be divided into three parts. In Part 1, we discuss the concept of consent and capacity; in Part 2 we investigate the issues of consent and informed consent; and in Part 3 we explore consent as it relates to children and the incompetent adult.

Before we embark upon this area, there are some fundamental principles which can be summarised as follows:

■ An adult patient who has capacity cannot be treated without his consent.
■ Any patient who does not have capacity is treated according to his or her 'best interests'.
■ An adult patient can refuse life-saving treatment if there is a valid Advance Decision.
■ A valid and applicable Advance Directive must be respected by a medical professional.
■ A *'Gillick* competent' child is able to consent to treatment.
■ A *'Gillick* competent' child's refusal of treatment can be overridden.

2.1 Part 1: Consent and capacity

AIMS AND OBJECTIVES

By the end of this section you should be able to:

■ Appreciate why consent is crucial to modern medical practice
■ Identify the key elements of a valid consent
■ Appreciate and demonstrate an understanding of the definition of competence with reference to both common law and statute
■ Understand how the common law principles and the law is applied to determine whether or not a patient has capacity
■ Demonstrate a clear understanding of the provisions of the Mental Capacity Act (MCA) 2005
■ Appreciate the important role which the principles of autonomy and paternalism have had to play in shaping the law in this area.

2.1.1 Why is consent important?

JUDGMENT

'Every human being of adult years and sound mind has a right to determine what shall be done with his own body.' (Cardozo J, *Schoelendorff v New York Hospital* [1914] 211 N.Y.125)

This well-known American quotation is often regarded as the foundation stone for the law on consent. Obviously this decision does not bind UK courts, but the courts have found it highly persuasive. The result of this is that the consent of a patient has become an essential prerequisite for any treatment. It is unlawful for a medical professional to touch a patient without their consent (express or implied) or statutory authority. The purpose of a patient's consent is to allow 'treatment or surgery which would otherwise be unlawful as a trespass is made lawful by the consent of the patient' (*per* Neill J in *F v West Berkshire Health Authority* [1990] 2 AC 1).

Any physical interference with a patient initiated without their consent can amount to the tort of trespass to the person (in civil law). In extreme cases such conduct could also amount to the criminal offence of ABH (actual bodily harm) contrary to s 47, Offences Against the Person Act 1861 or GBH (grievous bodily harm) contrary to ss 18 and 20, Offences Against the Person Act 1861.

In reality criminal liability would be hard to imagine as it would mean that *no* consent would have been obtained from the patient. This might be the case where the medical professional has simply proceeded with treatment without obtaining the patient's consent, acted against the patient's will or where they have obtained the patient's consent but it is vitiated as the result of a fraud.

2.1.2 Consent, the competent adult and the common law criteria

A patient is able to consent to treatment if they are competent. A patient is competent if they are found to have capacity to make decisions about their treatment. If a patient lacks capacity, he will be treated in his or her best interests.

CASE EXAMPLE

Re C (Adult: Refusal of Treatment) [1994] 1 WLR 290

The plaintiff was an in-patient at Broadmoor Hospital, suffering from paranoid schizophrenia. He had a gangrenous foot, and was advised that without amputation he would be likely to die. The plaintiff, however, believed he was a famous doctor and he could cure himself. He fully understood the doctor's advice, simply choosing to reject it, believing that God would not wish him to have his foot amputated. He applied for an injunction preventing the Health Authorities from removing his left foot.

The court held that there were three criteria for establishing competence:

- being able to comprehend and retain the information
- a belief in the information, and
- weighing up the advice in order to reach a decision.

Despite his irrational view, the plaintiff could fulfil the criteria; he could understand the advice he was given and, on the facts, he fully understood that it was likely he would die if he did not have his foot amputated; lastly, he was capable of weighing up the information. Miraculously, his foot largely recovered without medical intervention.

JUDGMENT

'I am satisfied that he has understood and retained the relevant treatment information, that in his own way he believes it, and that in the same fashion he has arrived at a clear choice.' (*per* Thorpe J)

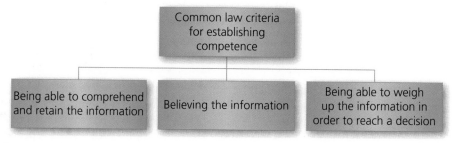

Figure 2.1 Common law test for establishing competence

ACTIVITY

Applying the law

Imagine the following scenario; you have just been told that you are suffering from some rare condition which may kill you. There is an operation which will enable you to make a full recovery but you must undergo this operation immediately, and the operation will 'put you out of action' for a long period. You can understand and retain the information but you are in such emotional turmoil you do not know what to do. You know that if you do not have the operation you may die, but you are understandably scared.

Would the law consider you competent to make a decision about your treatment in that scenario? A consideration of some relevant cases should help us decide.

CASE EXAMPLE

Re MB (Medical Treatment) [1997] 2 FLR 426

The plaintiff was pregnant and it was likely that she required a Caesarean section. She consented to the operation but withdrew her consent to the anaesthesia as she had a needle phobia. In anticipation of this possibility, the Trust had obtained a declaration for her to be treated as incompetent if she did require a Caesarean section and she appealed against the declaration.

Her appeal was dismissed. Although the court recognised that treating her without her consent was an assault, the presumption of consent was rebuttable. While a patient could refuse treatment even where it could lead to her and/or her baby's death, the Court of Appeal held her needle phobia rendered her temporarily incompetent and her appeal was dismissed.

JUDGMENT

'A person lacked capacity when some impairment or disturbance of mental function rendered that person unable to make a decision. Inability to make a decision occurred when a patient was unable to comprehend, retain and use information and weigh it in the balance.' (*per* Butler-Sloss LJ)

The Court of Appeal further stated that 'temporary factors such as shock, pain or drugs might completely erode capacity'. The impairment referred to in the above quote which could affect a patient's capacity (albeit temporarily) could, in theory, be something as basic as pain-relieving drugs. This does suggest that the test for competence is somewhat fluid.

The cases below illustrate where individuals have been deemed to suffer from a temporary lack of capacity.

CASE EXAMPLE

Rochdale Healthcare (NHS) Trust v C [1997] 1 FCR 274

The patient was in labour and refused to undergo a Caesarean section despite being told that without it both she and the foetus would die. The hospital questioned her capacity to refuse consent.

The court held that she was able to understand and retain the information she was given, as well as believing such information. However, the court said she was incapable of weighing up the information she was presented with, thus preventing her from making a reasoned choice. It was felt this inability was caused by the pain she was experiencing at the time she refused consent.

JUDGMENT

'The patient was in the throes of labour with all that is involved in terms of pain and emotional stress. I concluded that a patient who could, in those circumstances, speak in terms which seemed to accept the inevitability of her own death, was not a patient who was able properly to weigh up the considerations that arose so as to make any valid decision, about anything of even the most trivial kind, surely still less one which involved her own life.' (*per* Johnson J)

Consequently the patient was held to lack the requisite capacity to refuse consent, leaving the doctors free to treat the patient in her best interests.

CASE EXAMPLE

Bolton Hospitals NHS Trust v O [2003] 1 FLR 824

The patient was 39 weeks pregnant with her fifth child. All previous deliveries had been by Caesarean section and it was clear she would not be able to have this child by normal delivery. There was a high risk both to her and her baby's life. She initially consented to a Caesarean section but withdrew her consent on four occasions prior to being anaesthetised. It would appear that she was experiencing signs of post-traumatic stress disorder relating to previous deliveries. The Trust sought a declaration from the court declaring her to be temporarily incompetent and therefore lacking capacity. She was, the Trust alleged, so blinded by her emotional state that she was unable to process the information.

The court accepted that while a patient was entitled to refuse medical treatment, this was a situation where the patient was acting so irrationally that she was unable to process the information properly. Accordingly, it was acceptable to declare her incompetent and treat her against her will. It was further accepted that where:

- that patient lacks capacity to give a valid refusal to treatment, and
- treatment is deemed to be in their best interests,

it is lawful to use reasonable force to treat them.

It is no coincidence that many of these cases involve women in the throes of labour who, whether through anxiety, distress or pain, may express the desire to die rather than to undergo a Caesarean operation. If one was to ask the same question to the same woman when she was not in labour, it would be very likely that she would express incredulity at the thought of dying rather than undergoing a Caesarean section. In any event, the court held the patient to be temporarily lacking in capacity and the Trust proceeded to act in the patient's best interests; her baby was delivered by Caesarean.

Key facts on common law cases on capacity

Case	Judgment
Re C (Adult: Refusal of Medical Treatment) (1994)	Patient could comprehend and retain the information; he could believe the information; and he could weigh it up in order to reach a decision. He was competent and could refuse medical treatment if he so wished.
Re MB (Medical Treatment) (1997)	A patient with a fear of needles was held to be temporarily incompetent. Incompetence, however temporary, can be caused by shock, pain or the effect of prescribed drugs.
Rochdale Healthcare (NHS) Trust v C (1997)	The pain and emotional stress of labour temporarily compromised the patient's competence.
Bolton Hospitals NHS Trust v O (2003)	The patient was so affected by her emotional state while in labour that it was justifiable to declare her incompetent.

2.1.3 The Mental Capacity Act 2005

The MCA 2005 largely puts the common law decisions on a statutory basis. Hence while the common law is important for an understanding of the development of the law, the guiding principles are now contained in statute, and it is the MCA 2005 that must now be applied.

We begin with a presumption that a person has capacity to make decisions, and s 1(2) states that a person must be assumed to have capacity unless it is established that he lacks capacity.

As demonstrated with the common law decisions, it is worth recalling that we are concerned with a *specific* decision about the patient's medical treatment and *not* about teir *general* decision-making ability.

We have also seen that just because the patient makes a decision which appears to be odd or bizarre, this does not mean that the patient lacks capacity. Section 1(4) states that just because a person makes an unwise decision it does not mean he is unable to make a decision.

The common law test of capacity that we saw in *Re C* has now been encapsulated in s 2(1), MCA 2005 which explains that a person lacks capacity:

SECTION

2(1) 'if at the material time he is unable to make a decision for himself in relation to the matter because of an impairment of, or a disturbance in the functioning of, the mind or brain'.

Therefore, if he does have an impairment of, or a disturbance in the functioning of, the mind or the brain which affects his decision-making, he will lack capacity.

Section 3(1) provides that a person is unable to make a decision if they cannot:

- understand information relevant to the decision to be made
- retain that information
- use or weigh that information as part of the decision-making process, or
- communicate their decision (whether by talking, using sign language or any other means).

If the answer to both of those questions is 'Yes', then the patient will be deemed to lack the necessary capacity to make a decision.

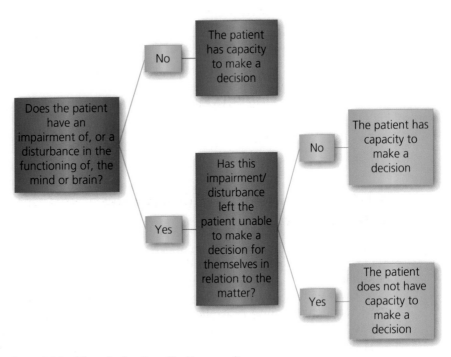

Figure 2.2 Deciding whether the patient has capacity

However, s 2(3) and the Mental Capacity Act 2005 Code of Practice states that any decision about the capacity of the individual to make a decision must never be based upon:

- their **age** – for example, an individual should not be deemed to lack capacity merely because they are elderly
- their **appearance** – for example, an individual should not be deemed to lack capacity merely because of the way they may look, whether it be untidy or scruffy, or because they exhibit the physical characteristics of conditions such as Down's Syndrome
- assumptions about their **condition** – for example, an individual should not be deemed to lack capacity merely because they suffer from long-term health conditions such as learning disabilities, or even if they appear drunk or withdrawn.
- any aspect of their **behaviour** – for example, an individual should not be deemed to lack capacity merely because they are shouting and gesticulating wildly or because they may appear withdrawn.

Key facts of the MCA 2005 relating to capacity

Section	Provision
S 1(2)	A person must be assumed to have capacity unless it is established that he lacks capacity.
S 1(4)	A person is not to be treated as unable to make a decision merely because he makes an unwise decision.
S 2	A person lacks capacity to make a decision if at the material time he is unable to make a decision for himself in relation to the matter because of an impairment of, or a disturbance in the functioning of, the mind or brain.
S 2(2)	The impairment or disturbance of the mind or brain experienced by the decision-maker can be temporary or permanent.
S 3(1)	A person is to be viewed as 'unable to make a decision for himself' (for the purposes of s 2(1)) if he is unable to: a) understand the information relevant to the decision b) retain that information c) use or weigh that information as part of the process of making the decision, or d) communicate his decision.

2.1.4 Patients demonstrating capacity and the consequences of their decision

CASE EXAMPLE

Re T (Adult: Refusal of Medical Treatment) [1993] Fam 95

The patient, a pregnant Jehovah's Witness, was involved in a car accident. Although she had been brought up as a Jehovah's Witness she was not now practising. She required a Caesarean section, but after a conversation in private with her mother she refused any blood products. After the Caesarean section her condition worsened significantly. Members of her family applied to the courts to order treatment and override her refusal, alleging that she had been under pressure from her mother.

The court ordered the transfusion as they found her decision to refuse treatment was not entirely her own, and she had been unduly influenced or pressurised by her mother. Her appeal to the Court of Appeal was dismissed. In rebutting the presumption of capacity the court was then able to allow the hospital to act in her best interests, and the blood transfusion was ordered. The case illustrates not only that the presumption of capacity is capable of being rebutted, but that a decision to refuse medical treatment must be made freely and not under any influence, pressure or coercion.

JUDGMENT

'This situation gives rise to a conflict between the two interests, that of the patient and that of the society in which he lives. The patient's interests consist of his right to self-determination – his right to live his own life how he wishes, even if it will damage his health or lead to his premature death. Society's interest is in upholding the concept that all human life is sacred and should be preserved if at all possible. It is well established that in the ultimate the right of individual is paramount ... the patient's right of choice exists whether the reasons for making that choice are irrational, unknown or even non-existent.' (*per* Lord Donaldson)

There are two crucial points made in his judgment which ought to be highlighted:

1. There is a presumption that every adult patient has the capacity to make decisions about their treatment. This is, however, a rebuttable presumption.
2. The mere fact that the patient's decision appears to be an unwise decision (or an 'irrational' reason to use the words of Lord Donaldson MR in *Re T*) does not automatically mean that the patient lacks capacity.

Lord Justice Staughton confirmed the same principle:

JUDGMENT

'An adult whose mental capacity is unimpaired has the right to decide for herself whether she will or will not receive medical or surgical treatment, even in circumstances where she is likely or even certain to die in the absence of treatment.'

Thus, following the decision in *Re T*, an adult who possesses the requisite capacity can refuse treatment even if they might die or suffer serious injury as a result of that refusal.

Moreover in the case of *Airedale NHS Trust v Bland* [1993] AC 789 (which we consider in more detail in Chapter 11), Lord Goff emphasised the fundamental principle that a medical professional must respect the wishes of a competent patient who refuses medical treatment even where a patient's refusal could lead to death.

JUDGMENT

'... if an adult patient of sound mind refuses, however unreasonably, to consent to treatment or care by which his life would or might be prolonged, the doctors responsible for his care must give effect to his wishes, even though they do not consider it to be in his best interests to do so.'

A similar view was expressed by Lord Mustill who stated that:

JUDGMENT

'A doctor has no right to proceed in the face of objection, even if it is plain to all, including the patient, that adverse consequences and even death will or may ensue.'

Therefore, the courts acknowledge that a patient can refuse life-saving or life-sustaining treatment and this must be a patient's autonomous decision but, when this conflicts with the sanctity of life and where there is any doubt about whether the patient has sufficient capacity to refuse life-saving or life-sustaining treatment, the sanctity of life principle will prevail and the patient's refusal in that case can be lawfully overridden. It is thus a balancing act, as shown in Figure 2.3.

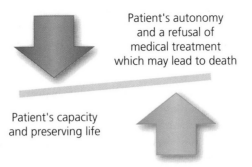

Patient's autonomy and a refusal of medical treatment which may lead to death

Patient's capacity and preserving life

Figure 2.3 Balancing capacity with autonomy

CASE EXAMPLE

Re B (Adult: Refusal of Medical Treatment) [2002] EWHC (Fam) 429

Ms B was a 43-year-old woman who was paralysed from the neck down. She was dependent on respiratory support. There was no prospect of Ms B recovering although steps could be taken to try and improve her quality of life. Ms B made numerous requests for her ventilator to be removed, knowing this would ultimately lead to her inevitable death. It was agreed that Ms B had the requisite capacity to make such a decision.

The clinicians treating Ms B, however, were unwilling to remove Ms B's ventilation in light of the inevitable consequences of those actions. Ms B, therefore, applied to the High Court for a declaration that she had the requisite capacity to refuse treatment and that her ventilator should be removed.

In an overwhelming respect for her autonomy, the court held that she was competent and any continued treatment would be unlawful. The fact that she had been ventilated despite her refusal was unlawful as a battery for which she was awarded £100 damages. There had been a question as to her competency but Dame Butler-Sloss indicated that the medical profession should seek to avoid overt paternalism in a severely disabled patient. If she was competent, which she was, then she had the same rights as everyone else, including the right to be taken off ventilation and reject referral to a spinal rehabilitation unit or other care alternatives.

Discussion point

There are some further points stemming from this case which are worthy of a brief examination.

It is clear from the judgment that Dame Butler-Sloss had a great deal of sympathy for the medical team who were directly involved in the day-to-day care of Ms B. They had been involved in the long-term care of Ms B and had been trained to save life, in contrast to Ms B's request to end her life.

Consequently Ms B's autonomous wishes were ignored. What Dame Butler-Sloss made clear, however, is that the fact that the patient's wishes go against the medical team's values and their beliefs about what is in that patient's best interests, is not a valid justification for not acting on the patient's request. If the team in charge of the patient's care are unwilling to comply with the patient's request, they must find somebody who will.

'If there is no disagreement about competence but the doctors are for any reason unable to carry out the wishes of the patient, their duty is to find other doctors who will do so.'

There was also some concern within the team responsible for Ms B's care that switching off Ms B's ventilator (a step that would inevitably result in her death) was tantamount to murder as the required elements would be fulfilled. However, this case followed the well-known decision in *Bland* where Lord Goff had stated *obiter* in that case that switching off a life-support machine should be viewed as an omission and therefore there could be no criminal liability imposed on any individual who performed that task.

Furthermore, it must not be thought that the decision in *Re B* (2002) has any application to 'right to die' cases. Dame Butler-Sloss makes this point where she states:

JUDGMENT

'It is important to underline that I am not asked directly to decide whether Ms B lives or dies but whether she, herself, is legally competent to make that decision. It is also important to recognise that this case is not about the best interests of the patient but about her mental capacity.'

The decision in *Re B* (2002), therefore, was not about whether Ms B should be allowed to die or not; rather it is solely about whether Ms B had sufficient capacity to refuse life-saving treatment. This limits the potential scope for using the principle in *Re B* and a parallel should not be drawn between *Re B* and later 'right to die' cases.

2.1.5 Rational and irrational decisions

We have seen in *Re T* that just because a decision appears to be irrational, it does not follow that the decision-maker is not competent.

We also know that s 1(4), MCA 2005 confirms, 'A person is not to be treated as unable to make a decision merely because he makes an unwise decision'.

This principle is subsequently reinforced by Butler-Sloss in *Re MB* (1997) who declared that 'A competent woman who has the capacity to decide for ... rational or irrational reasons or for no reason at all' can choose not to have medical intervention regardless of whether it may lead to her death and/or that of her baby.

It may be reasonable in light of these observations to conclude that one can make an unwise or irrational decision and still be competent in the eyes of the law, but consider the case below.

CASE EXAMPLE

St George's Healthcare NHS Trust v S, R v Collins and others [1998] 3 WLR 936

The patient was in the latter stages of pregnancy when she was diagnosed with pre-eclampsia, a condition which threatened the life of both her and her baby. She refused to be admitted to hospital in order for labour to be induced. She said she would not have any medical intervention, even if that meant that she and/or the child would die.

Her medical records showed some previous depression and there was a suggestion by her GP that her mental state could be affecting her capacity. An application was made and granted under s 2, MHA 1983 for her admission to a mental hospital against her will; shortly afterwards, she was transferred to a general hospital. She still refused treatment and application was made for her consent to treatment to be dispensed with. This was made possible by the fact that she was detained under the provisions of the Mental Health Act 1983 (MHA). The declaration was granted, a Caesarean section carried out and a baby girl was born. The patient's detention under the MHA 1983 ended. She left hospital and subsequently appealed against the court's findings.

The Court of Appeal ruled that her detention and the treatment she had forced upon her were both unlawful. Judge LJ's judgment in this case is of particular interest.

JUDGMENT

'Even when his or her own life depends on receiving medical treatment, an adult of sound mind is entitled to refuse it. This reflects the autonomy of each individual and the right of self-determination.'

The importance of a patient's autonomy has already been established in previous case law, but did the fact that her decisions were putting the life of her unborn baby at risk entitle the medical team to treat her against her will?

Lord Justice Judge said:

JUDGMENT

'In our judgment while pregnancy increases the personal responsibilities of a woman it does not diminish her entitlement to decide whether or not to undergo medical treatment. Although human, and protected by the law in a number of different ways ... an unborn child is not a separate person from its mother. Its need for medical assistance does not prevail over her rights. She is entitled not to be forced to submit to an invasion of her body against her will, whether her own life or that of her unborn child depends on it. Her right is not reduced or diminished merely because her decision to exercise it may appear morally repugnant.'

The decision in *St George's NHS Trust v S* therefore provides us with the strongest support for any contention that a patient must not be deemed as incompetent simply because '[their] thinking process is unusual, even apparently bizarre and irrational, and contrary to the views of the overwhelming majority of the community at large.'

SUMMARY

- The courts will respect a competent patient's right to make autonomous decisions such as a decision to refuse medical treatment. A patient's autonomous decision based upon religious conviction will be respected. However, if a patient's decision (not based on any religious conviction) is so irrational that it defies logic, the courts could intervene and declare that a patient temporarily lacks capacity, allowing doctors to take a more paternalistic approach and order treatment if it is deemed to be in the patient's best interests.
- We might question whether the courts have become more paternalistic in their approach to cases involving refusals of treatment. In *Re C* (1994), the patient was deemed to have capacity to refuse treatment (a decision which might have resulted in his death), even though he was clearly delusionary. In *Re MB* (1997) on the other hand, the court was willing to override the patient's refusal of treatment on the grounds that the patient temporarily lacked capacity (the patient had a needle phobia). This approach was applied in both *Rochdale Healthcare NHS Trust v C* (1997) and *Bolton Hospitals NHS Trust v O* (2003), despite the clear expressions of respect for a woman's autonomy expressed in *St George's Healthcare Trust* (1998).
- The question remains, whether such decisions demonstrate an increasing willingness on the part of the courts to override patient refusals, or whether cases such as *Re MB*

(1997) are to be viewed as isolated decisions limited to the particular facts of that case? Without doubt, a competent patient has a right of self-determination. However, it increasingly seems to be the case that the more irrational the decision in question is, the more likely it is that the courts will declare that the patient lacks competency, even if it only temporarily.

- The one area where the courts seem more ready to take this step is where a woman in labour declines treatment for what one may say are irrational reasons. It would appear that the courts are taking a common sense approach by declaring a woman temporarily lacking in competency in order to deliver the baby and save both the mother and the baby's life, rather than respecting their autonomy and watching them die. Many would say that despite an overtly paternalistic approach, this is the preferred approach.

ACTIVITY

Self-test questions

- With reference to case law, consider the legal presumption of competence. Why is it important? How can it be rebutted? Do you think that the threshold for capacity is set at an appropriate level?
- Accurately define the statutory criteria for capacity.
- With close consideration of case law, what approach have the courts taken when dealing with women in labour? Do you consider this to be a satisfactory approach? If so, why?
- Critically evaluate the decision in *Re B* (2002). Do you support the decision? Ensure that you explain your reasons clearly.

2.2 Part 2: Consent and the competent adult: the need for sufficient information

AIMS AND OBJECTIVES

By the end of this section you should be able to:

- Appreciate the importance of consent in modern medical law
- Appreciate the roles of paternalism and autonomy in shaping the development of the law governing consent issues
- Demonstrate an understanding of the development of informed consent and judicial opinion.

2.2.1 Introduction

Even if the patient is deemed to have the requisite level of capacity to consent to/ refuse treatment, and even if that decision has been made of the patient's own free will, that patient's decision will be meaningless if they were not provided with sufficient information to help them make an *informed* decision.

There are two major questions to address:

1. How much information must be provided to patients before their consent can be said to be valid?
2. What are the consequences of failing to give patients sufficient information to enable them to make an informed decision about their treatment?

This section of the chapter is devoted to answering these two questions.

2.2.2 Battery

We begin by looking at a number of cases where the defendants have been found liable in battery.

CASE EXAMPLE

Devi v West Midlands Health Authority [1981] CA Transcript 491 Unreported

The patient consented to an operation to repair a perforation of the uterus. The surgeon performed a sterilisation as well as the repair as he considered it was in the patient's best interests.

The defendants were liable for battery as she had not consented to the procedure. It was irrelevant that the surgeon had acted in her best interests.

Similarly, in the earlier case in the USA, *Mohr v Williams* (1950) 104 N.W. 12 the plaintiff consented to an operation on her right ear. Once she was anaesthetised, the surgeon discovered it was her left ear rather than her right ear that required surgery. The defendants were liable in battery as the surgeon did not have consent to operate on her right ear.

In the rather extreme civil case of *Appleton v Garrett* [1997] 34 BMLR 23 involving about 100 patients, a dentist treated patients unnecessarily for profit. The dentist had fully explained the procedures involved to each patient but was found liable in battery as none of the plaintiffs had given real and genuine consent.

It is however rather difficult for a claimant to succeed in a claim in battery. This is because the threshold test for avoiding a claim in battery is set at such a low level. This point is evident in the following case which represented the position of law in this area at that time.

CASE EXAMPLE

Chatterton v Gerson [1981] QB 432

The plaintiff was being treated for chronic pain around an operation scar from a hernia operation. She was given an injection of a substance to destroy the nerves that were giving her the pain, but the result was that her leg became completely numb, affecting her mobility. She did not allege negligence in the way the defendant carried out the operation but claimed in the tort of trespass, alleging that her consent was invalid as the defendant had not warned her of the danger and therefore she could not give 'informed consent'.

Bristow J stated, 'In my judgment once the patient is informed in broad terms of the nature of the procedure which is intended, and gives her consent, that consent is real.' Since the patient had consented in broad terms, consent was 'real' and there could be no action in battery. Further, the court confirmed that where the claimant is seeking to claim damages for failing to advise them of risks associated with their treatment, the correct basis for such an action was the tort of negligence and not the tort of battery.

The reluctance of the courts to find doctors liable in battery was apparent and demonstrated again in the case of *Hills v Potter* (1983) below.

CASE EXAMPLE

Hills v Potter [1983] 3 All ER 716

The patient suffered from a neck deformity and consented to an operation from which there was a risk that even if the operation were performed competently, paralysis could occur. Post-operatively, the risk materialised and she was paralysed from the neck down. Her action against the defendant was twofold: firstly, in battery as she alleged her consent was not real and effective; and secondly, in negligence for a failure to provide information about the risk.

As she had given real consent, the action for battery failed. The action in negligence also failed as the *Bolam* test (see Chapter 1) was applied to the information that was required to be disclosed. In order for adequate disclosure to be satisfied, all that was needed was to provide the patient with a global picture of the proposed treatment. There was no requirement to advise of the specific or particular risks.

JUDGMENT

'… he did not have to inform the patient of all the details of the proposed treatment of the likely outcome and the risks inherent in it but was merely required to act in accordance with a practice accepted as proper by a responsible body of skilled medical practitioners.'

2.2.3 Informed consent and negligence claims in England and Wales: the early years

The key issue that has arisen out of claims based on an alleged negligent failure to disclose risks associated with treatment has been the question of how the courts should determine what information the defendant must disclose to the claimant to avoid liability.

CASE EXAMPLE

Sidaway v Board of Governors of the Bethlem Royal Hospital and the Maudsley Hospital [1985] 1 AC 871

Mrs Sidaway was suffering from neck and back pain and underwent an operation to help relieve the symptoms. She did not allege negligence in relation to the operation but, rather, alleged that the neurosurgeon had negligently failed to warn her of a one to two per cent risk of paralysis associated with the treatment. She also alleged that, had she been warned of the risk, she would not have had the operation. Unfortunately, the risk materialised and Mrs Sidaway was left severely disabled.

The House of Lords agreed that Mrs Sidaway's claim should fail but their respective reasons for reaching such a conclusion differed. The House of Lords applied the *Bolam* test to the standard to be applied when deciding whether the information that was disclosed to the patient fell below an acceptable standard so as to amount to negligence. Here, the neurosurgeon was not liable in negligence as it was found there was a responsible body of neurosurgeons who agreed it was acceptable *not* to disclose the potential risk of paralysis in that case.

Lord Scarman dissented:

- He emphasised 'the right of self-determination', that is, the principle that a patient has the right to decide for herself whether to accept the medical treatment she is offered. The 'patient has a right to be informed of the risks inherent in the treatment'.
- It is not for the medical profession to override the patient's decision as to whether to undergo the medical treatment recommended. What is in the 'best interest' of the patient should not be the prevailing principle.
- The important question is 'whether in the particular circumstances the risk was such that this particular patient would think it significant if he was told it existed'.
- It would appear that it is significant if it is 'material', and it is material if 'a reasonable person in the patient's position would be likely to attach significance to the risk.'
- However, the court will not find the doctor liable if the doctor reasonably considers that disclosure of the risk would be harmful to the patient's psychological health and in such circumstances the risk need not be disclosed. This is referred to as 'therapeutic privilege'.

- The matter of risk disclosure is relevant to the tort of negligence (with respect to the duty of care) rather than the tort of battery.

As part of the majority decision, Lord Diplock considered that the *Bolam* test should be applied to decide whether a medical professional has provided a patient with sufficient information about the risks. The reasoning is that he regarded the act of advising a patient of a risk as part of a doctor's duty of care and, accordingly, *Bolam* would apply in the same way. Lord Bridge recognised:

JUDGMENT

'the logical force of the *Canterbury* doctrine, proceeding from the premise that the patient's right to make his own decisions must at all costs be safeguarded against the type of medical paternalism which assumes that "doctor knows best"' (see page 58 for the *Canterbury* (1972) doctrine).

This is precisely what Lord Scarman was advocating, but Lord Bridge (and also Lord Keith) dismissed this approach as 'impractical in application', preferring the application of the *Bolam* test as the appropriate standard but indicating that this would be subject to judicial approval. He said:

JUDGMENT

'I am of the opinion that the judge might in certain circumstances come to the conclusion that the disclosure of a particular risk was so obviously necessary to an informed choice on the part of the patient that no reasonably prudent medical man would fail to make it.'

The question which we now face is: what amounts to a risk that no reasonably prudent medical man would fail to make? Clearly, a one to two per cent risk was not sufficiently significant in this case, but in comparison Lord Bridge referred to the Canadian case of *Reibl v Hughes* [1989] 2 SCR 880, where a ten per cent risk was clearly sufficiently significant. In referring to this case he suggested that disclosure of a particular risk would be obvious where there was 'a substantial risk of grave adverse consequences'.

Lord Templeman added:

JUDGMENT

'a doctor ought to draw the attention of a patient to a danger which may be special in kind or special to that patient.'

The case of *Sidaway*, while containing a range of fascinating speeches, was clear in its decision: the *Bolam* test would be applied to cases alleging a failure to disclosure a risk, and it would be negligent not to warn a patient of a risk where there was a 'substantial risk of grave' outcome or where the danger may be 'special to that patient'.

In any event, the decision in *Sidaway* left us with two major questions, namely:

- Whose approach should be followed when deciding what level of disclosure the defendant should have met in any subsequent claims?
- If we follow the adapted *Bolam* test advanced by Lord Bridge and Lord Keith, how do we determine whether a risk 'was so obviously necessary to an informed choice on the part of the patient'?

On the second point, a one to two per cent risk of paralysis in this case was not sufficiently significant to warrant disclosure. On the other hand, Lord Bridge referred to the example of the Canadian case of *Reibl v Hughes* (1989), to make the point that a ten per cent risk of harm was clearly sufficiently significant. In referring to this case he suggested that disclosure of a particular risk would be obvious where there was 'a substantial risk of grave adverse consequences'.

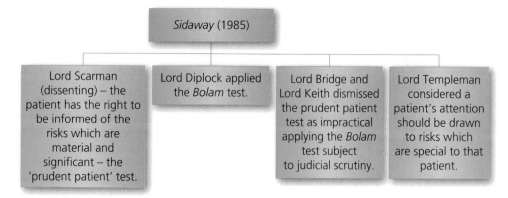

Figure 2.4 Judgments in *Sidaway* (1985)

Disappointingly, in *Gold* (1988) below the court failed to take sufficient consideration of the specific nuances of the judgment in *Sidaway*, and opted to adopt a straightforward application of *Bolam* instead.

CASE EXAMPLE

Gold v Haringey Health Authority [1988] QB 481

The plaintiff elected to have a non-therapeutic sterilisation operation. She then became pregnant and claimed damages for the upbringing of the child. She claimed that had she been advised of the risks of the sterilisation reversing or the greater success rate of vasectomies in men, her husband would have had a vasectomy instead.

At first instance the court found in Mrs Gold's favour, but the defendant's appeal was successful. One might think that following *Sidaway*, the risk of the sterilisation reversing itself was clearly 'special to this patient' (to use the words of Lord Templeman in *Sidaway*) and should therefore be disclosed. After all, Mrs Gold chose to have the operation precisely because she did *not* want to become pregnant again and it would follow that she would naturally wish to be informed of *all* the risks of the procedure. Therefore, the court could have adopted the more sophisticated interpretation of the *Bolam* test advanced by Lords Bridge, Keith and Templeman in *Sidaway*. Surprisingly, however, the Court of Appeal simply followed Lord Diplock's approach and applied the *Bolam* test with no amendments. The defendant was subsequently found to have disclosed sufficient information to the claimant. It almost appeared as if Mrs Gold's right to self-determination had disappeared.

A similar theme was repeated some five years later, where in the case of *Blyth v Bloomsbury Health Authority* [1993] 4 Med LR 151, Kerr LJ appeared to suggest *obiter* that the *Bolam* test would apply even to where a specific question was asked by a patient. The reliance on the *Bolam* test almost seems to imply that a doctor is not even required to respond directly to a specific question his patient may ask. Such a conclusion would sit uneasily with the *obiter* comments of Lord Bridge in *Sidaway*:

JUDGMENT

'When questioned specifically by a patient of apparently sound mind about risks involved in a particular treatment proposed, a doctor's duty must, in my opinion, be to answer both truthfully and as fully as the questioner requires.'

The courts appeared to be consistent in their approach. The case of *Poynter v Hillingdon HA* [1993] 7 BMLR 192 illustrates this further, where the parents of a 15-month-old boy consented to a heart transplant. Although they had not specifically asked, they were not told of a less than one per cent risk of permanent brain damage. The risk materialised and the child suffered brain damage. It was held by Sir Maurice Drake that there was no duty on the doctors to advise the parents of the risk.

KEY FACTS

Key facts on cases of consent

Case	Judgment
Sidaway v Board of Governors of the Bethlem RH and the Maudsley Hospital (1985)	*Bolam* standard was applied to information disclosure but note the dissenting judgments and *obiter* comments made. Found for the defendant.
Gold v Haringey Health Authority (1988)	The court followed Lord Diplock in *Sidaway* and applied an unmodified version of the *Bolam* test. Found for the defendant.
Blyth v Bloomsbury HA (1993)	*Bolam* standard was applied in relation to information disclosure. No duty to disclose information even to a question specifically asked. Found for the defendant.
Poynter v Hillingdon HA (1993)	No duty to inform patient of one per cent risk of brain damage. Found for the defendant.

2.2.4 Informed consent and negligence claims in England and Wales: the change in judicial opinion

The frustratingly slow pace of development of the law in this area in the UK quickened to an amble from 1998. Early signs of a gradual change in the attitude of the courts towards failure to warn claims were clearly evident in the following case.

CASE EXAMPLE

Smith v Tunbridge Wells Health Authority [1994] 5 Med LR 334

A young man underwent rectal surgery but was not warned of the risks of impotence associated with this type of surgery. Although the surgery was conducted competently, the risk materialised. The claimant alleged the defendant had been negligent in failing to warn him of the risks. Furthermore he claimed that, had he been advised of the risks, he would not have undergone the surgery. The expert evidence submitted by the defendant supported the decision not to advise him of this particular risk.

Despite the defendant's expert medical evidence, the High Court found for the plaintiff. In doing so, the court referred to Lord Bridge in *Sidaway* (1985), stating that the failure to advise of this particular risk to this particular patient was a decision that was not reasonable and therefore could not be supported. The court explicitly rejected the defendant's expert evidence in a way that was not expressed directly by the courts until *Bolitho* in 1997 some three years later. The case demonstrates a significant change of direction of judicial opinion, but perhaps the turning point in England and Wales can be identified in the case below.

CASE EXAMPLE

Pearce v United Bristol Healthcare NHS Trust [1998] 48 BMLR 118

A mother pregnant with her sixth child was 14 days beyond her expected delivery date. In desperation, she asked the consultant obstetrician either to induce the labour or perform a Caesarean section in order that her baby could be born. He explained the risks involved in induction and the longer recovery time associated with a Caesarean. She accepted his advice, but seven days later she was admitted to hospital where no foetal heart rate could be traced and the foetus was subsequently stillborn. There was a 0.1–0.2 per cent risk of a stillbirth which the defendants did not consider significant, but she alleged negligence in the failure to inform her of these risks.

The court held that it was not negligent to fail to inform the plaintiff of the risk of stillbirth as the risk was so insignificant. While the court still took the doctor's view as to whether in these circumstances *they* considered *this* risk to be significant, they appeared to be considering a far more patient-centred approach for the future. It was therefore not relevant that this woman in labour with her sixth child could not decide for herself whether the risk was one to accept, and therefore follow the doctor's advice for a natural birth or maintain her desperate demands for a Caesarean. Effectively, she had no autonomy.

The court held that it was not negligent to fail to inform the plaintiff of the risk of stillbirth as the risk was so insignificant. What is significant about the decision in *Pearce,* however, was that it was delivered not long after the pivotal case of *Bolitho* and, therefore, provides the courts with the first real opportunity to consider what impact the decision in *Bolitho* might have on *Sidaway.*

JUDGMENT

'In a case where it is being alleged that a plaintiff has been deprived of the opportunity to make a proper decision as to what course he or she should take in relation to treatment ... that if there is a significant risk which would affect the judgment of a reasonable patient, then in the normal course it is the responsibility of a doctor to inform the patient of that significant risk, if the information is needed so that the patient can determine for him or herself as to what course he or she should adopt.' (Lord Woolf MR)

> Was the risk of a type which if disclosed would have influenced the patient's decision whether to consent to treatment or not?

> If yes, the defendant may have breached his duty to disclose risks to the claimant.

Figure 2.5 The risk in *Pearce* (1998)

How relevant is the judgment of *Pearce*? It is fundamental to the shift of judicial opinion we can see in the House of Lords' case of *Chester v Afshar* (2004) (also examined in Chapter 1).

CASE EXAMPLE

Chester v Afshar [2004] UKHL 41

The claimant, Mrs Chester, suffered from severe back pain and sought the advice of the defendant, a neurosurgeon. He recommended surgery but failed to warn Mrs Chester of the one to two per cent risk of significant nerve damage that could occur. This risk was inherent in the procedure. As such it did not matter who performed the surgery, where it was performed or when it was performed; the risk was always there. Mrs Chester consented to the surgery and, although the surgery was carried out without the slightest hint of negligence on Mr Afshar's part, the one to two per cent risk materialised. This meant that Mrs Chester was left partially paralysed. Mrs Chester maintained that, had she been advised of the risk, she would not have undergone the operation that day but would have sought a second opinion. No finding of fact was made, however, about whether she would have undergone surgery at a later date.

In a particularly patient-centred judgment, the House of Lords found in favour of the claimant even though she accepted that she would have undergone the operation with the same surgeon, albeit probably at a later time, after she sought a second opinion. The duty of care was said to encompass a duty to warn the patient of 'possible serious risks' involved in the treatment.

Lord Steyn indicated in the clearest of terms that:

JUDGMENT

'in modern law paternalism no longer rules and a patient has a *prima facie* right to be informed by a surgeon of a small, but well established, risk of serious injury as a result of surgery'.

This statement is indisputably fundamental to modern medicine to ensure 'that due respect is given to the autonomy and dignity of each patient.'

The majority in *Chester* adopted a flexible approach to the rules governing causation on policy grounds and accepted that she had a right to make an informed decision about what happened to her body. They also realised that adopting a strict approach to the rules of causation would have denied her compensation, thereby rendering the duty to secure a patient's informed consent 'a hollow one, stripped of all practical force and devoid of all content.'

The decision in *Chester* will prove to be a tipping point in the move towards a more patient-centred approach in the future.

KEY FACTS

Key facts on leading cases

Case	Judgment
Smith v Tunbridge Wells HA (1994)	Rejected expert defendant evidence. Unreasonable not to advise this particular patient of this particular risk. Found for the plaintiff.
Pearce v United Bristol Healthcare NHS Trust (1998)	Not negligent not to warn the patient of a small risk of stillbirth which the defendant felt was insignificantly small. Found for the defendant. Lord Woolf stated that medical men are required to disclose significant risks that would affect the patient's decision to consent or decline the proposed course of treatment.
Chester v Afshar (2004)	Duty of care included a duty to warn of possible serious risks. Found for the claimant in a patient-centred judgment. The House of Lords recognised a need to compensate the claimant in recognition of the fact that her autonomous rights to make an informed decision about what happened to her body had been violated. Found for the claimant.

2.2.5 The approach in other jurisdictions

The above discussion represents the law in England and Wales, but much earlier in the United States of America, the courts had made similar progress. The earlier case of *Canterbury v Spence* (1972) 464 F 2d 772 (DC) saw the clear emergence of the doctrine of 'informed consent' in the USA.

CASE EXAMPLE

Canterbury v Spence (1972) 464 F 2d 772 (DC)

A young man who suffered from back pain underwent an operation. He had not been warned of a one per cent risk of paralysis associated with that operation. A day after the operation he developed paralysis and was operated on again, but never regained complete use of the lower half of his body.

The surgeon accepted he had not warned the patient of the possible risk of paralysis because 'he felt that communication of that risk to the patient was not good medical practice because it might deter patients from undergoing needed surgery and might produce adverse psychological reactions which could preclude the success of the operation'.

This was accepted by the lower courts who did not consider this practice to be negligent. Nor did they feel that the patient's consent was compromised by the withholding of information regarding the risk inherent in the treatment.

However, the United States Court Of Appeals for the District Of Columbia reversed this decision and, after quoting Cardozo J in *Schoelendorff*, commented:

JUDGMENT

'True consent to what happens to one's self is the informed exercise of a choice, and that entails an opportunity to evaluate knowledgeably the options available and the risks attendant upon each'. Given that the average patient has little understanding of their medical condition, it becomes necessary for them to rely on "a reasonable divulgence by physician to patient to make such a decision possible".'

The court then continued by explaining that the right to decide for oneself whether to proceed with treatment is related to the information to disclose, but what should be disclosed?

JUDGMENT

'Thus the test for determining whether a particular peril must be divulged is its materiality to the patient's decision: all risks potentially affecting the decision must be unmasked. And to safeguard the patient's interest in achieving his own determination on treatment, the law must itself set the standard for adequate disclosure ... a risk is material when a reasonable person in what the physician knows, or should know, to be the patient's position, would be likely to attach significance to the risk or cluster of risks in deciding whether or not to forego the proposed therapy.'

Therefore the 'prudent patient' standard seeks to determine what information the medical professional should have disclosed by reference to whether a reasonable patient, rather than the reasonable doctor, would view the information as significant.

2.2.6 GMC guidance to disclosure

The General Medical Council (GMC)'s most recent guidance on information to be disclosed is entitled *'Consent; patients and doctors making decisions together'*. While the guidance states that 'individual patients may want more or less information or involvement in making decisions depending on their circumstances or wishes', although not a definitive list, information that must be given to a patient must include:

a. the diagnosis and prognosis
b. any uncertainties about the diagnosis or prognosis, including options for further investigations
c. options for treating or managing the condition, including the option not to treat
d. the purpose of any proposed investigation or treatment and what it will involve
e. the potential benefits, risks and burdens, and the likelihood of success, for each option; this should include information, if available, about whether the benefits or risks are affected by which organisation or doctor is chosen to provide care.

Medical professionals can therefore adhere to the GMC guidance in order to ensure that adequate information disclosure is provided, as the common law appears to lack certainty in its approach. It is worth noting however that the GMC guidelines are extensive and require a greater degree of disclosure than the law itself requires.

KEY FACTS

Key facts on failure to disclose

- A failure to disclose risks associated with a recommended course of treatment has, in some limited cases, led to liability for trespass to the person, for example *Devi v West Midlands Health Authority* (1981).
- The decision in *Chatterton v Gerson* (1981) makes it clear that where a claimant is alleging that the medical professional failed to provide them with sufficient information about the treatment to allow them to make an informed decision, that action should be based in negligence and not in battery.
- A key decision in the development of negligence claims in this area is the decision in *Sidaway* (1985). Lord Diplock suggested that the level of disclosure required in such cases was to be determined by making reference to *Bolam*. Lords Bridge, Templeman and Keith however concluded that the risk should be disclosed if no reasonable medical man could have failed to disclose it. Lord Scarman (dissenting) preferred the 'prudent patient' test.
- Subsequent cases saw a straightforward application of the *Bolam* test although the case of *Smith v Tunbridge Wells Health Authority* (1994) followed the *Bolitho* approach favoured by Lord Bridge. One can see the changing shape of judicial opinion towards a more patient-centred approach, as in *Pearce v United Bristol Healthcare NHS Trust* (1998) Lord Woolf suggested that medical professionals were required to disclose 'serious risk[s] which would affect the judgement of a reasonable patient'.
- Importantly, in the House of Lords' case of *Chester v Afshar* (2004) the doctrine of informed consent was accepted without reservation and applied in a truly patient-centred judgment. According to their Lordships, paternalistic practice no longer had a place in the area of information disclosure. While clearly a policy decision, the case may herald a new dawn of patient-centred judgments where paternalism gives way to respect for patient autonomy.

Self-test questions

- What liability can a medical professional incur if consent is absent? Give common law examples.
- Why is consent considered to be so essential in the context of medical treatment?
- Evaluate the dissenting judgment of Lord Scarman in *Sidaway* (1985).
- How did the cases of *Gold v Haringey HA* (1988) and *Blyth v Bloomsbury HA* (1993) approach the issue of information disclosure?
- What is the significance of *Chester v Afshar* (2004)? How far do you consider this to be a policy decision?

2.3 Part 3: Consent and the incompetent patient; incompetent adults and children

AIMS AND OBJECTIVES

By the end of this section you should be able to:

- Demonstrate an understanding of how the principle of best interests is applied, both at common law and by statute
- Appreciate the meaning of advance decisions
- Understand the statutory provisions.

2.3.1 Introduction

The term 'incompetent patient' covers three classes of patient:

- an adult patient who has temporarily lost capacity
- an adult patient who has permanently lost capacity
- child patients.

You have already learnt that it is unlawful to treat an individual without their consent, but incompetent patients *are unable to provide a valid consent*. You will learn in this chapter that the law has developed a number of mechanisms to combat this difficulty.

2.3.2 The incompetent adult patient: the position under the common law

The treatment of incompetent patients used to be governed by the decision in the case of *Re F (Mental Patient: Sterilisation)* (1990) below.

CASE EXAMPLE

Re F (Mental Patient: Sterilisation) [1990] 2 AC 1

F was a 36-year-old woman who was a voluntary in-patient in a mental hospital. It was said that F had a mental age of between five and six years old. She had formed a relationship with a male patient. The hospital was concerned that her mental condition would be jeopardised if she fell pregnant and wished her to be sterilised as they felt there were no other suitable forms of contraception available for her.

A declaration permitting the sterilisation was granted. Lord Goff explained that in the case of treating incompetent patients:

JUDGMENT

'we are searching for a principle on which, in limited circumstances, recognition may be given to a need, in the interests of the patient, that treatment should be given to him... It is this criterion of a need which points to the principle of necessity as providing justification.'

What the decision in *F v West Berkshire Health Authority* (1990) effectively stated was that any treatment provided by medical professionals to incompetent adult patients may be excused on the basis of the defence of necessity. The defence of necessity however could only be raised successfully where the medical professional could demonstrate that the treatment in question was in the patient's best interests. In the words of Lord Goff, the action taken

JUDGMENT

'must be such as a reasonable person would in all the circumstances take, acting in the best interests of the assisted person.'

But how do we decide what is in the patient's best interests? There was no definition given in *F v West Berkshire Health Authority* (1990) to address this question; however what was in the patient's best interests was not to be determined by making reference to the *Bolam* test, but by taking into account all the surrounding circumstances including the interests of *all the parties* involved.

What is intriguing about the 'best interests' test is that it has occasionally been given a very wide ambit, as was the case in *Re Y (Mental Patient: Bone Marrow Donation)* (1997) below.

CASE EXAMPLE

Re Y (Mental Patient: Bone Marrow Donation) [1997] 2 FCR 172

Y was a young woman who had severe mental and physical disabilities. Y lived in a care home but received regular visits from her mother. Y's sister was in need of a life-saving bone marrow transplant and Y was a suitable donor but lacked the capacity to consent to such an operation. Clearly, this operation had no therapeutic benefit for Y; nevertheless the sister sought a declaration which would allow Y's bone marrow to be harvested on the grounds that such a procedure would be in Y's best interests.

In a difficult judgment Connell J allowed the declaration, making it lawful for the operation to harvest the bone marrow to proceed. How could this be in the donor's best interests? The operation, while straightforward, is not without its own risks and Y would receive no direct benefit. Moreover the *Department of Health Reference Guide to Consent for Examination or Treatment* (March 2001) specifically states that a bone marrow operation is not a 'minimal intervention' and that the operation should be in the best interests of the donor.

It was not relevant to the court's decision that the operation would save the sister's life. However, the court said that since the operation was low risk (although some small risk did exist) and there was some benefit to Y, it would be allowed. The benefit to Y was put in terms of general family benefit: it was a psychological and emotional benefit as her status quo would remain largely the same. Her sister would hopefully live and her mother would continue to spend the time with Y that Y valued considerably.

In contrast, in the case of *Re A (Medical Treatment: Male Sterilisation)* [2000] 1 FCR 193, the Court of Appeal refused to grant a declaration permitting a vasectomy on a male patient with acute learning difficulties. The court held in this particular case it was not in the best interests of this particular patient to undergo an irreversible, intrusive procedure from which he would receive no personal benefit.

The judges opined about where responsibility should lie for determining what is in a patient's best interests, and how the courts should set about performing that task. Dame Elizabeth Butler-Sloss LJ stated:

JUDGMENT

'in the case of an application for approval of a sterilisation operation, it is the judge, not the doctor, who makes the decision that it is in the best interests of the patient that the operation be performed'.

A similar sentiment was repeated in the case below.

CASE EXAMPLE

Re S (Sterilisation: Patient's Best Interests) [2001] Fam 15

A 39-year-old female patient with severe learning difficulties was severely distressed by her menstrual periods and had a phobia of hospitals. The patient's mother applied to the court for a declaration that it would be lawful for the hospital to perform either a sterilisation or a hysterectomy on her daughter. The judge considered the relative merits of these options and also considered the further option of inserting a contraceptive coil.

The judge concluded that the hysterectomy was the preferred course of action but that the insertion of a contraceptive coil might also be lawful even though it did not fully meet the patient's needs. The trial judge ultimately held that it was for the mother and the patient's doctors to decide which of those two options to adopt. The patient appealed against that ruling.

The Court of Appeal upheld the patient's appeal. While there may be a range of options that might meet the patient's needs, there must be *one best* course of action, and it was for the courts to decide what that was. The weight of medical evidence available supported the insertion of the contraceptive coil as it was the least invasive option and so only that method of treatment would be lawful. Thus, it appears it is for the court to decide what amounts to a patient's best interests.

The case of *R v Human Fertilisation and Embryology Authority, ex parte Blood* [1997] 2 All ER 687 raised similar issues. Mr and Mrs Blood were trying to start a family (of this there is no doubt) when Mr Blood contracted meningitis. He was left in a coma and his prognosis was very poor. Mrs Blood gained permission for his sperm to be taken and preserved in order that she might bear his children. It is difficult to see how obtaining sperm from an unconscious patient who is likely not to recover can possibly be in his best interests. Presumably, best interest in this context was given a wide interpretation and perhaps it could be fairly and reasonably considered in his best interests that Mrs Blood was eventually able to have the children they both so clearly desired.

2.3.3 Treating the incompetent adult patient: the position under statute

The common law approach has now been replaced by the provisions of the Mental Capacity Act 2005.

Under s 15 the court is empowered to make a declaration as to the lawfulness of any proposed act. When making any such declaration they must take into account the criteria for determining what is in the patient's best interests; the criteria is now contained in s 4, MCA 2005.

Section 4(4) makes it clear that any person must also:

SECTION

4(4) 'so far as reasonably practicable, permit and encourage the person to participate, or to improve his ability to participate, as fully as possible in any act done for him and any decision affecting him.'

Thus the views of the patient must, so far as is reasonably practicable, be taken into account.

Section 4(6) states that when a person is trying to determine whether the proposed course of action is in the patient's best interests,

SECTION

4(6) '... He must consider, so far as is reasonably ascertainable –

(a) the person's past and present wishes and feelings (and, in particular, any relevant written statement made by him when he had capacity),
(b) the beliefs and values that would be likely to influence his decision if he had capacity, and
(c) the other factors that he would be likely to consider if he were able to do so.'

There are difficulties with this section: could it be that there are conflicts between the patient's past and present wishes? How easy is it to determine the incompetent patient's current wishes, and what weight can be attached?

Section 4(6) needs to be read in conjunction with s 4(7) below which states that if it is both practicable and appropriate, views of others are to be taken into account.

SECTION

'4(7) He must take into account, if it is practicable and appropriate to consult them, the views of –

(a) anyone named by the person as someone to be consulted on the matter in question or on matters of that kind,
(b) anyone engaged in caring for the person or interested in his welfare,
(c) any donee of a lasting power of attorney granted by the person, and
(d) any deputy appointed for the person by the court,

as to what would be in the person's best interests and, in particular, as to the matters mentioned in subsection (6).'

KEY FACTS

Key facts for cases on the incompetent adult patient

Case	Judgment
Re F (Mental Patient: Sterilisation) (1990)	Treatment can be given without the patient's consent and the defence of necessity can be relied upon. Medical professionals can only act in the patient's best interests.
Re Y (Mental Patient: Bone Marrow Donation) (1997)	The bone marrow donation was not in Y's best interests but the anticipated result would be as her own status quo would remain. Best interests are not necessarily medical; here it was psychological together with all the circumstances of the case.
Re A (Medical Treatment: Male Sterilisation) (2000)	It was not in the best interests of the patient to have a vasectomy.
Re S (Sterilisation: Patient's Best Interests) (2001)	Best interest can be for the court to determine.

2.3.4 Advance decisions

An advance decision provides a competent person with a means to exercise some control over how they are treated in the event that they lose capacity. Effectively, it allows a person to dictate the manner in which they are treated when they are no longer able to do so.

The use of advance decisions is governed by ss 24–25, MCA 2005. The following are key points to note about advance decisions:

- The patient must be aged 18 (or over) and had capacity to make such a decision at the time it was made (s 24(1)).
- Advance decisions are made when the patient has capacity and refers to a time when he lacks capacity to consent to the carrying out of the continuation of treatment (s 24(1 (b)).
- Advance decisions do not normally need to be made in writing and witnessed unless the advance decision contains a refusal of life-saving treatment (s 25(6)).
- Any advance decision must specify the type of treatment that is being refused and it may specify the particular circumstances in which the refusal will apply (s 24(1) and (2)).
- Advance decisions only apply to *refusals* of treatment. They cannot be used to *demand* treatment as seen in *R (on the application of Burke) v The General Medical Council* [2005] EWCA 1003. It is acceptable however for individuals to use advance decisions to express their wishes/preferences in advance: 'Mental Capacity Act 2005 Code of Practice', paragraph 9.5.
- An advance decision will not be valid if:
  - it has already been withdrawn by the patient (s 25(2)(a)). An individual is free to withdraw any advance decision they might have made as long as they retain the capacity necessary to do so (s 24(3))
  - the patient has already granted power to make the decision in question to a donee under a Lasting Power of Attorney (s 25(2)(b))
  - the patient has since acted in any way which is inconsistent with the apparent wishes expressed in the advance decision (s 25 (2)(c)).
- An advance decision will not be deemed to be 'applicable to the treatment' in question if:
  - the treatment in question is not dealt with in the advance decision (s 25(4)(a))
  - the circumstances in which the patient finds himself are not the circumstances specified in the advance decision (s 25(4)(b))
  - there are reasonable grounds for believing that the current circumstances had not been anticipated by the patient and, if they had been anticipated by the patient, this would have affected their decision (s 25(4)(c)).

If the healthcare professional concludes that the advance decision is *not* valid and/or applicable to the treatment, this does not mean that the advance decision can be ignored altogether. Instead, the healthcare professional should take the content of that advance decision into account when making a decision about what is in that patient's best interests under s 4, MCA 2005.

If, on the other hand, the healthcare professional concludes that the advance decision *is* both valid and applicable, it must be respected even if that decision will result in serious injury or death (*Re T* (1993)). Failure to respect those wishes could result in a criminal charge (battery) or a civil action (battery/negligence).

Advance decisions in practice

While these cases were all heard pre-MCA 2005, the provisions of the Act are largely consistent with the approach taken by the courts in the past few years.

Earlier, we considered the case of *Re T* (1993), where the courts overrode the patient's advance refusal of a blood transfusion following an application to the courts from her father and brother, despite her mother steadfastly supporting her daughter's refusal. Although this case was fact-specific, there was a doubt in the court's mind as to whether the patient had been unduly influenced by her mother. The courts opined that, in the case of doubt, the courts should err on the side of preserving life. Despite this judgment, in *Re AK* [2001] 1 FLR 129, the courts allowed a declaration of a valid refusal of treatment in a young man suffering from motor neurone disease, who communicated his refusal by blinking his eyelid.

CASE EXAMPLE

HE v A Hospital NHS Trust [2003] EWHC 1017 (Fam)

The patient was a Jehovah's Witness who made an advance directive rejecting all forms of blood products. She was unconscious and required a blood transfusion in order to preserve life. Evidence showed that she had intended to convert to Islam and marry a Muslim man. Her mother however remained a Jehovah's Witness.

The court concluded that the advance decision was not valid, and furthermore that a withdrawal did not need to be in writing. Munby J explained that 'Any condition in an advance directive purporting to make it irrevocable is contrary to public policy and void'. Furthermore, he indicated that if there was any doubt it 'falls to be resolved in favour of the preservation of life.'

Although this case was heard pre-MCA 2005, s 24(4) confirms that 'a withdrawal (including a partial withdrawal) need not be in writing'.

For a valid advance directive, the maker must be *specific* about the treatment to be refused as s 25(4)(a) states:

SECTION

s 25(4)(a) 'an advance decision is not applicable to the treatment in question if (a) that treatment is not the treatment specified in the advance decision'.

Therefore, to be valid the maker must be particularly careful in the wording (layman's language is acceptable) so as to exclude specific treatment which the maker does not wish to have.

Obstacles or safety net?

The wording of s 25 presents a further obstacle or safety net for the maker, depending how one perceives the situation. Section 25(4)(c) states as above, that the advance decision will not be applicable to the treatment if:

SECTION

s 25(4) 'c) there are reasonable grounds for believing that circumstances exist which P did not anticipate at the time of the advance decision and which would have affected his decision had he anticipated them.'

Section 25(4)(c) means that the advance decision will not apply if there are reasonable grounds to believe that the person who made the decision with capacity and now lacks capacity did not anticipate the circumstances that now exist and, if he did, they would affect the decision that is now being considered. But what are 'circumstances'? It would appear that these might simply depend on the facts of the case in hand; it could mean personal circumstances or advances in medical treatment that were not known to the maker at the time at which the advance decision was made. If these circumstances were known, how would it affect the maker's advance decision? Maybe he would not have made it at all. The Mental Capacity Act 2005 Code of Practice 9.30 recommends that an advance decision is reviewed and regularly updated to ensure that the maker's wishes can be adhered to. The less frequently it is reviewed and considered, the more its validity may be questioned as 'views and circumstances may change over time'.

Section 25(5) refers to life-sustaining treatment. It provides that an advance decision will not apply unless the decision is in writing (s 25(6)), and the maker must acknowledge his decision applies to treatment even if 'life is at risk'. An advance directive must be in writing (s 25(6)(a)), must be signed by the person making it or by another but by his direction (s 25(6)(b)). The maker's signature must be witnessed (s 25(6)(c)) and the witness signed in the presence of the maker (s 25(6)(d)). The stringent provisions reflect the seriousness of the decision relating to the refusal of life-sustaining treatment.

The effect of an advance directive is that provided the medical professional is satisfied that the advance directive is both 'valid' and 'applicable' (s 26(1)(a) and (b)) he will not incur liability if he withholds or withdraws treatment from the patient. If he wishes to seek clarification, s 26(5) allows him to provide life-sustaining treatment or anything necessary 'to prevent a serious deterioration' in the patient's condition while he seeks guidance from the court. The Code of Practice states that in an emergency situation, he does not have to stop to check whether the patient has made an advance directive 'unless there is a clear indication that one exists' (para 9.56).

The ethics of advance decisions

Advance directives (ADs) give us the opportunity to have an element of control over our lives during a period when we lack the capacity to be able to control our lives in other ways.

The richness of their value is twofold:

1. We can exercise the right to refuse what we perceive to be futile, painful or meaningless treatment.
2. They provide us at the end of our lives with the same rights that we exercise during our normal day-to-day life: the right of self-determination and of autonomy. They allow us the sense of remaining in control in a time when we are clearly not.

How valid are these arguments? Buchanan argues that these observations may not be valid (2004). If one makes an advance decision about one's treatment in 2012, and it then becomes effective eight years later in 2020, medical treatment and life expectancy (including quality of life) may have changed so significantly since the advance decision was made, that to invoke the advance decision would be fundamentally wrong. We might also have different views and opinions from those which we originally held. Buchanan suggests in these circumstances we may not necessarily know what is best for us. Fagerlin and Scheider (2004) question whether it is at all possible even to envisage or properly assess how we would feel if illness befalls us and, if we are actually able to fulfil this task adequately, then how can we articulately express our own wishes? What words do we use and what are we really trying to say?

A difficulty of advance directives or decisions relates to determining the true intentions of the person who makes the advance decision. While we acknowledge a person's right to refuse medical treatment, is it ethically acceptable if these reasons concern worries about being a financial or emotional burden? Is altruism necessarily negative? Perhaps one can agree that providing these wishes reflect the person's true wishes, uninfluenced by others, the motivation behind the making of an advance decision is not necessarily relevant. There is certainly an undeniable satisfaction about determining the way one ends one life, if that end is to be rooted in illness, but the difficulties one would encounter are immeasurable. Just like the extent of one's illness is difficult to measure in advance, so might the accuracy of the contents of the advance decision.

Advance directives are valuable in the sense that they empower a person to determine the way in which their life may end. This may be particularly valuable if it is made at the beginning of a degenerative disease, where the patient can map out the future course of the illness. Even if the patient is careful to ensure its validity, the interpretation of s 25(4) may allow a medical professional to question whether circumstances which the patient did not anticipate have changed and would have affected his decision, had he known about them. If a person is adamant they wish to exercise their autonomy and have their wishes adhered to, they must ensure that they keep their advance directive under regular review.

Key facts of provisions of MCA 2005

Mental Capacity Act 2005	Provisions
Must be over 18 and have capacity	S 24(1)
Comes into force when patient lacks capacity	S 24(1)(b)
Must specify the type of treatment to be refused	S 24(1)
Does not need to be in writing unless the AD contains refusal of life-saving treatment	S 24(6)
Will not be valid if it has already been withdrawn by the patient	S 25(2)(a)
Can withdraw the AD provided he has capacity to do so	S 24(3)
Will not be valid if patient has acted in a way which is inconsistent with the wishes expressed	S 25(2)(c)
AD will not be applicable to treatment if the treatment is not dealt with within the AD	S 25(4)(a)
AD will not be applicable to treatment if the circumstances are different to those specified in the AD	S 25(4)(b)
AD will not be applicable to treatment if there are reasonable grounds for believing that the current circumstances would affect the provisions of the AD, had the patient been aware of them	S 25(4)(c)

2.4 Part 4: The child patient

AIMS AND OBJECTIVES

By the end of this section you should be able to:

- Appreciate the circumstances in which a minor can consent to medical treatment
- Understand the court's approach to a child's refusal of medical treatment
- Appreciate the role of the courts
- Understand the 'best interests' approach.

2.4.1 Introduction

We begin by exploring a child's capacity to consent to treatment. Section 1, Family Law (Reform) Act 1969 provides that a child is anyone under the age of 18. The law effectively divides child patients into three main categories when it comes to deciding whether they have the requisite capacity to give a valid consent, namely:

1. Children aged between 16 and 18 years.
2. Children aged below 16 who are 'Gillick competent' (see below).
3. Children aged below 16 who are not 'Gillick competent'.

Thereafter we will move on to look at the extent to which child patients are capable of refusing treatment, and how the law deals with authorising the treatment of a child who lacks capacity to consent to or refuse treatment. We will learn that some children may be found to have the requisite capacity to give a valid *consent* to treatment; yet those same children will normally not be deemed to possess the requisite level of capacity needed to give a valid *refusal* to treatment.

2.4.2 Children between 16 and 18 years

In England and Wales, s (8), Family Law (Reform) Act 1969 creates a statutory presumption in favour of competence where the child is aged 16–18. Section 8(1) of the Family Law Reform Act 1969 states:

SECTION

8(1) 'The consent of a minor who has attained the age of sixteen years to any surgical, medical or dental treatment which, in the absence of consent, would constitute a trespass to his person, shall be as effective as it would be if he were of full age; and where a minor has by virtue of this section given an effective consent to any treatment it shall not be necessary to obtain any consent for it from his parent or guardian.'

Therefore, a child patient who is older than 16 but younger than 18 is deemed to have sufficient capacity to give a valid consent to treatment.

Section 8(1) refers to decisions about surgical or medical 'treatment' but what is meant by 'treatment'? Section 8(2) of the Family Law Reform Act 1969 explains:

SECTION

8(2) 'In this section "surgical, medical or dental treatment" includes any procedure undertaken for the purposes of diagnosis, and this section applies to any procedure (including, in particular, the administration of an anaesthetic) which is ancillary to any treatment as it applies to that treatment.'

Those areas of medical treatment which are not specifically included such as cosmetic surgery are likely to be excluded. It must also be pointed out that:

- s 8(1) creates a presumption that a child aged 16–18 has the capacity necessary to consent to certain types of surgical and dental treatment. This presumption may be rebutted by evidence which demonstrates the child does not possess the capacity necessary for making the decision in question
- s 8(1) has no application to any attempts made by a child aged 16–18 to *refuse* treatment.

2.4.3 The *'Gillick* competent' child

The ground-breaking and highly controversial case of *Gillick v West Norfolk and Wisbech Area Health Authority* [1986] 1 AC 112 gave some children rights to control their treatment where previously they had none. Alarmed by pregnancy statistics in the young teenage years, the DHSS (Department of Health and Social Security) released a circular in 1980 which stated that in certain 'exceptional' circumstances, a doctor could lawfully prescribe contraception to a girl under the age of 16 without her parents' consent. The circular recognised that it would be desirable if the parents were involved in the decision but it imposed no specific requirement on doctors. Unsurprisingly, there was some public disquiet about the DHSS decision.

CASE EXAMPLE

Gillick v West Norfolk and Wisbech AHA [1986] AC 112

Mrs Gillick was the mother of five girls, all of whom were aged under 16. She objected to the fact that contraceptive advice and/or treatment could be provided to children under the age of 16. She sought reassurance from her health authority that no medical professional would be allowed to treat, advise or provide contraception to any of her children while they were under 16, without her knowledge and consent. The area health authority declined to give her any such reassurance. She then sought a declaration from the courts that the DHSS circular was unlawful. At first instance she was unsuccessful, but on appeal the court found in her favour. The DHSS then appealed to the House of Lords.

In a lengthy and complex judgment, the House of Lords allowed the appeal and declined to make the declaration requested by Mrs Gillick.

In a majority decision of 3:2, the House of Lords (more particularly Lord Fraser) set down five requirements that had to be satisfied before a doctor could treat or provide contraception to a child under the age of 16 without parental consent or knowledge. Mason and Laurie refer to children of this age as 'mature minors' (2010, page 71).

Lord Fraser explained that before a child under 16 could be given contraceptive advice and/or treatment without her parents' knowledge or consent, it was necessary to establish that:

- the child under 16 understood the advice
- the doctor cannot persuade the child to talk to her parents, or for him to advise her parents that she requires contraceptive advice
- she will carry on having sexual intercourse, whether it is protected or unprotected
- if she does not receive contraceptive advice, her physical or mental health will be affected
- it is in her best interests to receive contraceptive advice and/or treatment without her parents' consent.

Lord Scarman continued by stating that it would be a 'question of fact' whether a child has sufficient understanding to be able to provide a valid consent to treatment and, until that time, the parental right to make decisions on a child's behalf remained intact. He explained that it was not sufficient that she simply understood what she was being told; she also had to have the maturity to appreciate the significance of her decision.

While the court in *Gillick* was asked to focus on issues related to providing contraceptive advice and/or treatment, it has long been accepted that the principles derived from that case also apply to consent given by children under 16 to other forms of medical treatment.

In essence, the judgment from *Gillick* states that a child under 16 can (without the agreement or knowledge of his or her parents) consent to medical advice and treatment, provided they have a sufficient level of maturity and intelligence to understand the implications of the proposed course of treatment.

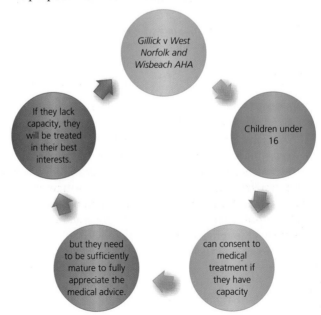

Figure 2.6 The judgment from *Gillick* (1986)

The *Gillick* decision was unsuccessfully challenged in the case of *R (Axon) v Secretary of State for Health* [2006] EWHC 37. Here, the parents challenged a child's right under

Department of Health guidelines to an abortion under the age of 16. Silber J confirmed the approach in *Gillick* and a mature minor's right to autonomy and confidentiality. Once a child reaches this stage, not only is a child entitled to confidentiality but the parents cannot rely on a potential breach of Article 8 and argue a violation of a private and family life.

2.4.4 Children under the age of 16 who are not '*Gillick* competent'

If the child patient does *not* possess the level of maturity, intelligence and understanding necessary to be considered '*Gillick* competent', they will not be able to give a valid consent to treatment.

This creates a potential problem for the medical professional. It was made clear during the discussion of the law governing adult patients that treating a patient without their consent can amount to the tort of battery or negligence and, in extreme cases, non-consensual touching can also be a crime. It was also made clear during the discussion of the law governing the treatment of incompetent patients that the law has developed mechanisms to enable such patients to be treated lawfully. As we are about to see, the same principles apply to child patients.

2.4.5 Treating children who lack capacity to consent

CASE EXAMPLE

Re R (A Minor) (Wardship: Consent to Treatment) [1991] 4 All ER 177

Due to a number of family problems R, a 15-year-old girl, had been placed in a children's home. Her mental health worsened while in care and she showed signs of extremely disturbed behaviour. It was necessary to transfer her to a psychiatric unit for young teenagers where they wished to prescribe anti-psychotic drugs to control her behaviour. Her state of mind varied and during lucid periods she refused consent to the drugs. She became psychotic but the local authority would not administer the drugs against her wishes and the unit would not keep her in the unit if she did not take them. The local authority wished to apply for leave to administer the anti-psychotic drugs regardless of her consent or refusal, and began wardship proceedings. The Court of Appeal approved the lower court's judgment that *R* was not '*Gillick* competent' and thus could not give a valid refusal of treatment. How might R be lawfully treated? The answer was provided by Lord Donaldson who stated:

JUDGMENT

'… [C]onsent by itself creates no obligation to treat. It is merely a key which unlocks a door. Furthermore, while in the case of an adult of full capacity there will usually only be one keyholder, namely the patient, in the ordinary family unit where a young child is the patient there will be two keyholders, namely the parents, with a several as well as joint right to turn the key and unlock the door. If the parents disagree, one consenting and the other refusing, the doctor will be presented with a professional and ethical, but not with a legal, problem because if he has the consent of one authorised person, treatment will not without more constitute a trespass or a criminal assault.'

It is clear therefore that there are a number of parties who can provide a valid consent to the child's treatment, namely:

- the child
- the child's parent(s)
- any other authorised person (such as an individual with parental responsibility for the child or even the court exercising its wardship jurisdiction).

This approach allows medical professionals to treat a child without fear of legal action (for trespass) providing they can obtain a 'key' (consent) from one of these 'keyholders'.

Arguably, this dictum rides roughshod over children's rights and cannot be reconciled with *Gillick*. Where *Gillick* gave rights, *Re R* has effectively taken them away. The fact that *Re R* effectively allowed parents to veto a child's refusal of treatment led Ian Kennedy to declare that *Re R* 'drove a coach and horses through *Gillick*' (Mason and Laurie (2010), page 71).

Nevertheless, Lord Donaldson subsequently revisited his 'keyholder' analogy in the case below.

CASE EXAMPLE

Re W (A Minor) (Medical Treatment) [1992] 3 WLR 758

A 16-year-old girl with anorexia nervosa was being cared for in a local authority unit. Her condition had deteriorated significantly to the point that she was critically ill. The local authority wished to move her into a more specialised unit where she could be force-fed. She refused consent and relied on s 8(1), Family Law (Reform) Act 1969, arguing that this gave her the same rights as an adult to refuse treatment.

The court, relying on their inherent jurisdiction, declared that the Act was not applicable to a child's right to refuse medical treatment. Reaffirming the position he took in *Re R* (1991) Lord Donaldson stated that a child's refusal of treatment can be overridden by the court or someone who has parental responsibility. In this instance it was the local authority and the court, acting in her best interests, who ordered her to be transferred to a specialised unit.

Referring back to his 'keyholder' analogy in *Re R* Lord Donaldson commented:

JUDGMENT

'On reflection I regret my use in *Re R (A Minor) (Wardship: Consent to Treatment)* of the keyholder analogy because keys can lock as well as unlock. I now prefer the analogy of the legal "flak jacket" which protects the doctor from claims by the litigious whether he acquires it from his patient who may be a minor over the age of 16, or a *"Gillick competent"* child under that age or from another person having parental responsibilities which include a right to consent to treatment of the minor. Anyone who gives him a flak jacket (that is, consent) may take it back, but the doctor only needs one and so long as he continues to have one he has the legal right to proceed ...'

In justifying how the courts could effectively dispense with a child's statutory right to refuse medical treatment, Lord Donaldson (stepping back from his 'key holder' analogy in *Re R*) drew a parallel between consent and a 'flak jacket'.

Although the language used has changed, the underlying principle remains the same. Providing the doctor treating the child receives consent from the child or someone with parental responsibility for the child (which can include the courts in some cases) then that treatment will be lawful.

2.4.6 The child patient who refuses treatment

If some children under 16 years are able to consent to medical treatment, is it not axiomatic that they must also be capable of giving a valid refusal of treatment? As a rule, the courts take a paternalistic approach and err on preserving life. Nowhere is this point illustrated with greater clarity than in the following case.

Re R   equals consent

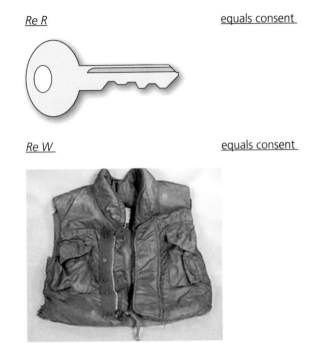

Re W   equals consent

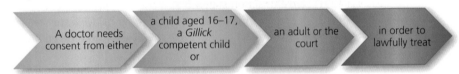

| A doctor needs consent from either | a child aged 16–17, a *Gillick* competent child or | an adult or the court | in order to lawfully treat |

Figure 2.7 Consent in *Re R* (1991) and *Re W* (1992)

CASE EXAMPLE

Re E (A minor) (Wardship: Medical Treatment) [1993] 1 FLR 386

This case involved a 15-year-old boy who was a Jehovah's Witness and suffering from leukaemia. The boy refused a blood transfusion on the grounds that it went against his religious beliefs. His refusal was supported by his parents. The health authority applied for a declaration to allow them to administer treatment lawfully. By the time the matter came to court, the boy was in a critical condition.

The court granted the declaration, allowing the hospital to treat A without his consent or that of his parents. While he was sufficiently intelligent to make general decisions about his own wellbeing, the court declared that he lacked sufficient capacity to refuse life-saving treatment. It was the court's view that A lacked a clear understanding of the effects of his refusal, in particular 'the manner of his death and the extent of his and his family's suffering'. Moreover, Ward J argued that the court 'should be very slow to allow an infant to martyr himself'.

The court took a similar approach in the case of *Re S (A Minor) (Consent to Medical Treatment)* [1994] 2 FLR 1065. This case involved a 15-year-old girl who suffered from thalassaemia. For many years S had been kept alive by a treatment regime which required monthly blood transfusions and daily, self-administered injections.

The child and her mother had become Jehovah's Witnesses and they eventually decided there would be no further blood transfusions as this was against their religious beliefs. An application was made to the court asking them for an order which would compel the child to undergo treatment.

The court held that S lacked *Gillick* competence as she failed to appreciate the nature and extent of her suffering and inevitable death which would result from her refusal. The court granted the order sought. In overriding S's refusal Mr Justice Johnson stated:

JUDGMENT

'It does not seem to me that her capacity is commensurate with the gravity of the decision which she has made. It seems to me that an understanding she will die is not enough. For her decision to carry weight she should have a greater understanding of the manner of the death and pain and the distress.'

Re L [1998] 2 FLR 810 involved a 14-year-old girl who was a Jehovah's Witness and had suffered severe burns. L required treatment which would necessitate blood transfusions. The court considered that although she was clearly intelligent, and her beliefs were sincere, she was influenced by her upbringing and as she grew older, might change her views. Accordingly, she was deemed not to be '*Gillick* competent' and the court could allow the hospital to treat her without her consent.

Discussion point

Although the cases we have just considered all involve refusals of life-saving treatment by children who were Jehovah's Witnesses, the principle we can derive from those cases is of general application in all of those cases involving refusals of treatment by child patients.

While many may regard the refusal of blood transfusion as defying logic, there are those, albeit a minority, for whom this is an expression of their religious freedom (Art 9, Human Rights Act 1998) which is not being respected.

However, as reported on 18 May 2010 in *The Telegraph*, a young man who was a Jehovah's Witness suffered appalling crush injuries after a car accident. He declined a blood transfusion. In this instance, the hospital respecting his wishes did not seek legal intervention, and he died later that same day.

Whatever the reasoning behind the refusal, the courts will always be reluctant to allow a child to refuse life-sustaining treatment and will act in the child's best interests. As Sir Mark Potter observed in *Re K (a child) (withdrawal of treatment)* [2006] EWHC 1007:

JUDGMENT

'it has to be borne in mind that English law placed a very heavy burden on those advocating a course which would lead inevitably to the cessation of a human life.'

A child will not be allowed to refuse treatment unless they are deemed to have sufficient capacity to make such a decision. In reality however it seems that where a child patient is seeking to refuse treatment, the court set the level of understanding required at such a high level that it seems as if 'no child could ever be deemed sufficiently competent (to make it)' (Jackson (2009), page 268).

Re E (1993)	*Re S* (1994)	*Re L* (1998)
• lacked capacity to refuse life-saving treatment • *per* Ward J the court 'should be very slow to allow an infant to martyr himself'	• lacked capacity to refuse life-saving treatment • *per* Johnson J 'It seems to me that an understanding she will die is not enough'	• court considered patient may change her beliefs as she became older • was not considered to be *Gillick* competent

Figure 2.8 Consent for children

2.4.7 Treating the child where the parents are in disagreement with each other

In *Re R (A Minor) (Wardship: Consent to Treatment)* (1991) Lord Donaldson said with reference to parents who disagree about a child's treatment:

JUDGMENT

'If the parents disagree, one consenting and the other refusing, the doctor will be presented with a professional and ethical, but not with a legal problem because, if he has the consent of one authorised person, treatment will not without more constitute a trespass or a criminal assault.'

Although Lord Donaldson changed his analogy in *Re W* from a key to a flak jacket, the principle remained the same. The case law which has followed on from *Re W* therefore illustrates two key points:

1. The medical professional does not normally have to obtain consent from both parents before they can lawfully administer treatment to the child; however
2. There are some types of treatment which can only be lawfully administered by the medical professional where both parents (and all parties with parental responsibility for the child) consent to it.

2.4.8 Treating the child where the parents and the medical team disagree

A consideration of case law where parents have disagreed with doctors over the proposed course of treatment shows us that the courts have been willing to override parental refusals where the court perceives that treatment would be in the child's best interests.

CASE EXAMPLE

Re B (A Minor) (Wardship: Medical Treatment) [1990] 3 All ER 927

B was a young girl with Down's syndrome who suffered from an intestinal blockage. It was operable and curable. Her parents however refused to consent to the operation, even though their action would inevitably lead to B's death. Her parents expressed their belief that it would be more considerate to allow her to die. She was made a ward of court and the local authority applied to the courts for a declaration allowing the operation.

The first instance court upheld the parents' wishes. An immediate appeal reversed the judgment. While the parents' wishes were taken into account, the court, taking the welfare of the child as '**the paramount consideration**', deemed it to be in the child's best interests to undergo the operation.

The outcome in *Re B* however stands in stark contrast to that in the case below.

CASE EXAMPLE

Re T (A Minor) (Wardship: Medical Treatment) [1997] 1 All ER 906

The infant suffered from a serious liver defect. It was clear that without surgical intervention he would die. Nevertheless, the child's parents (who were separated) both agreed that the operation should not go ahead. The local authority applied to the courts for a declaration allowing the operation to proceed.

The court of first instance granted the application requested by the local authority but the mother appealed. The Court of Appeal upheld the mother's appeal and overruled the earlier decision to allow the operation.

The contrast between the two cases could not be starker. In the second case it was considered significant that the infant would need many years of care from the mother, but the children in *both* cases would have required many years of parental support. The courts also took into account that the infant had suffered considerably after the previous operation, and that the family were not living in the UK at the time so would have to return for the operation.

Despite the apparent inconsistency with the decision in *Re B*, it should not be thought that the decision in *Re T* marks a departure from the **'best interests'** approach. The reader should not lose sight of the fact that both of T's parents were healthcare professionals. They were clearly in a position to make an informed evaluation about the level of suffering and distress which T was likely to experience as the result of the need for further surgery. This meant that they were better placed than most parents to make a decision about what would be in their child's best interests in the circumstances. Although the parents' views were relevant, they did not determine the issue.

Doubtless, *Re T* is a unique case and the judgment should be considered to be case-specific, the courts showing on numerous occasions that they will err on preserving life wherever possible.

Re B (1990)	Re T (1997)
• Parents refused child's operation • Welfare of the child was the paramount consideration and the courts overrode the parents' refusal to the operation	• Parents refused child's operation • Court allowed the parents' refusal of their child's life-saving operation • Considered to be a case-specific, unique judgment

Figure 2.9 Judgments in *Re B* (1990) and *Re T* (1997)

CASE EXAMPLE

Re C (a Minor) (Medical Treatment) [1998] Lloyd's Rep Med 1

In this case a child aged 16 months suffered from spinal muscular atrophy. Her condition was so acute that without ventilation she would die. The doctors responsible for her care decided it would not be in her best interests to continue to ventilate her as such treatment was futile and the benefits she gained from the process did not outweigh the suffering she continued to experience as a result. They wished to withdraw artificial ventilation and not ventilate in the event of respiratory failure. This would allow her to die peacefully and without pain.

Stephen Brown P acknowledged that while the principle of the sanctity of life was important, the child's welfare remained the court's paramount consideration. He noted that it was for the doctors, exercising their clinical judgment, with the help of experts, to determine what was in the best interests of the child.

In the view of Stephen Brown P it was evidently in C's best interests not to receive ventilation in the event of respiratory failure.

CASE EXAMPLES

Re C (HIV Test) [1999] 2 FLR 1004

Baby C's mother was HIV-positive. The mother had refused consent for the baby to be HIV tested; the local authority applied for an order to allow them to test the child as there was a 25 per cent chance that the baby was HIV-positive as well. The parents relied on what was then the newly introduced Human Rights Act 1998, arguing that forcing the child to undergo the test would be a breach of their right to a private family life under Art 8 of the European Convention on Human Rights.

The court, allowing the local authority's application for an order for a blood test, rejected reliance on Art 8, instead relying on Art 8(2), that the blood test was required '**for the protection of health**' or '**for the protection of the rights and freedoms of others**'. Ultimately this reflects the court's observation that the primary issue of concern in this case was the *child's welfare* and not the *parents' rights*. In any event, the court had to take into account that the child also had rights of her own which deserved respect.

It should be clear by this point that what is in a child's '**best interests**' is not always easy to determine. No clearer is this demonstrated than in *Re A (Children) (Conjoined Twins: Surgical Separation)* (2001) below where Ward J expressed the difficulty with which the courts were faced in light of '**the scale of the tragedy for the parents and the twins, difficult for the seemingly irreconcilable conflicts of moral and ethical values.**'

CASE EXAMPLE

Re A (Children) (Conjoined Twins: Surgical Separation) [2001] Fam 147

This well-known case involved conjoined twin girls, known as Jodie and Mary, who were born in Manchester in 2000. Their Roman Catholic parents, the Attards, had travelled from Gozo for the birth. Mary was undoubtedly the weaker of the two twins. They were fused along the lower end of their spines and shared a bladder. The twins also had a shared circulatory system and so Mary relied on Jodie for her supply of blood pumped by Jodie's heart.

It was apparent that this situation was placing an enormous strain on Jodie's heart and, if the twins were not separated, either both twins would die or Mary would die, which would raise the need for the twins to be separated in any event. The problem was that such an emergency procedure would place Jodie at greater risk than if the surgery was pre-planned and attempted while both twins were alive.

It was widely acknowledged that if the twins were separated then Jodie would go on to lead a relatively normal life but Mary would inevitably die. The parents would not make the most painful of decisions and, in light of their faith, stated they would leave the twins' fate in God's hand.

The Trust responsible for the twins' care applied to the High Court for a declaration that they could perform the separation lawfully without the parents' consent. The courts, by virtue of s 1, Children Act 1989, are able to rely on the principle that whenever a decision about a child is made, '**the child's welfare shall be the court's paramount consideration**' and can override the parents' refusal of consent.

At first instance, the court granted the Trust a declaration for the operation to proceed. Mr Justice Johnson argued that surgery would be in the interests of both the twins on the basis that Jodie would be able to lead a near normal life and Mary would be spared the pain, suffering and the significantly reduced quality of life that she would experience. The parents appealed.

In a lengthy and complicated (but ultimately) unanimous judgment, the Court of Appeal dismissed the parents' appeal.

A more recent example of the 'best interests' test in operation can be found in the case of *Glass v UK* (2004). This case illustrates the extent to which parents can disagree with doctors caring for their child.

CASE EXAMPLE

Glass v UK [2004] ECHR 102

David Glass, aged 12, suffered extensive physical and mental difficulties requiring 24-hour care which was provided by his mother. He was not suffering from any terminal illness. His condition deteriorated after a minor operation and the doctors felt that he should be treated with palliative care, that his condition was without hope and that their approach was in his best interests. The mother disagreed. Unbeknown to her, a 'Do Not Resuscitate' order had been placed on his notes.

So began a lengthy battle between the hospital and the mother, who even resuscitated him on one occasion herself. Having exhausted her options in the English courts, the mother took the case to the European Court of Human Rights, which found that the hospital's approach to treating David had been a substantial interference with David's Article 8 rights (the right to a private and family life).

The European Court of Human Rights confirmed that, where there is a dispute between the family and the treating medical professionals as to what is deemed to be in the best interests of the patient, applying to the courts to determine the issue is the only viable solution. Indeed, the point was made by the court that the doctors could have avoided breaching David's Article 8 rights simply by making a timely application to the court to authorise the disputed treatment.

Re A (2001)	*Glass v UK*
• Conjoined twins were separated. The children's welfare was the court's paramount consideration and this overrode the parents' refusal.	• Where there is a dispute between the parents and medical professionals it may be for the court to determine the best interests of the patient.

Figure 2.10 The judgments of *Re A* (2001) and *Glass v UK* (2004)

Discussion point

In November 2008 the newspapers were full of the story of Hannah Jones, a 13-year-old girl from Herefordshire (see, for example, *The Guardian*, Tuesday 11 November). Hannah had refused to consent to a heart transplant. She had the full support of her parents even though all parties knew that she would die as a result of this refusal. The local hospital instigated court proceedings requesting an order compelling Hannah to undergo the transplant. This application was subsequently withdrawn.

The courts seem more than willing to override a child's refusal of treatment, particularly where they have refused life-saving/life-sustaining treatment; however that only becomes an issue *if an application is made to the courts*. If all parties involved (the child, those with parental responsibility and the medical team) all agree that not treating the patient is in their best interests, then the child's wishes may well be respected. Of course, the medical team might want to make an application to the court requesting a declaration that not treating the child would be acceptable in that particular case.

Hannah subsequently changed her mind, consented to a heart transplant and made a good recovery.

Conclusion

The case of *Gillick* (1986) was revolutionary in terms of providing minors with the respect and the rights to make decisions about their own healthcare. To some extent, with parental responsibility in some guise or another lurking in the background, these rights rather than being eroded have been tempered with a judicial paternalism and protect ive measures. When considering the incompetent patient, the courts when acting in the patient's best interests will consider the wider picture, including the social and ethical implications of their decision.

ACTIVITY

Self-test questions on consent

Ensure that all your answers are supported by case law where appropriate.

- Clearly explain the principle in *Re F (Mental Patient: Sterilisation)* (1990). On what basis was the hospital permitted to proceed with the operation?
- Discuss, with reference to a range of case law, what amounts to a patient's 'best interests'. Are medical best interests the sole consideration?
- Have statutory provisions adopted the common law approach?
- What is an advance decision? When are they made? How can one ensure that an advance decision remains enforceable?
- What is *Gillick* competence?
- How is a medical professional able to treat a child who lacks capacity to consent?
- Can a child under 16 years of age have the capacity to refuse treatment? Illustrate your answer by reference to more than one case.
- In *Re A (Children) (Conjoined Twins Surgical Separation)* (2001) the concept of best interests was severely tested. Demonstrate a clear understanding of the judgment.

SUMMARY

- A patient who cannot consent can be treated by a medical professional according to their best interests.
- Case law has demonstrated that, in determining what amounts to a patient's best interests, all the circumstances of the case can be taken into account.
- The common law approach has now been replaced by provisions of the MCA 2005.
- An advance decision allows a competent person to make decisions about his future care should he lose competency. The maker should ensure that the requirements are closely adhered to and the AD is kept up to date so as to ensure its continuing validity.
- There is a rebuttable presumption that a child between the ages of 16 and 18 can consent to medical treatment.
- A child under the age of 16 can consent to medical treatment if they are considered '*Gillick* competent': that is, they have a sufficient level of maturity and intelligence to understand the implications of the treatment.
- Case law shows that a '*Gillick* competent' child is most unlikely to be able to refuse medical treatment, the courts erring on the side of paternalism until a child reaches majority.
- Extraordinary cases such as *Re A* (2001) show that determining a child's best interests can be extremely difficult.

Michael, aged 15, is in desperate need of a kidney transplant, and is likely to die within a year if this does not take place. Although he has been told that there is now a kidney available, he is refusing to consent to the operation. Sadly, he has already had the experience of a failed kidney transplant and does not want to go through the same level of suffering again. He does not want to spend his life on medication and fully understands that if he does not consent he will die. Michael's doctors believe he should have the transplant and do not believe he has the capacity to refuse. The Trust seeks your advice.

- Michael is 15 years old, and this is the first relevant point that should be identified. The relevance of the age is that it requires you to refer to the seminal case of *Gillick* (1986) and explain its implications. As he is under the age of 16, s 8, Family Law (Reform) Act which presumes competence in children aged 16–18 will not apply. It will be necessary to explain that as a result of *Gillick*, a child can consent to treatment if they can understand the nature and effect of the treatment.

- However, the question is about Michael, a child patient who refuses treatment rather than one who consents, and this is important.
- Close consideration should be paid to case law which illustrates that a minor patient's refusal to medical treatment is often overruled by the courts. You should explain how the courts take a paternalistic approach and err on the side of preserving life.
- Refer to case law to support your answer, for example *Re E* (1993) which held that the patient lacked a clear understanding of the effect of his refusal on both him and his family. Note particularly the words of Ward J which emphasise that the courts 'should be very slow to allow an infant to martyr himself'.

- Avoid limiting your answer to just one example of case law as this tends to show a lack of breadth of knowledge. There are a number of cases which illustrate a similar principle, including *Re S* (1994) and *Re L* (1998). Where you are able to, demonstrate wider reading with reference to academic opinion, or perhaps quote from the judgment. Most importantly, ensure that you focus on the principle: although a minor can consent to medical treatment, the courts are unlikely to permit a minor to refuse medical treatment.
- Although the courts can override a child's refusal of medical treatment, one should also explore who else can give consent. Turn now to explore how the courts can lawfully treat Michael.
- In these circumstances, Michael's parents can consent on his behalf and this allows medical professionals to treat him without fear of legal action.

- Remember that all the medical professionals need is a 'key'; reference to Lord Donaldson's dictum in *Re R* (1991) would be essential. Remember, however, that the keyholder analogy was revisited in *Re W* (1992) where the analogy to a flak jacket was made.
- The medical staff simply need consent from Michael's parents, the court or someone with parental responsibility in order to be able to proceed to treat him lawfully.

- It is now time to conclude: it should be clear that Michael will not be able to maintain his refusal.
- Ensure that you have covered the following:
  - Can a minor consent to medical treatment?
  - What is the authority?
  - Can he refuse medical treatment? Why not?
  - What are the authorities?
  - What happens next?
  - How can the medical staff treat him?
- Explain all aspects with clear reference to case law and statute.

Further reading

Buchanan, A. (2004) *Bioethics*, ed by John Harris. Oxford: Oxford University Press.

Fagerlin, A. and Scheider, C. E. (2004) *The Hastings Center Report*, 34(2) March/April, pages 30–42.

Jackson, E. (2009) *Medical Law: Text, Cases and Materials*, second edition. Oxford: Oxford University Press.

Mason, J. K. and Laurie, G. T. (2010) *Mason and McCall Smith's Law and Medical Ethics*, 8th edition. Oxford: Oxford University Press.

3

Mental health law

AIMS AND OBJECTIVES

After reading this chapter you should be able to:

- Understand the amendments to statutory definitions in the Mental Health Act (MHA) 2007
- Demonstrate an understanding of the statutory provisions for involuntary detention under the MHA 2007
- Demonstrate an understanding of the statutory provisions for voluntary detention under the MHA 2007
- Appreciate the complexity of judicial interpretation
- Understand the relationship between the mental health law and the European Convention of Human Rights (ECHR).

3.1 Mental health law: an introduction

Mental illness is a vast area of the law in itself, and a book of this nature cannot treat such an important and complex area in the depth it demands. It is therefore the intention of this chapter to provide an effective overview and to highlight the amendments in the new Mental Health Act (MHA) 2007. It is hoped that the reader will develop an appreciation of this vast area of law through the snapshot consideration of the topic.

The MHA 2007 was given Royal Assent in June 2007 and was implemented between 2007 and October 2008. Essentially, the MHA 2007 represents another building block on the MHA of 1959; nevertheless, the MHA 2007 introduced significant reforms to the MHA 1983 and also amended the Mental Capacity Act (MCA) 2005, many provisions of which we have already considered. One of the most significant reforms of the MHA 2007 was that it amended the MCA 2005 to introduce new provisions relating to the deprivation of liberty, which came into force in 2009.

When considering this topic it is important to bear in mind that just because a person has a mental illness, it does not mean that he lacks capacity to make a decision. We only need remind ourselves of the case of *Re C (Adult: Refusal of Treatment)* (1994) where C had been admitted to a secure hospital under Part 3 of the MHA 1983 because he had been diagnosed as a paranoid schizophrenic. He then refused potentially life-saving treatment but did not lack capacity to make a decision regarding his treatment because of his mental illness. One is simply not dependent on the other. Conversely, had he lacked capacity to make a decision, the medical professional would have treated him under the MCA 2005 on the basis of what was in the patient's best interests.

The MHA 2007 plays a different role, as it is used where the patient has capacity to make a decision about his or her treatment *but* that person refuses to consent to treatment. It is also used where a patient lacks capacity. In reality, one of the main purposes of the Act is to ensure that if a person suffers from a serious mental disorder which affects their health, their safety or the safety of the public, they can be treated regardless of whether or not they consent. Their consent is largely irrelevant as treatment is necessary to stop them from harming either themselves or another.

Statistics show that in 2006–2007 there were 48,083 formal detentions under the Mental Health Acts (representing all NHS facilities and independent hospitals). This represented a slight increase from 47,394 in 2005–2006 (source: National Statistics, The Information Centre).

3.2 What orders can be obtained under the Mental Health Act 2007?

Although we consider each of the following sections separately, it is probably helpful at the outset for the reader to appreciate how a patient may be detained under the MHA 2007: see Figure 3.1.

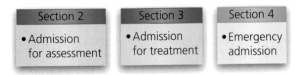

Figure 3.1 Sections 2–4, MHA 2007

3.3 Statutory definition of 'mental disorder'

Without doubt, one of the most important changes in the MHA 2007 is the fundamental change to the definition of mental disorder.

Section 1(1), MHA 2007 amends s 1(2), MHA 1983 and now redefines mental disorder as any 'disorder or disability of the mind', which provides a wider, more encompassing definition. It is worth noting that there is no statutory difference in the definition if the patient is to be detained for a short period or a longer period of time. The definition which is particularly broad is designed to ensure that a person with a personality order can be detained without reference to a particular disorder.

Subsections 1(2) and 1(3) remove the four categories of previously defined mental disorder which were applied to longer term admissions, and replace the four categories with one definition which applies continuously throughout the Act.

3.4 What amounts to a 'disorder or disability of the mind'?

The Code of Practice para 3.3 provides assistance as to what amounts to a 'disorder or disability of the mind'. The list below is non-exhaustive but specifically includes the following:

- affective disorder, such as depression and bipolar disorder
- schizophrenia and delusional disorders
- neurotic, stress-related disorders and somatoform disorders, such as anxiety, phobic disorders, obsessive compulsive disorders, post-traumatic stress disorder and hypochondriacal disorders
- organic mental disorders such as dementia and delirium (however caused)
- personality and behavioural changes caused by brain injury or damage (however caused)
- personality disorders
- mental and behaviour disorders caused by psychoactive substance use (see below)

- eating disorders, non-organic sleep disorders and non-organic sexual disorders
- learning disabilities
- autistic spectrum disorders including Asperger's syndrome
- behavioural and emotional disorders of children and adolescents.

Thus, the categories of mental disorder or abnormality are broad. One requirement that is now noticeably absent is that particularly aggressive or unpredictable behaviour is no longer a prerequisite to a person's detention.

Example

Umar suffers from obsessive compulsive disorder. Recently, it has appeared that his conditioning is worsening, and he is more depressed than normal. His family are concerned about the effect which this condition is having on his health. Umar can be admitted for treatment under s 2, MHA 2007 if there is a concern for his health, his safety or for the safety of others. As there appears to be some concern about his health, he can be admitted for treatment without his consent.

3.5 Mental and behaviour disorders caused by psychoactive substance use

Paragraph 3.8 of the Code of Practice states that alcohol or drug dependency is not considered a mental disorder or disability for the purposes of mental disorder under the Act. Therefore, a person cannot be detained for being simply dependent on either drink or drugs (paragraph 3.9) but could be detained if the disorder was related to dependence upon drink or drugs.

3.6 Sexual deviancy

An important amendment to the 1983 Act concerns removing the previously excluded reference to sexual deviancy. This was an issue highlighted by the Reed Committee in 1994. There was a concern that:

> 'as a consequence people who might benefit from medical care were at times, denied it and remained in prison or be left unsupported in the community. The implications for public safety were clearly matters of concern.'
> *(Report of the Department of Health and Home Office Working Group of Psychopathic Disorder (1994), para 10.16)*

The government expressed concern that the 1983 Act failed to allow a person to be considered to be suffering from a mental disorder if he displayed signs of 'promiscuity or other immoral conduct' or 'sexual deviancy'. They reasoned that it was more appropriate to bring sexual offences such as paedophilia under the umbrella of mental disorders. This would allow a person to be treated under the Mental Health Act if they posed a risk of re-offending once they were released from prison.

3.7 Learning difficulties

'Learning difficulties' are defined under MHA 1983 as amended. Section 1(2A) defines a learning disability as:

SECTION

> 'a state of arrested or incomplete development of the mind which includes significant impairment of intelligence and social functioning'.

A person with a learning difficulty is not considered to be suffering from a mental disorder *unless* that difficulty leads to behaviour which is 'abnormally aggressive or seriously irresponsible'. Unless they display such behaviour, they cannot be detained for treatment under s 3. This allows a clear distinction to be made between those who suffer from significant learning disabilities but should not be labelled as suffering from a mental disorder, and those who suffer from a mental disorder due to behaviour associated with a mental disorder.

3.8 Who can detain for treatment?

We have already established that a person with a mental disorder or disability can be detained without their consent under s 2, MHA 2007 where there is concern that that person's health is a risk or where there is a question about either his safety or the safety of others. We now have to consider who can apply for the order for detention without the person's consent:

1. the person's relative
2. an approved mental health professional.

3.8.1 The person's relative

Arguably relatives are often best placed to recognise that the mental condition from which their family member suffers is now a threat to their health, safety or the safety of others. However, there is also an inevitable difficulty with involving family members as the case of *JT v UK* [2000] 1 FLR 909 ECHR demonstrates. Here, a girl who had been sexually abused by her step-father did not want her mother involved at all in the decision-making process concerning her future care. Perhaps it is therefore appropriate that the role of the nearest relative (if applicable) is to make the application to the hospital managers rather than to the court.

Who is a relative? Section 26, MHA 1983 defines who can act as a nearest relative. Relatives of half-blood are also included in the list:

a. husband or wife
b. son or daughter
c. father or mother
d. brother or sister
e. grandparent
f. grandchild
g. uncle or aunt
h. nephew or niece.

The MHA 2007 amends the provisions that simply relate to 'man' or 'wife' so as to include the term 'civil partner'.

3.8.2 An approved mental health professional

Most applications for patients to be detained are made by approved mental health professionals, as they are the most likely to be involved with the patient's ongoing care, know the relevant procedures and seek to help the patient without recourse to the MHA 2007. Most approved mental health professionals are social workers, but may also be a mental health nurse or a psychologist who has had appropriate training.

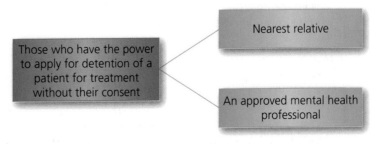

Figure 3.2 Who can detain for treatment?

3.9 The Mental Health Act 2007 Code of Practice

The revised Code of Practice which accompanies the 2007 Act was written further to s 118, MHA 1983, which allows the Secretary of State to revise guidance to interested bodies from time to time.

The Code itself is not legally binding but provides guidance for those seeking to implement the Act. While the Codes may not be binding, the House of Lords case of *R (Munjaz) v Mersey Care NHS Trust* [2006] 2 AC 14 confirmed that the Codes should be followed and applied unless there is a good reason for not following them in relation to a particular patient. Lord Bingham observed that 'great weight' should be given to the Codes; they are not instruction, but it is much more than mere advice ... from which it should depart only if it has cogent reasons for doing so.'

3.10 Guiding principles

While there are five guiding principles contained within the Mental Health Code of Practice paras 1.2–1.6 which should be taken into account when a professional makes a decision under the Act, these principles are not enshrined in statute and therefore lack the enforceability of the principles within the MCA 2005.

Purpose principle

This refers to the mental and physical safety and wellbeing of patients, promoting their own recovery and protecting others from harm. The Codes of Practice state in paragraph 1.2:

'Decisions under the Act must be taken with a view to minimising the undesirable effects of mental disorder, by maximising the safety and wellbeing (mental and physical) of patients, promoting their recovery and protecting other people from harm.'

Least restriction principle

When a person takes action without the patient's consent, consideration must be given to the restrictions placed upon a person's liberty. Paragraph 1.3 states:

'People taking action without a patient's consent must attempt to keep to a minimum the restrictions they impose on the patient's liberty, having regard to the purpose for which the restrictions are imposed.'

Respect principle

Every patient must be respected. There must be no discrimination with regards to a person's race, religion, culture, gender, age, sexual orientation and any disability. As far as possible, a patient's wishes must be taken into account. Paragraph 1.4 states:

'People taking decisions under the Act must recognise and respect the diverse needs, values and circumstances of each patient, including their race, religion, culture, gender, age, sexual orientation and any disability. They must consider the patient's views, wishes and feelings (whether expressed at the time or in advance), so far as they are reasonably ascertainable, and follow those wishes wherever practicable and consistent with the purpose of the decision. There must be no unlawful discrimination.'

Participation principle

It is important that, as far as possible, patients are given the opportunity to be involved in their treatment to ensure that it is as suitable for them as is possible. Views of those who also have an interest in the patient should be taken into account and given close consideration. Paragraph 1.5 states:

'Patients must be given the opportunity to be involved, as far as is practicable in the circumstances, in planning, developing and reviewing their own treatment and care to help ensure that it is delivered in a way that is as appropriate and effective for them as possible. The involvement of carers, family members and other people who have an interest in the patient's welfare should be encouraged (unless there are particular reasons to the contrary) and their views taken seriously'.

Effectiveness, efficiency and equity principle

Those who take decisions must ensure that the needs of the patient are met and that the purpose for which the decision was taken is met fairly and appropriately.

'People taking decisions under the Act must seek to use the resources available to them and to patients in the most effective, efficient and equitable way, to meet the needs of patients and achieve the purpose for which the decision was taken'.

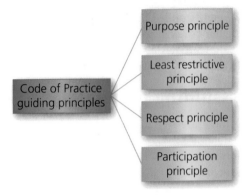

Figure 3.3 Code of Practice guiding principles

In contrast, s 1, MCA 2005 contains the following statutory obligations which are, unlike the guiding principles in the MCA 2007, enforceable.

They are as follows:

SECTION

(2) A person must be assumed to have capacity unless it is established that he lacks capacity.

(3) A person is not to be treated as unable to make a decision unless all practicable steps to help him to do so have been taken without success.

(4) A person is not to be treated as unable to make a decision merely because he makes an unwise decision.

(5) An act done, or decision made, under this Act for or on behalf of a person who lacks capacity must be done, or made, in his best interests.

(6) Before the act is done, or the decision is made, regard must be had to whether the purpose for which it is needed can be as effectively achieved in a way that is less restrictive of the person's rights and freedom of action.

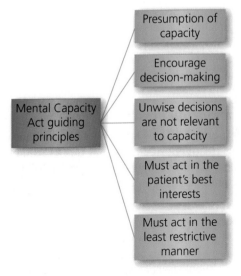

Figure 3.4 Guiding principles of MCA 2005

3.11 Involuntary admission to hospital

3.11.1 Mental Health Act 1983

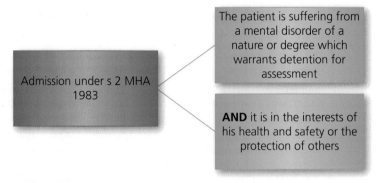

Figure 3.5 Section 2, MHA 1983

An application for admission for assessment for treatment for a period of 28 days (s 2(4)) can be made by virtue of s 2(2) on the grounds that:

SECTION

(a) he is suffering from mental disorder of a nature or degree which warrants detention of the patient in a hospital for assessment (or for assessment followed by medical treatment) for at least a limited period;
and
(b) he ought to be so detained in the interests of his health or safety or with a view to the protection of other persons.

An application for admitting a patient for assessment can be made either by a relative or a mental health professional, although the latter is preferable as they possess the necessary skills and expertise. If a relative applies on behalf of a family member it can naturally have adverse consequences on the relationship between the parties which would clearly be undesirable. Any application must be supported by two medical professionals, one of whom must have an appropriate qualification in mental health.

The maximum period that a patient can be detained under s 2 is 28 days, but the patient does have the option to apply to have his case reviewed at a Mental Health Review Tribunal (MHRT) after a 14-day period has elapsed.

The Codes provide guidance as to when s 2 should be used. A patient can be detained *without* their consent under s 2:

- if the full extent of the *nature* and *degree* of the patient's condition is unclear, or
- if there is a need to carry out an initial in-patient assessment in order to formulate a treatment plan, or
- if there is a need to carry out an initial in-patient reassessment in order to reformulate a treatment plan, or
- to reach a judgment about whether a patient will accept treatment on a voluntary basis following admission.

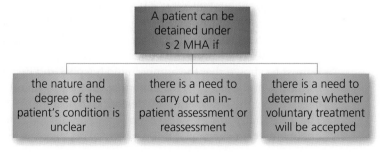

Figure 3.6 Detaining a patient under s 2, MHA 1983

3.11.2 What does *nature and degree* mean?

CASE EXAMPLE

R v Mental Health Review Tribunal for South Thames Region ex parte Smith [1998] 47 BMLR 104

The patient who was suffering from paranoid schizophrenia was subject to a hospital order under ss 37 and 41, MHA 1983. He applied to a MHRT to be discharged, and when he appeared was asymptomatic. In declining his application for discharge, Popplewell J drew a distinction between 'nature' and 'degree', explaining that while the two terms may appear to be inextricably linked, this was not necessarily the case. Here, the applicant's schizophrenia was not of a 'degree' that required detention as he was displaying neither 'positive' nor 'negative' signs of schizophrenia, but his condition was such that detention was required.

3.11.3 Section 3: longer term detention under MHA 2007

Section 3 differs from s 2 (above) and s 4 (below) in that it is intended that the patient detained under this section will be detained for the longer term. Section 3 states that:

SECTION

An application for admission for treatment may be made in respect of a patient on the grounds that

(a) he is suffering from mental disorder of a nature or degree which makes it appropriate for him to receive medical treatment in a hospital **and**

(b) it is necessary for the health or safety of the patient or the protection of other persons that he should receive such treatment and it cannot be provided unless he is detained under this section **and**

(c) appropriate medical treatment is available for him.

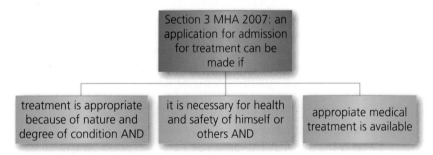

Figure 3.7 Section 3, MHA 2007

As with s 2, all the criteria *must* be met.

- Section 3 has been amended significantly. Since the former definitions of mental illness have been replaced, patients can only be detained if they are suffering from a 'disorder or disability' of the mind.
- The patient's mental disorder must be such that treatment in hospital is appropriate.
- Section 3 continues to require the application to be approved by written recommendations of two registered medical professionals, one of whom must have experience in the diagnosis of treatment of mental disorder.
- It must be shown that the admission to hospital and detention is necessary either for the health or the safety of the patient or for the protection of others, and the only way of providing the treatment is by detention in hospital.
- The 'treatability test' has also been replaced with the criteria of appropriate medical treatment being available for the patient. This suggests that if there is no appropriate

treatment, the patient cannot be detained even if there is a risk to his health or his safety or for the protection of others' safety.

- The consent of the patient is *not* required.
- Detention under s 3 can be for up to six months and can then be extended with the appropriate authority for a further six-month period. In turn, extensions for a year can be made.

Detention under section 3

CASE EXAMPLE

R (M) v South West London Mental Health NHS Trust [2008] EWCA 1112

A 44-year-old woman with a history of mental illness had been detained under s 2, MHA 2007 but had been taken to accident and emergency on two occasions on non-related medical issues. Having been detained on a surgical ward the psychiatrist sought to detain her under s 3. She asked for the assessment to be delayed as she did not feel well enough to be assessed. She was detained nonetheless. She applied for *habeas corpus* alleging her detention was unlawful.

The court held that she had been adequately assessed and deemed it was in her own interests and the interests of others that she be detained. It was clear, the court said, that she was highly uncooperative in the assessment. The medical practitioners were not obliged to postpone the assessment and, accordingly, she could be assessed for the purposes of s 3 and detained without her consent.

3.11.4 Treatment under s 3(4), MHA 2007

The often criticised 'treatability test' has been replaced with s 3(4) which states:

SECTION

'references to appropriate medical treatment, in relation to a person suffering from mental disorder, are references to medical treatment which is appropriate in his case, taking into account the nature and degree of the mental disorder and all other circumstances of his case'.

The removal of the 'treatability test' is regarded as a positive move forward. As Fennell J observes:

QUOTATION

'It is not overdramatic to say that opinion leaders within the psychiatric profession see the issue as crucial in preserving their role as doctors rather than agents of the state policies of preventative detention.' (2007, page 25)

Previously, under the 1983 Act, it would be necessary to certify that the proposed treatment of a patient would be 'likely to alleviate or prevent deterioration in the patient's condition'. This was extremely difficult for any doctor to be able to certify if the patient was refusing to cooperate. The new provision therefore only requires that treatment is *available* for the patient – he does not need to certify that the patient will accept it. The introduction of the new test has its own inherent risks as it 'risks increasing compulsory power unnecessarily for people who will have no therapeutic benefit' (Paul Farmer, Chair of Mental Health Alliance). It may be that use of the word 'appropriate' creates too wide an ambit, and without more specific definition may allow medical professionals to detain a patient to treat where there may be no clear benefit for the patient.

Treatability test replaced with ⟶ appropriate treatment test

3.11.5 Section 4: emergency treatment under MHA 1983

Under s 4, the Act allows a patient to be detained for emergency assessment. In order to satisfy these emergency powers, the patient's condition must be so serious that the need to be urgently assessed and treated justifies detention for emergency assessment on just a single medical professional's recommendation. It is not required that the doctor who detains by this procedure is a mental health specialist. This is relevant as if the doctor is faced with a suicidal patient, the doctor can take necessary and urgent steps without waiting for an appropriately qualified medical practitioner.

The Codes of Practice assist in determining what amounts to 'sufficiently urgent', and evidence of the following is deemed to be adequate:

- an immediate and significant risk of mental or physical harm to the patient or to others
- a danger of serious harm to property or
- a need for physical restraint of the patient.

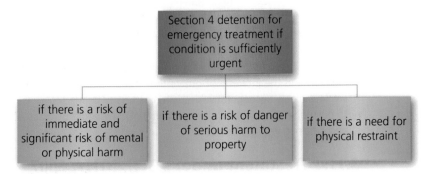

Figure 3.8 Provisions of s 4, MHA 1983

In urgent circumstances, the application for detention can be made by one of two interested parties, an approved mental health professional or a relative. If it is made by the relative then the applicant must have seen the potential patient within the previous 24 hours. If either party seeks to apply for emergency treatment then they must be able to state that the application is of 'urgent necessity' and prior compliance with the procedures set down in s 2 of the Act would lead to 'undesirable delay'.

Under s 4 the maximum period for which a person can be detained under this period is 72 hours. Thereafter the patient must either be released or considered under another section of the Act. Under s 4, patients must be treated only with their consent.

A further provision allowing emergency detention can also be found in s 136. Here, a police officer can remove a person to a place of safety if he finds 'a person who appears to him to be suffering from mental disorder and to be in immediate need of care or control' in a public place. The person can be taken to a police station or a hospital, although a police station should only be used in exceptional circumstances. A person can only be detained for a period of 72 hours for the purposes of examination by an appropriate mental health professional and for arrangements to be made for his treatment.

3.12 Section 63, MHA 1983

Section 63 states:

SECTION

'the consent of a patient shall not be required for any medical treatment given to him for the mental disorder from which he is suffering, not being a form of treatment to which ss 57, 58 or 58A applies, if the treatment is given by or under the direction of the approved clinician in charge of the treatment.'

Section 63 allows a patient to be treated for his mental disorder *without his consent* and without the need for a second opinion. A patient's autonomy is overridden by paternalism and while a competent patient can refuse treatment for physical conditions even if their refusal leads to their death as demonstrated in *Re C (Adult: Refusal of Medical Treatment)* (1994), the same level of autonomy is not afforded to a competent patient who also suffers from a mental disorder. It is even acceptable to use a reasonable degree of force to ensure that the patient complies with treatment allowed under s 63.

The fact that a degree of force can be used to ensure compliance with treatment is also shown in common law below, where the court ordered medical intervention even though the patient was not suffering from a mental disorder within the meaning of s 63.

CASE EXAMPLE

Norfolk and Norwich Healthcare Trust v W [1997] 1 FCR 259

A woman presented herself at hospital in labour. She had had three previous pregnancies and on all occasions had the baby delivered by Caesarean section. She had a history of psychiatric treatment and denied she was pregnant. The Trust sought authority to deliver her baby by Caesarean section if necessary. Failure to deliver in this way (if the baby could not be delivered by forceps) could result in the death of the baby, the mother or both.

Although it would appear that she was not suffering from a mental disorder, the court held that she lacked the necessary capacity to make decisions about her treatment. The court therefore held that it was in her best interests that the baby was delivered, to ensure that the health and wellbeing of both mother and baby were preserved, and authorised treatment.

3.13 The interpretation of s 63, MHA 1983

The courts have been asked to adjudicate on the interpretation of 'any medical treatment given to him for the mental disorder from which he is suffering'. Unsurprisingly, this section has been given a wide and liberal interpretation.

CASE EXAMPLE

Re KB (adult) (mental patient: medical treatment) [1994] 19 BMLR 144

KB was an 18-year-old woman who had been suffering from anorexia for several years and was rapidly deteriorating. She had been detained for treatment under s 3, MHA 1983. She was refusing to eat and the health authority sought a declaration that it would be lawful to feed her via a naso-gastric tube. The health authority argued that feeding by naso-gastric tube was part of the treatment itself.

It was held that naso-gastric tube feeding was covered by s 63, MHA 1983 and could be carried out without the patient's consent. Ewbank J held that force-feeding a patient who was suffering from anorexia fell within s 63 because 'relieving the symptoms was just as much a part of the treatment as relieving the underlying cause'.

Naso-gastric tube

A naso-gastric tube can be used as a method of feeding, by inserting a plastic tube through the nose, down the throat and into the stomach.

Of course, it is widely recognised that force-feeding a patient (often adolescent girls) suffering from anorexia does not necessarily resolve the long-term problem. However, the justification and academic approval appears to be, as Cameron-Perry observes:

QUOTATION

'as the provision of nourishment is required for the restoration of autonomy, force-feeding is a legitimate basic treatment for anorexia nervosa.' ((2000) *British Medical Journal*, 321, 510)

In a similar decision and only slightly later, the Court of Appeal in *B v Croydon Health* (1995) below allowed s 63 to be invoked to force-feed a patient who had a tendency to self-harm.

CASE EXAMPLE

B v Croydon Health Authority [1995] Fam 133

B was a woman of 24 years of age who suffered from a psychopathic disorder and had a tendency to self-harm. She was detained under s 3, MHA 1983 and had refused to eat. She had been threatened with feeding via a naso-gastric tube and her condition had improved slightly as a result. She then made an application to the court to restrain the health authority from feeding her without her consent. She was granted the application pending a full hearing. On the latter occasion, Thorpe J held that naso-gastric feeding amounted to treatment for the condition from which she was suffering and thus, under s 63, her consent was not required. She appealed.

Her appeal was dismissed: the term 'medical treatment' within the meaning of s 63 included and referred to treatment, the purpose of which was to treat the condition from which the patient was suffering. Feeding by way of tube was such a treatment and accordingly could be given without the patient's consent. Her deprivation of food was part of her act of self-harming, and in permitting her to be force-fed would 'alleviate the symptoms of the disorder as well as treatment to remedy its underlying cause'. (*per* Neill LJ)

This approach was also followed in the Scottish courts in *Reid v Secretary of State* (1999) (below) where provisions in the Mental Health (Care and Treatment) (Scotland) Act 2003 that referred to 'treatment for the condition' could also refer to treatment that would ease the symptoms of the patient's illness, thus creating a parity between the jurisdictions' application of mental health law.

CASE EXAMPLE

Reid v Secretary of State [1999] 1 All ER 481

Reid was a long-serving prisoner having been convicted in 1967 of culpable homicide. He was diagnosed as suffering from a psychopathic disorder, had been detained under MHA 1983 and was subject to a restriction order without time limit. He sought a discharge from the order. Under s 17 of the Mental Health (Scotland) Act 1984 there were three statutory criteria to be applied to determine whether a patient could be admitted and detained:

1) the nature and degree of the psychopathic order – the appropriateness test
2) whether the treatment was likely to alleviate or prevent worsening of the condition – the treatability test
3) whether treatment was necessary for his health or safety or for the safety of others – the safety test.

If the above conditions were not satisfied then the patient should be discharged under s 64. At first instance, the court found that the treatment he had received had alleviated his symptoms and that, if released, he could pose a real danger to society. The respondent appealed which was allowed on the basis that the medical treatment which he had received may have helped to alleviate his condition but it did not follow that it would continue to do so. Therefore, his condition could not be considered treatable, hence he should be discharged. The Secretary of State for Scotland appealed to the House of Lords.

In the House of Lords, the court adopted a wider meaning of 'medical treatment' and held that treatment which alleviated or prevented deterioration could refer to the symptoms of the disorder rather than the actual disorder itself. On the evidence before the lower courts, the House of Lords concluded it was not reasonable to say that the treatment had alleviated his condition and thus he could not be discharged from hospital. Although this was a Scottish case, the House of Lords accepted that the principles would apply to English law.

3.14 Wider interpretation of the Mental Health Act 1983

CASE EXAMPLE

Tameside and Glossop Acute Services Trust v CH [1996] 1 FCR 612

Here, the patient was a 41-year-old schizophrenic who had been sectioned under s 3, MHA 1983 and then became pregnant. At 37 weeks' gestation, it was felt that the foetus was in some difficulty and that labour needed to be induced. A Caesarean section was considered necessary if the foetus suffered further distress. There was some concern that although she consented to the induction she might withdraw her consent, and while this could have fatal consequences for the foetus, there was also concern for her mental wellbeing if the foetus was not delivered by Caesarean. The hospital sought a declaration under s 63 for a Caesarean to be carried out without her consent and with a reasonable degree of force if necessary.

Having considered the case of *B v Croydon Health Authority* (1995), the court took the extraordinarily wide view that a possible Caesarean section, by force if necessary, was within the perimeters of the treatment of her disorder. The court accepted the applicant's case that her mental state would deteriorate significantly if the baby was not born alive and it was therefore deemed to be part of her treatment that a Caesarean could be carried out by force.

Dolan and Parker observe that there must be a direct link between the physical symptoms and the mental disorder to fall within s 63 (2000, British Medical Journal, 7088; 314). In this case, the patient's pregnancy was not either symptomatic or a direct consequence of her mental condition. How can this case be distinguished from *Re C (Adult: Refusal of Medical Treatment)* (1994) where the patient was not forced to have his gangrenous foot amputated, despite the advice that he would surely die if he did not? It surely cannot and, while in *Re C* the patient who was competent could refuse medical treatment, the patient here cannot. The paternalistic approach authorising invasive treatment is reminiscent of the courts' approach in *Re MB (Medical Treatment)* (1997). There appears to be an inconsistency in the judicial approach, and in those cases which involve women in late stages of pregnancy or labour the women are considered to have little understanding of their own condition. Common law chooses to ignore a woman's autonomy altogether and replaces it with paternalism that authorises invasive procedures. It may be understandable but it introduces double standards that should not be perpetuated.

However, shortly afterwards, the courts retreated from this expansive approach in *St George's Hospital v S* [1998] 3 WLR 936 and held that a woman detained under the Act for mental disorder cannot be forced into medical procedures unconnected with her mental condition unless her capacity to consent to such treatment is diminished'. Moreover, Judge LJ specifically upheld the principle of autonomy, stating that the mere fact that a woman was pregnant did *not* reduce her right to decide whether or not to undergo a Caesarian section, and her right was not reduced because her decision may seem to others to be 'morally repugnant'. This may be a significant departure from *Tameside and Glossop Acute Services Trust v CH* (1996) but particularly hard to reconcile with the dictum of Butler-Sloss LJ in *Re MB* (1997) who considered the refusal of a Caesarean section as one that amounted to temporary incompetence under s 2(2), MCA 2005.

Key facts of cases relevant to s 63

Case	Judgment
Norfolk and Norwich Healthcare Trust v W (1997)	Although not suffering from a mental disorder, she lacked the necessary capacity to make decisions about her treatment.
Re KB (adult) (mental patient: medical treatment) (1994)	Force-feeding could be carried out without the patient's consent.
B v Croydon Health Authority (1995)	Force-feeding was a form of treatment and could be given to the patient without her consent.
Reid v Secretary of State (1999)	A wider definition of medical treatment was given. He could not be discharged because treatment had not alleviated his condition.
Tameside and Glossop Acute Services Trust v CH (1996)	Treatment for the patient's condition could also include a Caesarean section as this would relieve her symptoms.

3.14.1 Section 57, MHA 1983

This section (which admittedly is infrequently used) permits certain forms of medical treatment to be carried out on people with mental illness with the patient's consent and the agreement of a second opinion appointed doctor (SOAD). The treatment refers to psychosurgery, defined in s 57(1)(a) as 'any surgical operation for destroying brain tissue of for destroying the functioning of any brain tissue'. The section also applies to chemical castration, that is, 'surgical implantation of hormones for the purpose of reducing male sex drive'.

These requirements can actually be dispensed with if the application is urgent, as outlined in s 62. Thus in theory, chemical castration could be carried out without the patient's consent if it was:

SECTION

'immediately necessary and represents the minimum interference necessary to prevent the patient from behaving violently or being a danger to himself or to others.'

3.15 Section 58, MHA 1983

Section 58 requires the consent of the patient or a second opinion for administering electroconvulsive therapy or related medication. This section only applies to patients that are detained. In patients who lack capacity or refuse treatment, an opinion from a SOAD must be obtained and it must be deemed appropriate for the treatment to be given. In circumstances where the patient does not consent or lacks capacity to consent, once a SOAD is obtained, there is no necessity to obtain a further SOAD for up to three months.

3.16 Section 62, MHA 1983

This section removes the safeguards contained in ss 57 and 58, and enables treatment to be given without the patient's consent or without a second opinion. Section 62 is worded in such a way which states that the treatment must be 'immediately necessary'. In reality it is hard to envisage such a situation, but it does allow ECT to be administered without either the patient's consent or a second opinion. The section however does not permit treatment which is 'irreversible or hazardous' without consent or a second opinion.

ACTIVITY

Self-test questions

Please ensure that all your answers are supported by case law where appropriate.

- What is the statutory definition of mental disorder in MHA 2007?
- How can a patient be detained under s 2, MHA 2007?
- How does this differ from s 3?
- What are the four guiding principles contained in the Mental Health Act Code of Practice?
- Explain the significance of s 63, MHA 1983.
- Consider the subsequent interpretation. Has it been widely or narrowly interpreted?

3.17 Voluntary admission to hospital under MHA 1983

Section 131(1) states as follows:

SECTION

'Nothing in this Act shall be construed as preventing a patient who requires treatment for mental disorders from being admitted to any hospital or (registered establishment) in pursuance of arrangements made in that behalf and without application, order or direction rendering him liable to be detained under this Act, or from remaining in any hospital or (registered establishment) in pursuance of such arrangement after he has ceased to be so liable after he has been detained.'

Section 131, MHA 1983 provides for voluntary admission to hospital. Many patients would see this provision as infinitely preferable and far less stressful than the statutory powers of formal detention we have seen above. Since January 2008, a child aged 16–17 who has sufficient competence can also consent to their own informal admission to hospital.

CASE EXAMPLE

R v Kirklees Metropolitan Borough Council, ex parte C [1993] 2 FLR 187

A young girl aged 12 years was admitted to a mental hospital for assessment after being taken into care. She applied for judicial review of the decision and alleged she had been unlawfully imprisoned. She argued that since she had not been compulsorily admitted under Part 3 of MHA 1983 and she did not need treatment within the meaning of s 131 of the Act, there was no power to arrange her voluntary admission.

Her application was dismissed. She was not '*Gillick* competent'; the local authority was acting in *loco parentis* and could consent to her treatment under their inherent powers. Even though it was clear that the wording in s 131 referred to 'treatment' and not 'admission' as would have been more accurate in this case, the law was such that a person who consents could be admitted to hospital for assessment. Although she did not consent, the local authority on her behalf could. Therefore it could not be unlawful under common law since admission with an adult's consent was all that was required.

3.18 How informal is voluntary admission, and how free is the patient to leave hospital?

Patients are theoretically free to leave hospital and can indeed do so, *unless* the power under s 5 is invoked. As Fennell (1986) explains, s 131 does not necessarily entitle the patient to leave hospital. Despite the wording of the accompanying Codes of Practice to the 1983 Act which emphasise the patient's right to leave hospital, the right is in reality subject to 'significant limitations' as ss 5(2) and 5(4) provide doctors with a power to detain a patient for up to 72 hours.

Section 5(2) allows a registered medical practitioner or approved clinician to report that a patient who is already an in-patient can be detained for a period up to 72 hours from the time that the report is furnished. Furthermore, s 5(4) provides that a nurse may record that a patient is suffering from mental disorder to such a degree that it is necessary for his health or safety or for the protection of others that he be immediately restrained from leaving hospital without the immediate knowledge of the registered medical practitioner or approved clinician. In these circumstances, the patient may be detained for a period of six hours from the time that the fact is recorded.

The effect of s 5 appears to be that there were no procedural safeguards for a voluntarily admitted patient, in contrast with a detained patient whose detention is required by law to be regularly reviewed. This point was specifically tested in the seminal House of Lords case below which was first heard shortly before the introduction of the Human Rights Act 1998 (HRA).

CASE EXAMPLE

R v Bournewood Community and Mental Health NHS Trust, ex parte L [1998] 3 All ER 289

Mr L had suffered from autism since birth, had limited understanding and was unable to speak. He lacked the capacity to consent or otherwise to medical treatment. He had been treated by Bournewood Hospital for many years and had spent a period of time at the hospital's intensive behaviour unit. However, he had lived with paid carers for a period of three years and attended a day care unit at the hospital. On one occasion, he became extremely agitated and demonstrated such aggressive behaviour that he was admitted as an in-patient under the common law doctrine of necessity rather than under the provisions of MHA 1983. Staff were instructed that should he attempt to leave (although he never attempted to), he should be stopped. His carers were however refused access to him, in case he decided he wanted to return with them. His condition deteriorated; he became unhappy and withdrawn and required more significant medication than he had ever needed when he was living in the community with his carers. His carers challenged the grounds of his detention, stating that the procedure had not been followed under MHA 1983; he had instead been detained under the common law.

The Court of Appeal agreed with the carers' argument that no procedure had been followed; hence his continued detention was unlawful. He was discharged and returned home to the carers. Although the court rejected the carers' argument of false imprisonment and accepted that he had been detained unlawfully, they opined that there was a common law defence of necessity (as had been invoked in *Re F* (1990)), the purpose of which in these circumstances was to detain a patient who lacked capacity if it was deemed in his best interests to do so.

However, the case continued to the European Court of Human Rights (*HL v United Kingdom* (2004) 40 EHRR 76) where Lord Steyn stated that it was both 'stretching credulity to breaking point' and 'a fairy tale' that a patient in the applicant's position was free to leave. Since the patient was under the hospital's control and supervision and, despite not wishing to, was not able to leave if he so desired, the hospital was depriving the patient of his liberty. The court recognised that there were no procedures to be adopted, followed or considered, and accordingly ... this absence of procedural safeguards fails to protect against arbitrary deprivations of liberty on grounds of necessity and, consequently, to comply with the essential purpose of Article 5 of the Convention'. The patient's rights had been violated.

The judgment which concerns patients who lack capacity but are not resisting suggests that Art 5, ECHR is violated if they are detained in hospital on the basis of necessity. However, this detention could be justified under Art 5(4) for those who have a mental order within the definition of the MHA but only if the detention is legitimate and they have early recourse to the courts. The difficulty here was that the Trust was relying on the defence of necessity and neither of the safeguards applied.

3.19 The effect of *Bournewood*

As a result of the judgment from the ECHR, there was an obvious need to fill the '*Bournewood* gap' as it then became known. It was necessary to legislate to ensure that there were procedural safeguards for incapacitated patients who do not object but do not specifically consent to being admitted to hospital.

There were two significant responses. The first was to introduce a new s 64 into MHA 2007, and the same Act attached Sched A1 and 1A to MCA 2005.

Furthermore, there is guidance on what amounts to the deprivation of liberty in the Mental Capacity Act Codes of Practice paragraph 2.5 following a number of cases. Some of the factors that can be taken into account to indicate whether liberty has been deprived include (but is not limited to) where:

- staff exercise complete control and effective control over the care and movement of a person for a significant period
- staff exercise control over assessments, treatment, contacts and residence
- a request by carers for a person to be discharged into their care is refused
- the person loses autonomy because they are under continuous supervision and control.

Under the new Sched 1A there are six requirements that must be satisfied before a deprivation of liberty will be satisfied:

- The patient must be at least 18 years of age.
- The patient must be suffering from a mental disorder within the meaning of the MHA 2007.
- The person must lack capacity.
- It is in the best interests of the relevant person to be deprived of liberty and it is necessary for them to be deprived of liberty in order to prevent harm to themselves, and deprivation of liberty is a proportionate response to the likelihood of the relevant person suffering harm and the seriousness of that harm.
- They must not be detained under the Act or subject to restrictions on their freedom in the community.
- There must not be a valid and applicable advance refusal of the treatment for which the deprivation of the liberty authorisation is sought.

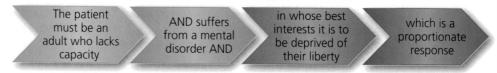

Figure 3.9 The requirements under Sched 1A

The Mental Capacity Act Deprivation of Liberty Safeguards (MCA DoLS) were introduced by MHA 2007. They seek to ensure that people are only deprived of their liberty where there is no alternative. In its first annual report (dated July 2010) statistics showed that the total number of applications was 7,160. This was considerably lower than expected, although the percentage of applications that resulted in depriving a person of their liberty was high, at 46 per cent.

Key facts on cases for voluntary admission

Case	Judgment
R v Kirklees Metropolitan Borough Council, ex parte C (1993)	The child lacked Gillick competence and could be treated without her consent as the local authority could consent on her behalf.
R v Bournewood Community and Mental Health NHS Trust, ex parte L (1998)	The patient had been detained under the common law doctrine of necessity.
HL v United Kingdom (2004)	The patient's rights had been violated under Art 5 as he had been deprived of his liberty.

3.20 Section 64, MHA 1983

This provides that a patient who lacks capacity but does not resist treatment can be treated provided the conditions in s 64D are met:

(2) The first condition is that, before giving the treatment, the person takes reasonable steps to establish whether the patient lacks capacity to consent to the treatment.

(3) The second condition is that, when giving the treatment, he reasonably believes that the patient lacks capacity to consent to it.

(4) The third condition is that —
   (a) he has no reason to believe that the patient objects to being given the treatment; or
   (b) he does have reason to believe that the patient so objects, but it is not necessary to use force against the patient in order to give the treatment.

(5) The fourth condition is that —
   (a) he is the person in charge of the treatment and an approved clinician;
   (b) or the treatment is given under the direction of that clinician.

(6) The fifth condition is that giving the treatment does not conflict with —
   (a) an advance decision which he is satisfied is valid and applicable; or
   (b) a decision made by a donee or deputy or the Court of Protection.

While the newly introduced provisions may seem to resolve the lacuna in the law, there are situations where use of MHA 2007 may be more appropriate than the amendment to MCA 2005. These terms of guidance can be found in the Code of Practice paragraph 13.12, which states that MHA 2007 could be used instead of MCA 2005 if the following apply:

- it is not possible to give the person the care or treatment they need without carrying out an action which might deprive them of their liberty
- the person needs treatment that cannot be given under MCA 2005 (for example, because the person has made a valid and applicable advance decision to refuse all or part of that treatment)
- the person may need to be restrained in a way that is not allowed under MCA 2005
- it is not possible to assess or treat the person safely or effectively without treatment being compulsory (perhaps because the person is expected to regain capacity to consent, but might then refuse to give consent)
- the person lacks capacity to decide on some elements of the treatment but has capacity to refuse a vital part of it – and they have done so, or
- there is some other reason why the person might not get the treatment they need, and they or someone else might suffer harm as a result.

Recent case law demonstrates some continuing issues with the application of deprivation of liberty orders.

CASE EXAMPLE

Hillingdon London Borough Council v Neary and others (2011) All ER 57

The respondent S was autistic and suffered from severe learning disability. He needed constant support and supervision which had been supplied by his father. His father fell unwell and requested that S went to stay at overnight respite care simply to allow him to recover. He did not agree to S remaining there for the long term. The unit signed an urgent deprivation of liberty order. They then issued proceedings in the Court of Protection to enable them to make long-term care decisions regarding his care. Meanwhile, his father still wanted S to return home in order that he might carry on caring for him. It was alleged that the period of S's deprivation of liberty which amounted to nearly a year breached S's right to a private and family life under Art 8 of the Convention. Furthermore, in depriving S of his liberty, it was contended that Art 5 had been violated.

There is a positive obligation to respect for family life and, subject to evidence to the contrary, patients who lacked capacity were better off cared for by their families. If the State was to remove an incapacitated adult, it could only be on the basis that they could provide better care than the family could. The court held that keeping S away from his family for so long violated Art 8. There had been no attempt at any time to determine what was in S's best interests.

Before it could be established whether Art 5 was engaged, it was necessary to establish whether there was a deprivation of liberty and whether the safeguards against a deprivation of liberty were effective. The relevant question was whether 'the restraint of liberty was of such a degree or intensity that it amounted to deprivation'. The court held that having taken all the circumstances of the case into account, keeping S at the unit for the amount of time that he had been detained amounted to a deprivation of his liberty and a violation of Art 5, ECHR. Furthermore, there had been an inadequate process put in place for S to be able to challenge the deprivation of liberty order, hence breaching Art 5 (4).

Only a week after the above case was reported, the Court of Protection ruled on the case below.

CASE EXAMPLE

C v Local Authority [2011] EWHC 1539 (Admin)

C was resident at a special school. He was an 18-year-old man with severe learning difficulties and autism; his behaviour was challenging, often aggressive and he was prone to self-harm. He had been in local authority care since the age of six and had been at the relevant unit for a period of two years. The school managed his behaviour by the use of a 'blue room' which was a padded room where he was taken when he was either aggressive or naked. He often chose to walk around naked as a sensory impairment meant that touch was particularly relevant to him. The time he spent in the room was considerable and evidence showed that he was placed there 192 times in a single month. There was however no statutory authority for such measures to be taken and judicial review of his care was sought with clarification as to 'best practice' to care for C as he moved into adulthood.

The relevant deprivation of liberty safeguards did not specifically include schools or children's homes, but it was deemed that they should apply. The policy of the school needed to give greater recognition to C's sensory needs and, while C should not be encouraged to walk around naked, he should not be punished by seclusion if he did. If seclusion was to be lawful then it had to comply with the Mental Health Act 1983 Codes of Practice and had to meet guidance set out by the Department of Health. If seclusion was to be sought then it should only be used when it was both necessary and proportionate to achieve the aims, and it had to be the least restrictive option. While the blue room could be somewhere C could choose to go to, he could not be detained there and had to be free to leave.

KEY FACTS

Key facts on deprivation of liberty cases

Case	Judgment
Hillingdon London Borough Council v Neary and others (2011)	S's detention amounted to a deprivation of his liberty and his rights under Art 5 had been violated.
C v Local Authority (2011)	Although the deprivations of liberty safeguards were not intended to cover schools, they were extended to include them. C's detention in a safe-style room could not be a place of seclusion and exclusion, and he could not be detained there.

3.21 Electro-convulsive therapy (ECT)

During ECT an electric current is passed briefly through the brain via electrodes applied to the scalp, in order to induce a therapeutic seizure in the patient. The procedure is carried out under general anaesthetic, and muscle relaxants are given to the patient to alleviate harm caused.

ECT was introduced in the 1930s and was widely used during the 1950s and 1960s. In modern medicine it is used far less frequently and is regarded by many as a controversial treatment. There are now only a small amount of mental disorders that are treated by ECT.

The National Institute of Clinical Excellence's (NICE) guidelines updated in May 2010 recommend that ECT is only used for the treatment of severe depressive illness, catatonia or a prolonged or severe manic episode. It is recommended that ECT is only used where other treatment has not resulted in an improvement in the patient's condition and is used to 'achieve rapid and short-term improvement of severe symptoms'.

Use of ECT is governed by s 58A(1), MHA 1983. ECT can be used by virtue of s 58A(3) if the patient consents, is above 18, the procedure has been certified by an approved clinician or a registered medical practitioner, and the patient is 'capable of understanding the nature, purpose and likely effects of the treatment'. If the patient is under the age of 18 then under s 58A(4) he can still consent to ECT, provided he is 'Gillick competent'. If the patient lacks competency, then s 58A(5) provides that ECT can still be administered provided it is appropriate for the treatment to be given, does not conflict with a valid and applicable advance decision or a decision made by a donee or deputy or by the Court of Protection. While the same authorisation must be obtained as for a competent patient, in addition two other people are required to be consulted. Neither can be the responsible clinician or the approved clinician who is in charge of the treatment. One should be a nurse but the other should be neither a nurse nor a registered medical practitioner. The requirements for further authorisation in the case of an incompetent patient highlight the controversial nature of the treatment and the necessity to ensure that, as far as possible, the benefits outweigh any potential risks.

3.22 The effect of the Human Rights Act 1998 on mental health law

Since HRA 1998 came into force on 2 October 2000, it has been necessary for the courts to play close attention to its provisions and its possible impact on mental health law. The ECHR has two important consequences on mental health law. Firstly (as with all other areas of law), the courts must interpret mental health legislation in light of HRA 1998 and in a way that is compatible with its Articles and, secondly, it is incumbent upon public authorities to ensure that they act in a way that is compatible with the Convention rights.

One of the most significant European judgments on mental health law was handed down in the case of *Winterwerp v The Netherlands* (1979) 2 EHRR 387 where criteria were introduced for the lawful detention of those of unsound mind. The courts stated that prior to detention and except in emergency cases:

- it is necessary to establish by objective expert assessment that the person is suffering from a mental disorder, and
- the established disorder is of a kind or degree that justifies confinement, and
- the patient cannot be lawfully detained if he is no longer suffering from the disorder.

Furthermore, the detention must not be a disproportionate response to the patient's mental disorder.

With reference to the last criterion, the detention must be reviewed in order to ensure that it is lawful. The statutory provisions in both MHA 1983 and 2007 adequately reflect these requirements.

3.22.1 Article 2 and the right to life

Article 2 states 'Everyone's right to life shall be protected by law'. Unusually in the area of mental health law, Art 2 became relevant in the following case.

CASE EXAMPLE

Savage v South Essex Partnership NHS Foundation Trust [2008] UKHL 74

The deceased was a paranoid schizophrenic who had been detained as an in-patient from where she absconded and committed suicide by throwing herself in front of a train. The proceedings were brought by her daughter who alleged that the Trust violated her right to life by allowing her to escape.

The House of Lords held that where there was a real and immediate risk of a patient committing suicide, Art 2 imposed an 'operational' obligation on the Trust to do all that was reasonably expected to prevent her from doing so. In referring to *Osman v United Kingdom* (1998) 29 EHRR 245 the court explained that this obligation was in addition to the health authorities' more general obligations. The operational obligation would apply where members of staff knew or ought to have known that a patient was a *real and immediate* risk of suicide. In these circumstances, Art 2 imposed an obligation to do all that is reasonably necessary to prevent the patient from committing suicide, and if they failed to do so would violate the operation obligation under Art 2 to help protect the patient's life.

However, the more recent case of *Rabone v Pennine Care NHS Trust* (2010) below reconsidered the extent to which unit providers are under an 'operational obligation' towards those who are at risk.

Rabone v Pennine Care NHS Trust [2010] EWCA 698

M had suffered from a depressive disorder and had been informally admitted to the defendant's hospital. She had suicidal and self-harm tendencies but she was allowed to return home for two days, during which time she committed suicide. Her parents claimed that the Trust had been negligent in allowing their daughter to return home. Further, they alleged that the Trust had acted in a way that was incompatible with Art 2.

The Trust accepted it had breached its common law duty of care by allowing her to leave the unit and settled damages in this respect. However, in relation to the claim under Art 2, the Trust maintained that as the deceased was a voluntary patient and was not detained under s 3, MHA 1983, the Trust did not have an operational obligation to her under Art 2. The Court of Appeal stated that there had to be some additional element over and above 'the real and immediate risk of death' before the operational obligation under Art 2 became effective. As the deceased was a voluntary patient, the Trust did not owe her the same operational obligation and the case failed in this respect.

3.22.2 The compatibility of s 2, MHA 1983 with Art 5

CASE EXAMPLE

MH v Secretary of State for Health [2005] UKHL 60

The patient who had Down's Syndrome had severe mental disabilities, and had been cared for at home by her mother. She was admitted to hospital under s 2, MHA 1983 for assessment when her behaviour became increasingly unpredictable, possibly in part as a result of her mother's ill-health. The grounds under which she was detained are set out above in s 2(2). Statute provides that a patient can be detained for 28 days (s 2 (4)) but can be discharged at an earlier time either by a medical professional or a relative. She could also by virtue of s 66(1) apply to the MHRT within 14 days of her admission to hospital, but no application was made. The hospital wished to make her 'received into guardianship' under s 7 so that the guardian, usually the local social services, could provide for her needs. Her mother objected. In circumstances where the relative objects, application must be made to court. Meanwhile, her detention was extended.

The crux of this case is that the patient who was unable to apply to the MHRT herself therefore became subject to court hearings and detention beyond the statutory 28-day period. The issue was whether this amounted to an infringement of her rights under Art 5(4), ECHR. This states:

ARTICLE

'Everyone who is deprived of his liberty by arrest or detention shall be entitled to take proceedings by which the lawfulness of his detention shall be decided speedily by a court and his release ordered if his detention is not lawful.'

It was argued that since she did not have the capacity to apply to the MHRT herself there was inadequate protection of her rights. Furthermore, she argued that s 29(4) was incompatible with Art 5(4) because her detention without review was unlawful. The unlawfulness arose from the fact that while a patient who was detained under s 3 would have a right of review, she did not.

The House of Lords held that s 2 was not incompatible with the provisions in Art 5(4) and does not need every case to be determined by a court. The patient should have the right to instigate proceedings, which becomes nonsensical if she does not possess the ability to do so.

The court continued by saying that the Convention exists to ensure rights are 'practical and effective' rather than 'theoretical and illusory'. However, despite this compelling argument, it did not follow that s 2 was incompatible with the convention or that the answer was to resort to court proceedings. The way forward was to help ensure that 'every sensible effort' should be made to help assist the patient to exercise her right if there was reason to consider she would wish to.

3.22.3 Article 3, ECHR and the MHA 1983

Article 3, framed as an unqualified right, states 'no-one shall be subjected to torture or to inhuman or degrading treatment or punishment'. The cases below illustrate the potential impact of Art 3 and circumstances that can amount to Art 3 being a qualified right.

CASE EXAMPLE

Herczegfalvy v Austria (1992) 15 EHRR 437

A Hungarian man living in Austria was transferred from prison to a psychiatric hospital when his physical condition worsened due to hunger striking. He was forcibly given drugs and food, was isolated and handcuffed to a security bed. He alleged violations of his human rights, among them Art 3 which prohibits inhumane or degrading treatment.

The ECHR opined that the very nature of patients in psychiatric hospitals, their 'inferiority and powerlessness' required increased vigilance when deciding whether the Convention had been complied with. There was no derogation from Art 3. However, there were cases, and this was just such one, where treatment which is 'therapeutic' in nature and can be justified as a medical necessity cannot be considered to be an infringement of Art 3. Given the facts here, there was no infringement of Art 3. Despite Art 3 being an unqualified right, it is apparent that therapeutic medical necessity effectively acts as a qualification of an unqualified right!

This case was applied more recently in the UK in the case of *R (Wilkinson) v Broadmoor Special Hospitals* [2001] EWCA Civ 1545, where the claimant had been detained for manslaughter under MHA 1983 at a secure hospital. He sought judicial review of the prison hospital's decision to treat him with anti-psychotic drugs despite his lack of consent, alleging that Art 3 had been breached. The court had little hesitation in concluding that having applied *Herczegfalvy,* his rights had not been violated.

CASE EXAMPLE

Keenan v UK (2001) 33 EHRR 38

The deceased was a prisoner with recognised mental health problems serving a relatively short sentence. Due to an incident in the prison he was sentenced to an additional 28 days within a matter of days prior to his release. He committed suicide the day after the sentence was handed down.

The European Court held that the timing and the manner of the additional sentence and the effect it would have on a mentally ill patient amounted to inhuman or degrading treatment. Article 3 had been violated. The prisoner's mental health had not been kept under close supervision and, given that seven days of the new sentence was to be in solitary confinement, this was highly unsatisfactory and showed a level of total disregard for prisoners with mental health problems.

Given that more than 70 per cent of the prison population has two or more mental disorders at any one time (Social Exclusion Unit (2004), quoting *Psychiatric Morbidity Among Prisoners in England and Wales 1998*), the effect of this decision is clear: there has to be a closer degree of care given to mentally ill patients who are detained in prisons.

CASE EXAMPLE

R (B) v Dr SS [2005] EWHC 86

Mr B was a prisoner serving a sentence for rape at Broadmoor Hospital, having been detained under ss 37 and 41, MHA 1983. He was appealing against a judgment where the lower court dismissed claims for judicial review which challenged a decision to impose medical treatment to which he did not consent. Applying the principles in *Herczegfalvy v Austria* (1992) the court accepted that the treatment can be considered to be a medical necessity for a non-competent person.

Interestingly enough, the general principles in *Herczegfalvy* have also been applied in cases where the complainant was not veven suffering from mental illness. In *Nevmerzhitsky v Ukraine* (2006) 43 EHRR 32, treatment against the patient's will was approved. The court held that:

JUDGMENT

'a measure which is of therapeutic necessity … cannot in principle be regarded as inhuman and degrading. The same can be said about force feeding that is aimed at saving the life of a particular detainee who consciously refuses to take food'.

Provided that the treatment can be proved to be a medical necessity, consent is not a prerequisite.

CASE EXAMPLE

R (PS) v (1) Responsible Medical Officer (Dr G) (2) Second Opinion Appointed Doctor (Dr W) [2003] EWHC 2335 (Admin)

The prisoner was detained under ss 37 and 41, MHA 1983 following a conviction for manslaughter on the grounds of diminished responsibility. He had capacity and alleged that his human rights under Arts 3 and 8 were being violated since he was to be given anti-psychotic drugs against his will.

The High Court held, after considering the principles in *Herczegfalvy*, that the level of severity of his treatment did not even engage Art 3 and therefore the court did not need to consider whether the treatment was a medical necessity. Furthermore, it was deemed to be in his best interests that he be treated with anti-psychotic drugs. Article 8 was not engaged as the interference was proportionate to achieve its aims.

It is interesting to note that although both prisoners in the above cases had capacity and therefore could make an autonomous decision, and in the ordinary course of events would be able to, the courts determined that in these cases capacity was not an overriding factor, just one of the factors to be taken into account.

Key facts on the effect of European human rights legislation

Case	Judgment
Winterwerp v The Netherlands (1979)	It is essential to establish that the person is of unsound mind which justifies detention, and must not be a disproportionate response to the patient's condition.
Savage v South Essex Partnership NHS Foundation Trust (2008)	An operational obligation was imposed on the Trust to do all that was reasonably necessary to prevent her suicide.
Rabone v Pennine Care NHS Trust (2010)	The patient was a voluntary patient and the Trust did not owe her the same operational obligation in order to prevent her from committing suicide.
MH v Secretary of State for Health (2005)	Art 5, ECHR had been violated as she was unable to apply for review to the MHRT.
Herczegfalvy v Austria (1992)	No infringement of Art 3. Although Art 3 is an unqualified right, therapeutic medical necessity acted as a qualification of Art 3.
Keenan v UK (2001)	The additional sentence added on just days prior to his release combined with the manner and nature of the sentence resulted in a violation of Art 3.
R (B) v De SS (2005)	Treatment can be considered a medical necessity and, if so, does not need the patient's consent.
Nevmerzhitsky v Ukraine (2006)	If treatment is a therapeutic necessity it cannot be regarded as inhuman and degrading.
R (PS) v Responsible Medical Officer (Dr G) Second Opinion Appointed Doctor (Dr W) (2003)	Art 3 was not engaged: it was therefore unnecessary to consider whether treatment was a necessity.

3.23 Discharge

Article 5, ECHR states that 'no one shall be deprived of his liberty'. As we saw in the criteria set down in *Winterwerp* (1979), a person can be detained further under the exceptions to Art 5(1)(e) and is dependent upon 'the persistence of such a disorder'. In order to ensure that there is some procedure to continued detention, Art 5(4) provides as follows:

ARTICLE

Everyone who is deprived of his liberty … By detention shall be entitled to take proceedings by which the lawfulness of his detention shall be decided speedily by a court and his release ordered if the detention is not lawful.

The violation of Art 5(4) has been tested through the use of the word 'speedily'. In *R (on the application of C) v Mental Health Review Tribunal* (1998) it was held that the listing of MHRT hearing some eight weeks after the applicant had applied for a hearing date was insufficiently speedy. While eight weeks in itself was not excessive, the practice of listing hearings with an eight-week date was one of mere convenience and it was incompatible with HRA 1998 not to provide an earlier date if one was requested.

The courts have also held in *R (on the application of H) v Ashworth Hospital Authority* [2002] All ER (D) 252 that even where the MRHT has authorised a patient's discharge, this can be delayed pending the hospital's application for judicial review of the MHRT's decision.

A patient can only be detained under s 2 for a period of 28 days. Under s 3, a patient can only be detained for a period of six months before a review must be made to the MHRT (s 68, MHA 1983).

Section 66, MHA 1983 provides that a patient who has been compulsorily detained under ss 2 or 3 has a right to apply to a MHRT to be discharged. The case of *R (on the application of H) v Secretary of State* [2005] UKHL 60 confirms that this is simply a patient's right, not an obligation on behalf of the hospital to bring every case before a MHRT.

Section 72, MHA 1983, places the burden on the tribunal to justify the reasons why the patient should not be discharged, and states that the patient should be discharged unless the following apply.

If he is detained under s 2 that:

SECTION

- 'he is suffering from mental disorder of a nature and degree which warrants his detention in a hospital for assessment for at least a limited period;
- or that his detention … is justified in the interests of his own health or safety or with a view to the protection of other persons;'

If he is detained under a section other than s 2, the patient shall be discharged unless the tribunal is satisfied that:

SECTION

- 'he is then suffering from mental disorder of a nature and degree which makes it appropriate for him to be liable to be detained in a hospital from medical treatment, or
- that it is necessary for the health or safety or the patient or for the protection of other persons that he should receive treatment, or
- that appropriate medical treatment is available for him'

or if the MHRT cannot satisfy the criteria for detention, the patient must be discharged and the MHRT must give reasons for its decision.

3.24 Conditional discharge

However, if a patient is subject to a conditional discharge and the conditions cannot be met so he is detained, his rights under HRA 1998 will not be breached.

CASE EXAMPLE

R v Secretary of State for the Home Department ex parte IH [2003] *3 WLR 1278.*

The patient was detained at Rampton Hospital under ss 37 and 41, MHA 1983 for severely mutilating his three-year-old son. Although the patient was considered to be no longer suffering from mental disorder so that he needed to be detained, his discharge was conditional on psychiatric supervision. The health authority attempted to comply with the conditions set down but was unable to do so. He therefore remained detained and argued that the continuing detention was unlawful and breached Art 5.

The House of Lords held that every attempt had been made by the health authority to meet the conditions of his discharge, but they were unable to. The court chose to distinguish *Johnson v UK* (1997) 27 EHRR. Here, the applicant had assaulted a woman and was detained in a psychiatric institution. He suffered from schizophrenia but also had a psychopathic personality. A time came when he was considered suitable for rehabilitation but not quite ready for a discharge. Strenuous but unsuccessful efforts were made to secure hostel accommodation. He could not be released and he argued that his continued detention violated his rights under Art 5. The Tribunal had no power to ensure that the condition was met within a specified period of time and there was no provision for judicial review of this decision.

The European Court of Human Rights held that while it was responsible to exercise an element of discretion when deciding whether it was appropriate to order the immediate discharge of this particular patient, the excessive delay which had led to the 'indefinite deferral of the applicant's release' and the lack of adequate safeguards to ensure that the patient's release would not be unreasonably delayed meant that the continued detention violated Art 5(1)(e), ECHR.

3.25 Community care

Section 117(2), MHA 1983 provides a duty on the primary health care trusts (PCTs) or the local social services to provide the patient who has been released with after-care services in conjunction with relevant voluntary agencies until such time that the services are no longer required.

In *Clunis v Camden and Islington Health Authority* [1998] QB 978 the claimant had been an in-patient detained under s 3, MHA 1983. It was planned that he was to receive after-care services under s 117, MHA 1983 in the community. While in the community, he stabbed a stranger. He was convicted of manslaughter on the grounds of diminished responsibility but then brought a claim against his local authority. He alleged negligence in that the health authority had breached their statutory obligations towards him under s 117. However, the local authority could not, despite their considerable efforts, find a psychiatrist to supervise him. The court held that there was no cause of action for the health authority to answer. Apart from rejecting the argument that anyone apart from the defendant should be responsible for his own criminal act, the court held that the health authority's statutory obligations did not give rise to an 'absolute obligation' on the part of the local authority.

CASE EXAMPLE

K v Central and North West London Mental Health NHS Trust [2008] EWHC 1217 (QB)

The patient sought to have his claim reinstated after it was struck out. The patient alleged that the local authority was negligent in failing to provide after-care in accordance with the statutory duty under s 117, MHA 1983. The patient was suffering from paranoid schizophrenia among other mental disorders, and was an in-patient in a psychiatric unit. The local authority undertook to care for him in the community, but while he was in accommodation provided by the local authority, he jumped from a second storey building and suffered significant injuries. He claimed in personal injury and alleged that his human rights under Arts 2, 3 and 8 had been violated. The question was whether or not there was a right of action for breach of after-care obligations.

The court held that there was a far closer relationship than in *Clunis v Camden and Islington Health Authority* (1998), and this case should no longer be regarded as the definitive decision in determining whether a duty of care existed. King J stated:

JUDGMENT

'*Clunis* [is] no longer to be regarded as a definitive ruling on the question of a common law duty of care in the context of s 117 functions.'

Of course, the court emphasised that the case was still fraught with difficulties, but that this was not a case that was automatically doomed to failure.

KEY FACTS

Key facts on cases of discharge

Case	Judgment
R v Secretary of State for the Home Department ex parte IH (2003)	The patient's release was unreasonably delayed as there was a lack of safeguards to ensure a speedy discharge. Violation of Art 5.
Clunis v Camden and Islington Health Authority (1998)	Section 117 did not impose an absolute obligation on the health authority. They could not be held liable for any failure to receive after-care.
K v Central and North West London Mental Health NHS Trust (2008)	This judgment is now deemed to be the definitive judgment on the application of s 117. There was a far closer proximity of relationship than in *Clunis*, and the court was wrong to strike out the claim.

ACTIVITY

Self-test questions

Ensure that your answers are supported by case law where appropriate.

* Explain the significance of the seminal case of *Bournewood* (1998).
* What is a deprivation of liberty order?
* Illustrate the above with case law.
* How has HRA 1998 affected mental health law?

SUMMARY

- This chapter provided an overview of mental health law.
- The Mental Health Act (MHA) 2007 applies where the patient has capacity to consent to treatment but refuses to consent to appropriate mental health treatment. The aim of the Act is to enable a person who suffers from a mental disorder or disability of the mind to be treated, regardless of their consent.
- Sections 2 and 3 allow a patient to be treated where he or she is suffering from a mental disorder of a nature of degree which warrants detention for assessment, and it is in the interests of the health and safety of the patient or the protection of others. Section 3 allows the patient to be detained for a longer period. Urgent detentions are contained within s 4.

- Case law has already demonstrated the considerable judicial interpretation since the enactment of MHA 2007, with occasionally a wider interpretation than was perhaps originally envisaged.
- The complexity of some statutory provisions is illustrated by s 131, MHA 1983 where the law was severely tested in the case of *Bournewood* (1998), as a result of which further legislative amendments were made.
- Mental health law remains both an extensive and highly complex arca of law. Most importantly, it is a vitally important area of medical law affecting thousands of patients every year. It is hoped that this snapshot will entice the reader to enquire further.

Further reading

Dolan, B. and Parker, C. (1997) 'Caesarean Sections: A treatment for mental disorder? *Tameside and Glossop Acute Services Unit v CH (a patient)* (1996) 1 FLR 762', *British Medical Journal*, 7088, page 314.

Fennell, P. (1998) 'Doctor Knows Best? Therapeutic Detention under Common Law, the Mental Health Act and the European Convention', *Medical Law Review*, 6, 322.

Fennell P, (2007) *Mental Health: The New Law*. Bristol: Jordans.

4

Resource allocation

AIMS AND OBJECTIVES

After reading this chapter you should be able to:

■ Appreciate the significance of resource allocation on the National Health Service (NHS)
■ Understand the ethical considerations of resource allocation
■ Appreciate the statutory provisions' relation to the NHS
■ Understand the judicial approach towards cases of judicial review
■ Appreciate the relevance of the exceptionality criteria
■ Understand the application of the Human Rights Act (HRA) 1998
■ Be able to apply the law and ethics to a hypothetical scenario.

4.1 Introduction

The study of resource allocation involves a consideration of how and why rationing of drugs and/or services occur. Here, we are concerned with both ethical and legal considerations. We will consider the effectiveness of the process of judicial review together with the exceptionality criteria, and conclude by assessing whether the only avenue available to aggrieved patients is adequate for their purpose.

Sir Thomas Bingham MR stated in *R v Cambridge Health Authority, ex parte B* [1995] 1 WLR 898:

JUDGMENT

'I have no doubt that in a perfect world any treatment which a patient … sought would be provided if doctors were willing to give it, no matter how much it cost, particularly when a life was potentially at stake. It would however, in my view, be shutting one's eyes to the real world if the court were to proceed on the basis that we do live in such a world. It is common knowledge that health authorities of all kinds are constantly pressed to make ends meet.'

Unfortunately, the quote above accurately reflects the harsh reality of this subject area. In an ideal world, a perfect utopia, this topic would not exist. However, resource allocation or rationing (as it is more plainly called) is a real and distressing problem. There is simply insufficient money to finance every patient's medical needs, so some patients cannot be prescribed drugs, even if there is every clinical indication that it would benefit their health.

According to *UK Public Spending*, estimated figures for healthcare spending in the fiscal year 2010 amounted to £119.8 billion, a significant 17.91 per cent of total government spending and far in excess of public spending on education, housing or defence. If public spending was increased to reflect the needs of the population in terms of healthcare then this would be the ideal scenario, but it is also unrealistic. The reasons are twofold:

1. The extra money has to have a recognisable source, and what is given with one hand is very often taken with the other. It would be likely that another public sector's budget would be adversely affected if additional money were to be diverted to healthcare.
2. How do we define a 'healthcare need'? Does this and should this include cosmetic surgery? Some may consider cosmetic surgery to be simply vanity while others might maintain that the need for cosmetic surgery amounts to a medical condition.

In a continuing climate of finite resources, there is a painful inevitability that not all patients will get the treatment they want or need all of the time. In terms of basic micro economic principles: human want is infinite; resources are finite. Just before we embark upon this topic, it is essential to remember when studying this area that rationing refers to a situation in which a patient is refused a drug due to lack of available funds, not because it is deemed to be clinically ineffective.

Decisions on the size of the NHS budget are made by central government who also have to take into account other public sector services such as education or transport. It has to be remembered that the government of the day may not only have specific political priorities and goals they wish to achieve, but they may also be constrained by deficits from previous government overspending. For any political party, it would be an unpopular policy to cut the NHS budget as the NHS has an immediate, all-encompassing effect. While some people may have the luxury of private health insurance, almost all of us rely at some time or another on the valuable service provided by GPs free of charge. Those from significantly working class backgrounds and socially deprived areas tend to rely more heavily on the services than those in the middle classes, and the NHS must be able to meet those needs. Importantly, the scarce resources of the NHS that are available should be distributed equally and fairly among all, so that the basic principles of the NHS are satisfied (see below).

Within the NHS, there are competing demands for finance, as consideration needs to be given to the different bodies within the NHS and how the available money is to be allocated. Should more money be allocated to expensive cancer screening equipment, which from a purely financial view may save valuable resources in the long term, or should more money be allocated to local services provided by GPs?

4.2 The National Health Service Constitution

Since its inception, the NHS has always been free to the general population. It 'belongs to the people' and according to its Constitution:

QUOTATION

'it exists to improve our health and wellbeing, supporting us to keep mentally and physically well, to get better when we are ill and when we cannot recover, to stay as well as we can to the end of our lives'.

The principles underlying the NHS are set out its Constitution, last reviewed and updated in 2009. The Constitution sets out the following guiding seven principles:

1. The NHS provides a comprehensive service, available to all irrespective of gender, race, disability, age or sexual orientation.
2. Access to NHS services is based on clinical need, not an individual's ability to pay.
3. The NHS aspires to the highest standards of excellence and professionalism.
4. NHS services must reflect the needs and preferences of patients, their families and their carers.

5. The NHS works across organisational boundaries and in partnership with other organisations in the interest of patients, local communities and the wider population.
6. The NHS is committed to providing best value for taxpayers' money and the most effective, fair and sustainable use of finite resources.
7. The NHS is accountable to the public, communities and patients that it serves.

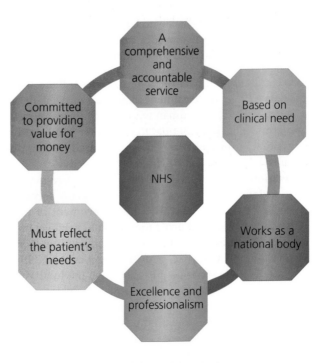

Figure 4.1 The principles of the NHS Constitution

The Constitution still reflects the values prevalent when the NHS was first established as part of the new visionary Welfare State in 1948. While the vision and the ethos may not have changed significantly, the society which this quite extraordinary institution serves has changed beyond recognition.

In 1960, the average life expectancy of the population according to the World Bank, World Development Indicators 2010 was 71.1 years. In 2010 the average life expectancy is 79.9 years. While this is a positive and pleasing trend, the increasingly ageing population places an increasing burden on the NHS which, according to the Office of National Statistics, serves a population in excess of 62 million people.

The NHS Constitution sets out what rights we as patients have. Furthermore, the Constitution contains pledges or commitments which, while not legally enforceable *per se*, are described as being above and beyond legal rights as they are described in terms of commitments between the NHS and the patient. The rights are lengthy, but a few of them are listed below. UK citizens have the right to:

▨ receive NHS services free of charge
▨ access NHS services
▨ expect their local NHS to assess the health requirements of the local community and to commission and put in place the services to meet those needs as considered necessary
▨ not be unlawfully discriminated against in the provision of NHS services including on grounds of gender, race, religion or belief, sexual orientation, disability (including learning disability or mental illness) or age.

One of the more relevant rights to the topic of resource allocation is phrased as follows:

QUOTATION

'You have the right to drugs and treatments that have been recommended by NICE for use in the NHS, if your doctor says they are clinically appropriate for you.'

This right also explains that the National Institute for Health and Clinical Excellence (NICE) is an independent NHS organisation which is responsible for producing guidance on drugs and treatments. The use of the word 'recommended' means recommended by a NICE technology appraisal.

QUOTATION

'You have the right to expect local decisions on funding of other drugs and treatments to be made rationally following a proper consideration of the evidence. If the local NHS decides not to fund a drug or treatment you and your doctor feel would be right for you, they will explain that decision to you.'

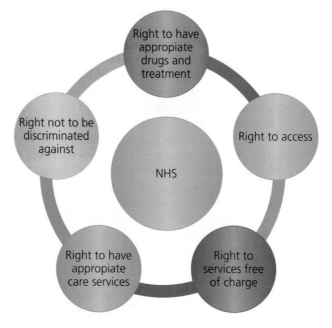

Figure 4.2 The rights of UK citizens within the NHS Constitution

Are the rights enforceable?

Section 2 of the Health Act 2009 states that bodies that are listed in section 2(2) must, in performing its NHS functions, 'have regard to the NHS Constitution'.

The bodies in s 2(2) are:

a. Strategic health authorities
b. Primary care trusts
c. NHS Trusts
d. Special health authorities
e. NHS Foundation Trusts
f. The Independent Regulator of NHS Foundation Trusts
g. The Care Quality Commission.

The term 'have regard' is without definition. It could mean that bodies need to do all that is reasonable to take into account the principles when performing their NHS functions, but the *extent* to which they are obliged to do so is yet to be defined. Undoubtedly, courts will have to take the principles of the NHS constitution into account when considering any claim a patient may have, but they do not appear to be sufficiently enforceable for a patient to rely on them as an adequate means of redress.

4.3 The role of the National Institute for Health and Clinical Excellence (NICE)

Health Secretary Frank Dobson assured the public in 1998 that access to healthcare would be accessible to all, regardless of their sex, income or ethnicity. Moreover, healthcare would be accessible regardless of where a person lived, undertaking that postcode lotteries would be a thing of the past. While the reality may be that there is insufficient money to fund every person's treatment, there was a recognition that decisions on funding could no longer be made according to where a patient lived. It was regarded as a failing of the provision of healthcare that a patient living on one street could receive funding, but if another patient lived a mile down the road and hence in a different county or borough, that funding may be refused.

Largely as a direct result of the government's desire to avoid this postcode lottery, NICE was set up in April 1999 as a special health authority with the responsibility of providing guidance on care and treatment for patients living in England and Wales. Its objective was to ensure that all patients had equal access to medical care and treatment regardless of where they lived. Part of their remit was to make allocation of resources more transparent in order to avoid the 'postcode lottery' issues of previous years and relieve the political pressure on government from potentially sensitive political decisions. Realistically, all the government was doing was setting up an organisation without any powers of enforcement, to carry out the most unpopular, but unavoidable, allocation of resources.

However, the role of NICE is extensive, and despite the impression given by frequent media reports, its role is not limited to whether new drugs should be granted to patients following an economic–health analysis (Clinical Guidelines). NICE also considers the use of new technologies in order to be able to advise medical professionals on new treatments which may benefit their patients (Technology Appraisals) and also assesses whether procedures are sufficiently safe. This role of 'Interventional Procedures' was added to NICE's role after the Kennedy Report following the Bristol Royal Infirmary Enquiry in 2001.

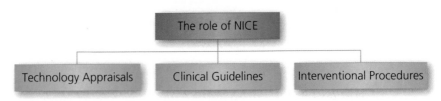

Figure 4.3 The role of NICE

Our focus, however, is with allocation of resources rather than the other roles which NICE undertakes. Since 1999 when NICE was first established, there have been regular media reports in which NICE has still been accused of rationing of resources.

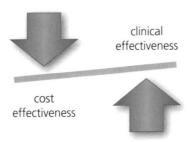

Figure 4.4 NICE's balance between cost and clinical effectiveness

Examples

1. Headlines such as 'Bowel cancer patients must do without life-extending drugs, says Nice' (*The Guardian*, 12 November 2010) have continued to damage the reputation of NICE. Here, it was reported that a drug, commonly known as Avastin, which can typically give a patient another six weeks of life, was denied to patients. The drug which was estimated to cost £21,000 per patient and could benefit approximately 6,500 patients in the UK, was considered to be too high a cost when balanced against the potential benefit.

2. 'Hundreds of liver patients denied drug lifeline' (*The Daily Mail*, 26 May 2010) presents a further example where NICE refused an appeal to approve the use of a cancer drug Nexaver, despite compelling evidence that it can double life expectancy. Statistics showed that it provided patients with a further 2.8 extra months of life but cost £27,000 per patient. NICE refused to fund the drug on the basis of its lack of economic viability.

In 2008 NICE on at least six occasions refused cancer drugs on the grounds that the cost was too high based upon a Quality-Adjusted Life Year (QALY) assessment (see page 119). Changes were then announced which allowed patients to purchase drugs privately without being deprived of healthcare on the NHS. Payment for drugs acts entirely contrary to the principles of the NHS which unequivocally express the right of access to free healthcare to all, together with the right to have appropriate access to drugs and treatment if a clinician recommends it is in the interests of the patient to receive them. Since we can ascertain that NICE is not achieving its aims and objectives in terms of allocation of resources, what steps can be taken to remedy this significant failing? The Labour Government was politically unable to make any significant changes as NICE was the brainchild of Prime Minister Tony Blair's Labour Government, and any detailed review could be regarded as a political failure.

4.4 The future of the National Health Service: A new Cancer Fund?

As a result of a change of government in 2010, the new Conservative–Liberal Democrat Coalition sought to address the inequality of access to both drugs and treatment for cancer. According to statistics produced by the Department of Health's consultation document, *The Cancer Drugs Fund*, October 2010, in 2007 245,300 people in the UK were diagnosed with cancer resulting in 127,800 deaths.

In a report entitled *Extent and causes of international variations in drugs usage*, July 2010, produced for the Secretary of State, statistics revealed that the UK has a relatively low rate of approving use of drugs when compared with a number of EU counties, New Zealand, the USA and Australia. The UK ranked particularly low among cancer drugs launched in the past five years, and those launched more than ten years ago. Not exclusive to the allocation of cancer drugs, this study also suggested that drugs for multiple sclerosis and other conditions were also prescribed far less in the UK than in other countries. As always, statistics should be treated cautiously, as these figures do not necessarily take into account whether there were clinical indications for these drugs to be prescribed. However, as an overall observation, the UK's allocation of drugs and in particular cancer drugs, is considerably lower than other countries, and the government has sought to redress this balance.

The Cancer Drugs Fund is proposed to be an interim measure with a lifespan of three years until a new value-based approach towards allocation of resources to medicines is established. The government has pledged £50 million to date and a further £200 million per year until the end of the fund's lifespan. This will not take place until the end of the Pharmaceutical Price Regulation Scheme in 2013.

The Cancer Drugs Fund's aim is to transfer the power from an organisation to clinicians at a grass roots level who can take decisions about a patient's treatment in consultation with them, as both patients and clinicians are at the core of the decision-making process. It will provide clinicians with greater flexibility to decide whether a particular treatment or drug is in the best interests of a patient. The Cancer Drug Fund is intended to give patients greater access to drugs which would not otherwise be available on the NHS. This will include access to drugs not yet approved by NICE, together with those drugs which are approved but not recommended on the basis of their cost-effectiveness. There are concerns of insufficient money in the fund to provide all the treatment required, while other critics identify many other diseases that are in desperate need of additional funding.

The consultation document explains that strategic health authorities will be abolished once the new NHS Commissioning Board is established from April 2012 and, once the Cancer Drugs Fund comes to an end, it will be evolved into the new-style NHS.

 ## 4.5 The future of the NHS: The Health and Social Care Bill 2011

The White Paper 'Equity and Excellence – Liberating the NHS' was presented to Parliament in July 2010, and the Health and Social Care Bill was introduced to Parliament in January 2011.

The White Paper's aim is to provide an NHS with a

CLAUSE

'coherent, stable and enduring framework for quality and service improvement. The debate on health should no longer be about structures and processes but about priorities and progress in health improvement for all'.

It is intended that the new NHS will be 'a more responsive, patient-centred NHS'. It is the government's intention to develop a more cost-effective NHS and while it has announced that spending will not be cut in real terms, the aim is to cut management costs by more than 45 per cent in four years.

According to the Department of Health, the Bill contains provisions covering five main themes:

- strengthening commissioning of NHS services
- increasing democratic accountability and public voice
- liberating provision of NHS services
- strengthening public health services
- reforming health and care arm's-length bodies.

It is proposed that the NHS be reorganised into a body that provides not only fairness but excellence. The White Paper pledges to increase health spending, put patients first and create one of the best health services in the world. With its emphasis on an equal service provided to all, its intention is to allow patients more freedom of choice: a choice of GP, healthcare provider, hospital and team. It will allow patients to rate their hospital according to their experience.

Its aim is to encourage a culture of openness and transparency with patient safety a priority. Its long-term vision is to be accomplished by:

CLAUSE

- 'Putting patients and the public first
- Focusing on improvement in quality and healthcare outcomes
- Autonomy, accountability and democratic legitimacy and
- Cutting bureaucracy and increasing efficiency'.

4.5.1 The issues of GPs and resource allocation

At the local level, it is problematic for GPs alone to make decisions about where best to allocate funds. Arguably, it should not be the doctor's role to consider rationing, as his first priority is the care of his patient not the competing interests of allocation of resources. There is a natural conflict between the doctor serving his patient and the need to consider where best to place available funds as what is given with one hand must be taken from another. At the risk of potential litigation, the reality is that doctors can be put in the invidious position of telling a patient that treatment exists but there are no available funds.

This acknowledgment is demonstrated in *R v North Derbyshire HA, ex parte Fisher* [1997] 8 Med LR 327 where Dyson J observed:

JUDGMENT

'when deciding whether to prescribe treatment to a patient, a clinician has to have regard to many factors, including the resources available for that treatment and the needs of a likely benefit to that patient, as compared with other patients who are likely to be suitable for that treatment during the financial year'.

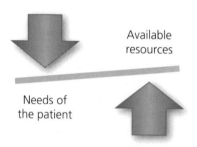

Available
resources

Needs of
the patient

Figure 4.5 The GPs' balancing act

With particular reference to 'Autonomy, accountability and democratic legitimacy', the government initially proposed to shift the balance of power from politicians to a GPs' Consortia. In order to simplify NHS organisations, the role of the primary care trusts (PCTs) and strategic health authorities would be replaced by 300–500 GPs' Consortia which would be empowered among other roles with the allocation of resources. It was suggested that the GPs' Consortia would take full financial responsibility by 2013.

It was envisaged that a GP's practice would be a member of a Consortium and then GPs' practices would have flexibility within that arrangement to form consortia in a way which they feel would benefit their local patients and their specific community. The GPs' Consortium would be given statutory powers in the new Health and Social Care Bill and would be responsible for purchasing health services for their patients. It is thought that the GP, being on the frontline of services provided to patients, would be better placed to evaluate what services are required. The GPs' Consortium would be the responsibility of the new NHS Commissioning Board who would calculate practice level budgets and then allocate them to the Consortia. It would be up to the consortia to determine where funds will be allocated and in partnership with whom.

The NHS Commissioning Board would be assisted with the transition by the strategic health authorities. The NHS Commissioning Board would have five distinct roles:

- providing national leadership on commissioning for quality improvement
- promoting and extending public and patient involvement and choice
- ensuring the development of GPs' Commissioning Consortia

- commissioning certain services that cannot solely be commissioned by Consortia, for example GPs, dentistry, community pharmacy and primary ophthalmic services, national specialised services and maternity services
- allocation and accounting for NHS resources.

One criticism of the NHS in the White Paper is that the NHS is not only bureaucratic but also that management costs are too high; there is therefore a clear commitment to reducing management costs significantly. However, it is also recognised that there would be significant costs, albeit one-off costs in establishing the new framework of the NHS. The new framework would be extremely costly; it is estimated that the removal of the PCTs and the strategic health authorities and their replacement with up to 500 GPs' Consortia will cost approximately £2–3 billion (Walshe, K. (2010) 'Reorganisation of the NHS in England', *British Medical Journal*, 341).

A criticism highlighted by Whitehead, Hanratty and Popay relates to the structure and purpose of the reorganisation itself (*The Lancet*, Vol. 376, Issue 9750, pages 1373–5). It is argued that the White Paper seeks to move the focus from 'population-based responsibility', which was the focus of the PCTs, to more localised responsibility. GPs' Consortia would be responsible for those registered patients (and only those who are registered) within their individual locality. Thus, the reforms seem to be replacing a far-sighted nationwide vision of healthcare with a more fragmented local picture. While it is expected that those who provide healthcare services on a local basis are those who can meet local needs, there is the concern that 'proper distribution of services will be lost'. Where services are allocated to private contractors, the fear is that the new proposals could in fact create the opposite of what they seek to achieve and create a two-tier system of health provision.

At this point in discussion we need to mention the NHS Future Forum. It was introduced as part of a government exercise and was an independent group to 'pause, listen and reflect' on the provisions on the Health and Social Care Bill in the light of unprecedented opposition. In reality, the forum acted as a break in the legislative process while an attempt was made to address significant and numerous concerns about the Bill. The forum gained a considerable amount of valuable views, and as a result made a number of recommendations to government in June 2011 which were subsequently adopted as amendments to the Bill. The amendments include:

- varying the pace of change
- ensuring that ultimate responsibility lies with the Secretary of State
- local decisions regarding commissioning of care will not just be made by GPs but by nurses, specialist doctors and other clinicians (therefore it appears unlikely that GPs will be solely responsible for resource allocation)
- competition should not be used as a means to an end but to increase patients' choice and allow them greater choice
- the focus on promoting competition should be removed and motivation behind the need for change should be the patient's power or right to challenge the provision of healthcare.

(Department of Health, Modernisation of Health and Care, 2011)

The concept is, however, that patients will be empowered and emboldened. They will have greater choice and access to more information, and it is believed this will make GPs more accountable as they, together with other health service providers, will have to be more directly responsive to the needs of the local community. One of the government's stated aims is that those providing services will be under a duty to ensure that any inequality in the provision of healthcare is reduced.

Doubtless, the reforms are supposedly well intentioned and, in principle, putting patients first is highly commendable. Critics suggest that an entire overhaul of the NHS is simply not needed and that the proposed reforms, which will be costly in themselves, may introduce unhealthy competition for a fundamental right to healthcare.

We can only wait and see whether the Health and Social Care Bill is deeply flawed and requires to be resigned to the draftsman's drawer, or whether this Bill, struggling in its embryonic form, reaches maturity and seeks to deliver an NHS fit for the twenty-first century.

ACTIVITY

Self-test questions

Please ensure that your answers are supported by case law where appropriate.

- What is rationing?
- Why does it exist?
- Are the rights contained in the NHS Constitution enforceable?
- Explain the role of the National Institute of Clinical Excellence.
- Do the proposed reforms in the Health and Social Care Bill appear encouraging for the future of the NHS? You may wish to do some independent up-to-date research in order to address this question.

4.6 Ethical considerations

4.6.1 Introduction

We have established thus far that there exists a limited pool of healthcare resources, whether this limitation is defined in staff, facilities, operating theatres or drugs. One must consider how these complex and difficult decisions are made and who should receive these limited funds.

Discussion point

Patient A and Patient B are both suffering from the same condition and both require the same drugs in order to help cure their condition. Without treatment they will die. How do we decide whether Patient A or Patient B receives the drugs? Patient A is a young man with no dependants; he is unemployed, often abuses drugs and is a petty criminal. He does however care for his ailing and elderly parents. Patient B is married with three young children and is a renowned heart surgeon. Only one of these patients can be treated. Which one?

If we are very honest with ourselves, our automatic response may be to consider Patient B; after all, he appears to have the most to lose and therefore by definition the greatest need, and there are many who are dependent on him both personally and professionally. The problem with this is that it does not produce a fair and just result and appears to be based on a social class analysis more than any equitable assessment. Maybe what we are asking is, who has the greatest *right* to treatment, patient A or patient B? However, if we adopt a rights-based approach, how are these rights to be balanced? All patients have a right to medical treatment, and given that both patients are in similar position, no one patient has a particular right over the other.

In other words, even in this most simplistic of examples, there are no simple solutions. Therefore, it is necessary to apply a more mathematical and sophisticated approach to this very real problem.

4.6.2 The Quality-Adjusted Life Year (QALY)

The Quality-Adjusted Life Year (QALY) is used as a means of calculating the cost-effectiveness of a medical procedure. This method is perhaps the most often applied means of calculating healthcare rationing. The QALY calculates not only the quantity of additional life as a result of any healthcare given, but also the quality of life.

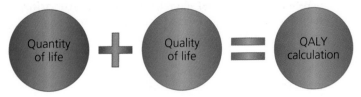

Figure 4.6 Calculating the QALY

A healthcare activity which can be considered as high priority is one where the cost per QALY is as low as possible. This explanation below of QALY is given by Alan Williams ('The Value of QALYs', *Health and Social Services Journal*, July 1985, 3):

QUOTATION

'The essence of a QALY is that it takes a year of healthy life expectancy to be worth 1, but regards a year of unhealthy life expectancy as worth less than 1. Its precise value is lower the worse the quality of life of the unhealthy person (which is what the 'quality adjusted' bit is all about). If being dead is worth zero, it is, in principle, possible for a QALY to be negative, that is, for the quality of someone's life to be judged worse than being dead.'

Steps to calculation

■ Assess the quality of life before and after treatment: 0 = deceased and 1 = full health.
■ Calculate the patient's life expectancy before and after treatment.
■ Multiply the above life expectancy with the quality of life score.
■ Deduct these two figures. The result is the QALY score.

Example

Patient C has a life expectancy of 1 year *without* treatment with a quality of life of 0.5. The QALY score is 0.5. *With* treatment she has a life expectancy of ten years with a quality of life of 0.9. The QALY score is 9. The value of her treatment in terms of QALY is 8.5. The cost of her treatment is £2,000. The QALY is 8.5; therefore the cost per QALY is £235.29.

We are saying that this particular treatment in terms of QALY is £235.29.

Commentary

Now it can be seen how a cost can be applied to treatment A; QALYs for different treatments can be compared in order to ascertain the most cost-effective forms of treatment. The economic value is that each medical treatment can be valued and funds allocated. The economic reality is that each QALY is metaphorically stretched in order that as much is achieved from each QALY as possible.

The advantage of QALY-operated resource allocation is that funds are distributed on a utilitarian style approach with distribution of funds based upon what is the best possible result for society as a whole, which is the greatest happiness for the greatest number of people. The reasoning is that the QALY approach maximises the greatest good for the greatest number of people.

The difficulty with the QALY approach is that it ignores the notion of fairness as it fails to take into account the individual needs of each particular patient. However, if *we* were asked who *we* felt had the greater need, one patient who needed life-saving drug treatment or 100 or even 1,000 patients requiring a much cheaper health provision such as cholesterol testing or blood pressure monitoring, it would be likely that we would opt for the patient whose need was immediately the greatest.

Frequent stories reach the tabloid and broadsheet newspapers, highlighting situations in which NICE has refused to fund drug treatment. Look back to page 115, *The Guardian* story about the bowel cancer drug, Avastin. This drug is an expensive proposition for NICE. In applying a 'cost versus benefit' exercise, NICE considered that it was not sufficiently cost-effective to fund treatment. Their refusal to fund Avastin to patients who could receive an increased life expectancy (albeit limited) creates injustice that is difficult to accept. The UK is one of the few developed countries that does not prescribe Avastin, and refusals of this kind do a disservice to the reputation of the NHS.

This story demonstrates consequentialism in practice; there are limited resources, and in order to achieve a potential of maximum benefit to the maximum number of people there will invariably be difficult decisions to make. Arguably, an application of utilitarian principles denies justice and creates unfairness.

4.6.3 Criticisms of the QALY approach

QALYs appear to be discriminatory in nature as the elderly (or disabled) patient who invariably has the lowest life expectancy and consequently the lower QALY score makes allocation of resources less economically attractive. Patients such as these are being treated with less value – not as people, but as economic commodities.

The lack of economic viability in treating patients such as these is emphasised by John Harris (1987) as he states that the 'ageism of QALY is inescapable' and explains how it would be considered more QALY-efficient to channel funds away from areas such as geriatric medicine and terminal care and towards neonatal care and paediatrics. On the other hand, there are those who argue that QALYs are not ageist as it is not the age of the patient that is being taken into account but their life expectancy. This argument has some merit as a person aged 80 who has treatment and is given a life expectancy of five years is considered the same in terms of QALY as the patient who is 20 and following treatment is given the same life expectancy.

Inequality

If the life expectancy of two patients is the same, they should be treated equally regardless of age or disability. If a person with disabilities has the same life expectancy as a person without disabilities, and the priority is to treat the latter, what does that say about the person with disabilities? It suggests that that person's life has less value: a concept extrinsically wrong.

One might argue that the nature of life reflects inequality itself. Regardless of specific illness, life expectancy in the UK is higher in more affluent areas and lower in the most deprived areas, and hospital waiting lists vary significantly throughout the country. The same is reflected outside the health system. The worst performing schools are by no coincidence in the poorest areas of the country, which arguably are the areas that deserve better education to help raise the next generation out of poverty. However, this too is simplistic as inequality runs deeper, as reflected in difficulties experienced by religion, race and gender.

Social value and age

One might consider whether age or a person's value to society should be considered when allocating resources. On page 119 we thought about Patient A and Patient B. Superficially, Patient B can offer more to society and could be treated in preference to Patient A, but what does this say about our society if we judge people in this way? If we were to adopt this approach, the discrimination would be immeasurable. NICE states:

QUOTATION

'NICE should not recommend interventions on the basis of individuals' income, social class or position in life. Nor should individuals' social roles at different ages affect decisions about cost effectiveness'.

(Social Value Judgments: Principles for the Development of NICE Guidance, 2008)

As far as age is concerned, NICE states that patients should neither be denied nor restricted treatment because of their age. The elderly patient should be treated the same as the young patient where their life expectancy and quality of life is the same. However, age can be taken into account where:

QUOTATION

'There is evidence that age is a good indicator for some aspects of patients' health status and/or the likelihood of adverse effects of the treatment.

There is no practical way of identifying patients other than by their age (for example, there is no test available to measure their state of health in another way).

There is good evidence, or good grounds for believing, that because of their age patients will respond differently to the treatment in question.' (2008)

Patient's behaviour

Earlier we looked at Patient A, a person who often abused drugs. How far should we hold patients responsible for their own condition? Should we allow an obese patient life-saving surgery when a sensible diet and exercise could have saved the NHS thousands of pounds, or a smoker treatment for lung cancer? Naturally, we may feel less inclined towards patients who have positively contributed to their ill-health rather than patients who are not authors of their own misfortune but innocent and unlucky bystanders. The NHS Constitution refers to 'rights'. Arguably with the privilege of rights comes obligations and we, as patients, have obligations. Indeed, the NHS Constitution states that in order that resources are used responsibly:

QUOTATION

'You should recognise that you can make a significant contribution to your own, and your family's, good health and wellbeing, and take some personal responsibility for it'.

While a patient's actions and lifestyle are not deemed to be relevant to whether they do receive treatment, it can be relevant to the effectiveness any treatment may have (see below). This in turn will have a bearing on any allocation of resources.

NICE avoids guidance that results in care being denied to patients with conditions that are, or may have been, dependent on their behaviour. However, if the behaviour is likely to continue and can make a treatment less clinically effective or cost-effective, then it is appropriate to take this into account.

Patient autonomy

When considering how to allocate resources either for patients with specific conditions or for the benefit of the entire community, the hallowed principle of patient autonomy is problematic. There is a clear conflict between an individual's choice regarding his or her treatment and allocating resources. Is a patient at liberty to ask or even demand a more expensive drug, and how is this to be measured against other patients' needs? A patient cannot demand specific treatment, as we have already mentioned in Chapter 2 in the case of *R (on the application of Burke) v General Medical Council* (2005), although in this case the issue was about specific life-prolonging treatment. Allocation of resources is often not far from the court's mind. In the case of *Re J (A Minor) Medical Treatment* [1992] 2 FCR 753, a sad case solely about the withdrawal of medical treatment from a severely sick child, Lord Donaldson made the following observation:

'the sad fact of life that health authorities may on occasion find that they have too few resources, either human or material or both, to treat all the patients whom they would like to treat in the way in which they would like to treat them. It is then their duty to make choices … I would also stress the absolute undesirability of the court making an order which may have the effect of compelling a doctor or health authority to make available scarce resources (both human and material) to a particular child, without knowing whether or not there are other patients to whom those resources might more advantageously be devoted.'

It is important to appreciate that this particular case was not about the allocation of resources but about whether continuing treatment was in a child's best interests. However, the observations of the court make one appreciate that where resources are limited, medical professionals may have to consider where those resources are best placed.

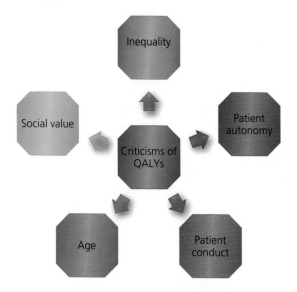

Figure 4.7 Criticisms of QALYs

Summary: ethical considerations

- Resources in the NHS are limited, therefore rationing is a reality.
- The NHS Constitution's guiding principles refer to providing a comprehensive service where access is based solely upon a patient's clinical need.
- While s 2, Health Act 2009 states that bodies performing NHS functions must have regard to the NHS Constitution, there is no statutory obligation to do so.
- QALYs exist as a means of assessing the economic viability of treatment.
- Other ethical considerations include principles of equality – all patients should be treated equally.
- A patient's social value should not be taken into account.
- A person's age should not be taken into account unless it is relevant to the patient's health or response to treatment.
- A patient's adverse behaviour is not taken into account unless the conduct is continuing and would make the treatment either less clinically- or cost-effective.

4.7 Legal considerations

4.7.1 Statutory provisions

The National Health Service Act 1977 provides statutory authority for the obligations of the State towards its citizens. It is written in terms of 'promotion' of the health service rather than an absolute duty to provide, and while there is an emphasis on the free-of-charge services, this is tempered by the use of words such as 'reasonable.'

Sections 1–3 of the National Health Service Act 1977 describes the Secretary of State's duty to the health service as follows:

SECTION

'Section 1 (1) It is the Secretary of State's duty to continue the promotion in England and Wales of a comprehensive health service designed to secure improvement —

(a) in the physical and mental health of the people of those countries, and

(b) in the prevention, diagnosis and treatment of illness,

and for that purpose to provide or secure the effective provision of services in accordance with this Act.

(2) The services so provided shall be free of charge except in so far as the making and recovery of charges is expressly provided for by or under any enactment, whenever passed.

Section 2 Without prejudice to the Secretary of State's powers apart from this section, he has power —

(a) to provide such services as he considers appropriate for the purpose of discharging any duty imposed on him by this Act; and

(b) to do any other thing whatsoever which is calculated to facilitate, or is conducive or incidental to, the discharge of such a duty.

Section 3 (1) It is the Secretary of State's duty to provide throughout England and Wales, to such extent as he considers necessary to meet all reasonable requirements —

(a) hospital accommodation;

(b) other accommodation for the purpose of any service provided under this Act;

(c) medical, dental, nursing and ambulance services;

(d) such other facilities for the care of expectant and nursing mothers and young children as he considers are appropriate as part of the health service;

(e) such facilities for the prevention of illness, the care of persons suffering from illness and the aftercare of persons who have suffered from illness as he considers are appropriate as part of the health service;

(f) such other services as are required for the diagnosis and treatment of illness.'

The wording of s 3(1) is particularly interesting as the duty refers to the provision of services 'to such extent as he considers necessary to meet all reasonable requirements'. Not only is there an element of subjectivity but the duty is restricted to meeting all *reasonable* requirements. The interpretation of s 3 was specifically challenged in the case of *R v Sec of State for Social Services ex parte Hinks* (1980).

CASE EXAMPLE

R v Secretary of State for Social Services ex parte Hinks [1980] 1 BMLR 93

In 1971, the Secretary of State had authorised plans for additional services to be made available at a local orthopaedic hospital. Given the cost of the plans, it became clear that the projects simply could not proceed as there were insufficient funds. Four patients, three of them elderly and a young girl, had been on the waiting list for surgery for some considerable time, and with support from senior orthopaedic clinicians they sought a declaration from the court that the Secretary of State had not fulfilled his duty to provide a comprehensive health service.

At first instance, Wien J held that s 3, National Health Service Act 1977 does not impose an absolute duty. As there is an element of discretion, it allows financial resources to be evaluated and this, he stated 'is the root of the problem'. Where funds are limited, voted on and approved by parliament, 'the health service has to do the best it can with the total allocation of financial resources'. Since the wording of s 3 is interpreted as imposing no absolute duty, it follows there is no positive requirement on the Secretary of State to provide the services. On appeal, Lord Denning observed how it was necessary for the Secretary of State to plan for the future and that the statutory provisions need to have an implication read into them as follows 'to such extent as he considers necessary to meet all reasonable requirements such as can be provided within the resources available'.

He continued thus:

JUDGMENT

'... it cannot be that the Secretary of State has a duty to provide everything that is asked for in the changed circumstances which have come about. That includes the numerous pills that people take nowadays: it cannot be said that he has to provide all these free for everybody'.

There was a judicial recognition that not all resources in the form of treatment could be provided to every patient. It was further considered whether it was possible to look at a particular area or hospital as a separate entity instead of considering the NHS as a whole. In concluding that it was not, Lord Denning agreed with the lower court, saying it is not possible to pinpoint precisely one hospital's needs against another. In this particular case, there were 12 hospitals within the particular area concerned. What it was necessary to establish was whether the Secretary of State was doing all that was required of him with the necessary resources available, and in this case he was.

A similar interpretation of s 3 was taken in *R v North and East Devon Health Authority, ex parte Coughlan* [2001] QB 213 in which the court confirmed that the duty which is contained in s 3 allows the Secretary of State discretion in exercising his judgment as to how he will provide the services, taking into account current government policy and restraints. In some circumstances he will be at liberty to exercise his judgment and decline to provide services, provided he does not consider that they are either reasonably required or necessary to meet a reasonable requirement.

The Court of Appeal stated at para 25:

JUDGMENT

'When exercising his judgment he has to bear in mind the comprehensive service which he is under a duty to promote as set out in s 1. However, as long as he pays due regard to that duty, the fact that the service will not be comprehensive does not mean that he is necessarily contravening either s 1 or s 3. The truth is that, while he has the duty to continue to promote a comprehensive free health service and he must never, in making a decision under s 3, disregard that duty, a comprehensive health service may never, for human, financial and other resource reasons, be achievable. Recent history has demonstrated that the pace of developments as to what is possible by way of medical treatment, coupled with the ever-increasing expectations of the public, mean that the resources of the NHS are and are likely to continue, at least in the foreseeable future, to be insufficient to meet demand.'

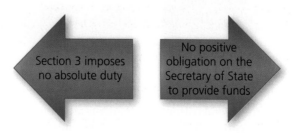

Figure 4.8 The provisions of s 3, National Health Service Act 1977

The judgment above illustrates that provided the Secretary of State does not lose sight of the provisions of s 3 and the duty he is under to provide services, an all-encompassing provision of healthcare is simply not achievable. This recognition of the impossibility is highlighted by the increasing pace of medical development and treatment, combined with patient expectations.

KEY FACTS

Key facts on interpreting s 3, National Health Service Act 1977

Statute or case	Provision or judgment
S 3, NHS Act 1977	Duty to provide services 'to such extent as he considers necessary to meet all reasonable requirements'.
R v Secretary of State for Social Services ex parte Hinks (1980)	S 3 does not impose an absolute duty to provide services; the provision of services was subject to available resources.
R v North and East Devon Health Authority, ex parte Coughlan (2001)	The wording of s 3 allows the Secretary of State discretion as to how services will be provided.

4.7.2 Judicial review

Judicial review provides an individual with the opportunity to challenge the exercise of power by a public body. If a public body such as the NHS breaches a principle of public law, their decision may be deemed unlawful by the courts. It could be that the NHS or any other public body makes a decision which it does not have the power to make, or makes an irrational decision, or indeed a decision which the courts consider is unfair. If the decision is considered unreasonable or irrational, it is referred to as **Wednesbury unreasonableness** (after the case, *Associated Provincial Picture Houses Ltd v Wednesbury Corporation* [1947] 2 All ER 680) as it would be deemed to be so unreasonable that no reasonable person acting reasonably could have made it.

While judicial review is the only available course of action in public law, a patient may take this course if they believe that their healthcare provider has deprived them of treatment which they consider to be appropriate. It may also be possible for an action to be brought on the grounds that a patient's human rights have been breached, a topic we will consider a little later.

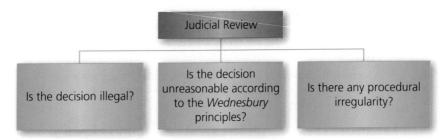

Figure 4.9 Cause for a judicial review

Challenges to NHS decisions are a recently new phenomenon as will be seen shortly. There are several reasons why patients are more willing to take actions in judicial review. Since the early 1980s patients have been more willing to challenge and question medical professionals' opinions. Compensation culture travelled across the Atlantic from the USA around this time or even earlier. Patients have become less deferential towards clinicians, in turn becoming more assertive, less fearful of demanding second opinions and more willing to make demands for treatment. This has coincided with patients having greater access to relevant medical information via the internet and the media exposing more scandalous stories about lack of resources and patients being denied healthcare. Lastly and perhaps most significantly, neither the NHS nor any statutory provision suggest anything other than a clear acknowledgment that their resources are limited and there are insufficient funds to treat everyone.

The courts' approach to a challenge of an NHS decision to refuse funding of treatment is illustrated below.

CASE EXAMPLE

R v Central Birmingham Health Authority, ex parte Walker [1987] 3 BMLR 32

An operation was required to repair a baby's heart defect. The baby's life was not in any danger and the operation had been cancelled on a number of occasions due to staffing shortages caused by a lack of resources. The mother sought judicial review of the decision to postpone the baby's operation.

Macpherson J revealed the difficulty for the courts when considering public law cases such as those involving resource allocation.

JUDGMENT

'The fact that the decision is unfortunate, disturbing and in human terms distressing, simply cannot lead to a conclusion that the court should interfere in a case of this kind.'

The court held that unless the decision was unreasonable, it would not become involved with the decisions of the executive who are responsible for allocating resources.

JUDGMENT

'It is not for this Court, or indeed any Court, to substitute its own judgment of those who are responsible for the allocation of resources. This court could only intervene where it was satisfied that there was a *prima facie* case, not only of failing to allocate resources in the way others would think that resources should be allocated, but of a failure to allocate resources to an extent which was "*Wednesbury* unreasonable".' (*per* Lord Donaldson MR)

Within the year the court had to consider a very similar issue.

CASE EXAMPLE

R v Central Birmingham Health Authority, ex parte Collier (unreported, 6 January 1988)

A four-year-old boy was in need of urgent surgery to repair a hole in the heart. The condition of his health could not be underestimated as his consultant considered he desperately required surgery. Due to a lack of resources of both staff and beds, the child's operation was postponed on a number of occasions. His father applied for a judicial review of the hospital's decision.

The application was unsuccessful. Stephen Brown LJ, while sympathetic to the plight of the child, was unequivocal that the father's application was 'wholly misconceived' and continued as follows:

JUDGMENT

'. . . even assuming that medical evidence does establish that there is an immediate danger to health, it seems to me that the legal principles to be applied do not differ from *Walker* (1987). This Court is in no position to judge the allocation of resources by this particular health authority . . . there is no suggestion here that the health authority have behaved in a way that is deserving of condemnation or criticism. What is suggested is that somehow more resources should be made available to enable the hospital authorities to ensure that the treatment is immediately given.'

If the health authority's decision was a reasonable one (even if entirely regrettable), applying *Wednesbury* reasonableness, then 'the courts cannot and should not, be asked to intervene'.

The decision, one of judicial passivity, makes it clear that the courts will refuse to intervene in a decision which although may be considered to be sufficiently reasonable to satisfy the *Wednesbury* criteria, may also be considered blatantly ethically unreasonable. However, as was observed in the *Collier* case above, the courts have no control over waiting lists, and patients cannot hope to seek executive decisions from the courts in the absence of unreasonableness. Little hope is offered to patients, not even judicial comment as to *why* the resources were not available, simply an acceptance that the decision was reasonable. If patients pin their hopes on judicial review to force NHS hospitals to provide what has been refused, they are likely to be extremely disappointed.

It took until the mid-1990s for a case concerning a lack of resources to attract media attention and for the courts to consider intervening.

CASE EXAMPLE

R v Cambridge Health Authority, ex parte B [1995] 1 WLR 898

Child 'B' (whose identity was originally prohibited by court order so as to shield her from the knowledge of the severity of her illness) was originally diagnosed with acute lymphoblastic leukaemia when she was five years old. At ten years old she developed acute myeloid leukaemia. The treating hospitals, Addenbrookes and the Royal Marsden Hospitals, gave her only eight weeks to live, having concluded that further chemotherapy and a second bone marrow transplant would be unlikely to be successful and it would be in the child's best interests not to treat her. Her father, exploring every avenue, sought alternative advice in both the USA and in the UK and found a doctor at another hospital who would treat his daughter privately. The father sought an extra contractual grant for £75,000 for the private treatment from the Cambridge and Huntingdon Health Commission, but it was refused and the father sought judicial review of the decision.

A significant shift in judicial policy can be detected at first instance as the court found in favour of the child and advised the health authority to reconsider their decision, stating that it was necessary for health providers to explain the priorities that led them to refuse funding. However, this intervention was short-lived and swiftly overturned by the Court of Appeal who explained that since the health authority had acted fairly and rationally, court intervention would be wrong.

JUDGMENT

'Difficult and agonising judgments have to be made as to how a limited budget is best allocated to the maximum advantage of a maximum number of patients. This is not a judgment that the court can make.' (*per* Bingham MR)

Although the health authority vehemently denied that the decision had anything to do with rationing and everything to do with what was in the best interests of Child B, the health authority was damned in the tabloid press. Headlines such as 'Condemned by bank balance' and 'What state is the country in when a girl's right to life hinges on the size of a hospital bank balance?' (*The Sun*, 11 March 1995) portrayed the callous NHS as denying a child life-saving treatment when in reality the decision was a clinical one. It is likely that the case drew media attention simply because this was a desperately ill little girl and there is a natural compulsion to try to do anything to save a young girl's life. However, this was also a clinical decision and it was felt that there was little hope. The money was raised to treat her privately after a news conference when an anonymous donor came forward to fund the treatment. She was never given the second bone marrow transplant, being treated instead with further chemotherapy and an experimental therapy which together lengthened her life until May 1996 when she died.

The case below demonstrates the courts' willingness to consider closely the lawfulness of the unit provider's action according to the *Wednesbury* criteria, even though they may be unwilling to become involved in the merits or otherwise of resource allocation.

CASE EXAMPLE

R v Derbyshire HA ex parte Fisher [1997] 8 Med LR 327

The patient suffered from relapsing remitting multiple sclerosis and was assessed as a suitable candidate for therapy of a new drug named beta-interferon. During this period, the NHS Executive had issued a letter or circular, EL (95) of 97 which had asked health providers to manage entry of the drug into hospitals. It stated that 'where the treatment with beta-interferon is appropriate, it is suggested that treatment should be initiated and the drug prescribed by the specialist'. The North Derbyshire health authority said that it would only fund beta-interferon as part of a clinical trial if they received extra funding. There was, however, no planned clinical trial and the health authority refused the patient treatment.

While the circular was not mandatory, it should have been taken into account as it was national policy. The court held that the health authority had acted unreasonably (in the *Wednesbury* sense) in failing to take the contents of the circular into account. They opined that the health authority's refusal to provide the beta-interferon amounted to a blanket ban and was unlawful.

Dyson J stated:

JUDGMENT

'The Trust knew that their own policy amounted to a blanket ban on beta-interferon treatment. A blanket ban was the very antithesis of national policy, whose aim was to target the drug appropriately at patients who were most likely to benefit from treatment.'

While the outcome of this case allowed the patient to receive the treatment previously denied to him, this is not a case where the courts have allowed themselves to become embroiled in issues of allocation of resources, hence one should not read too much into this case. It simply illustrates where an application has been successful on the grounds of unreasonableness, and as a direct result a patient has been allocated funds by way of treatment which was previously denied to him.

A similar decision was reached in the case below.

CASE EXAMPLE

R v North West Lancashire Health Authority, ex parte A and others [2000] 1 WLR 977

The applicants were transsexuals who wished to have gender reassignment surgery. The health authority refused to fund treatment, arguing that such surgery was a low priority for funding unless there was either an overriding need based upon clinical opinion or there were exceptional circumstances. The three applicants applied for judicial review of the decision.

Auld J who gave the leading judgment agreed that health authorities were free to prioritise types of treatment and furthermore agreed that reassignment surgery was a lower priority when compared with more urgent and pressing surgery such as cancer or heart disease or kidney failure. He acknowledged that the decision on how to prioritise is a matter of judgment for every authority, while bearing in mind the statutory obligation to meet the reasonable requirements of all those for whom it is responsible. This was acceptable and the policy was not irrational provided that it genuinely recognises a patient's need. He concluded that the health authority failed to do so as they did truly recognise **transsexualism** as an illness rather than a state of mind. While the health authority stated that provision would be made in exceptional cases, their policy amounted to a 'blanket ban' against funding the treatment.

transsexualism
where a person of one gender strongly identifies him or herself as a member of the opposite sex

What is the relevance of this decision? It simply appears to mean that unit providers can still refuse to provide treatment provided that they are sufficiently transparent about their reasons for refusal. The judgment requires health authorities or trusts to carefully consider the reasons for their refusal rather than reconsider their refusal *per se*.

A similar decision was reached in the more recent case of *AC v Berkshire West Primary Care Trust* [2010] EWHC 1162 (Admin) where the court considered an application for judicial review from the refusal of the PCT to fund breast augmentation surgery in a **gender dysphoria** case. Primary care trusts have an absolute obligation to break even financially every year by virtue of ss 229(1) and 230(1), National Health Service Act 2006. Against this background, PCTs have to balance clinical need and cost-effectiveness, making the most of their limited resources.

gender dysphoria
a condition where a person feels a lack of certainty about his or her birth gender

We have already seen from the dictum of Auld J that it is lawful to have policies about which treatments will be funded and those which are likely to be a lower priority. NHS policy classifies breast enlargement surgery as cosmetic surgery or 'non-core procedure', and the relevant issue was whether it was irrational for it to be categorised as such. Given that the clinical effectiveness of this surgery was uncertain, the court concluded that the decision not to fund the treatment was not irrational. Bean J concluded:

JUDGMENT

'I am satisfied that the defendants had due regard to the need to eliminate discrimination against transsexuals and to the need to promote equality of opportunity between transsexuals and non-transsexuals. Their gender dysphoria policy was drafted with great care and after extensive consultation.'

The courts are however willing to address issues of irrationality and abuse of power in clear and unequivocal terms in cases where unit providers have acted unreasonably.

CASE EXAMPLE

R v North and East Devon Health Authority, ex parte Coughlan [2001] QB 213

The applicant was severely injured in a road traffic accident in 1971, as a result of which she suffered from tetraplagia along with other severe physical disabilities. In 1993 she and seven other patients with similar disabilities were moved from a hospital to Mardon House, a NHS residence for long-term care. The patients had all agreed to this move; the hospital was closing and Mardon House was promised to be their home for life. Only six years later, the health authority decided to close the facility. The decision was taken following the publication of new eligibility criteria three years earlier which distinguished between providers of specialist healthcare and general healthcare. Mardon House no longer met the new criteria and it was proposed to transfer the patients' care to a different facility although one had not been identified. The applicant sought judicial review of the decision.

At first instance the court quashed the decision to close Mardon House. The applicant, together with the other patients, had been promised that this facility would be their home for life and the health authority had failed to demonstrate an overriding public interest which would justify breaking this promise. Furthermore, the court held that the decision was flawed as no alternative home had been found. The health authority appealed.

The Court of Appeal held firstly that the decision to close Mardon House in the first instance was wrong. The reasoning for this was due to the eligibility criteria itself, as it was flawed in its interpretation of its responsibilities under the National Health Act 1977. Secondly, the promise which the health authority made to the patients created a legitimate expectation which, if frustrated, would be so unfair as to amount to an abuse of power. The court when considering this latter point took into account whether there was any clear justification for denying the legitimate expectation and concluded there was none. There was no identified alternative accommodation and the court concluded the decision to close the unit was 'an unjustified breach which amounted to an abuse of power'.

KEY FACTS

Key facts on judgments of judicial review cases

Case	Judgment
R v Central Birmingham Health Authority ex parte Walker (1987)	Macpherson J: 'the decision is unfortunate, disturbing and … distressing' but 'cannot lead to a conclusion that the courts should interfere in a case of this kind'.
	The court indicated that it would only interfere if there was a failure to allocate resources unreasonably according to the Wednesbury criteria.
R v Central Birmingham Health Authority ex parte Collier (1988)	If the health authority's decision was a reasonable one (applying Wednesbury reasonableness), then the courts should not intervene.
R v Cambridge Health Authority ex parte B (1995)	The health authority had acted fairly and rationally. The court cannot assess whether the health authorities had allocated funds properly. Bingham MR: 'difficult and agonising judgments have to be made as to how a limited budget is best allocated to the maximum advantage of a maximum number of patients. This is not a judgment that the court can make'.
R v Derbyshire Health Authority ex parte Fisher (1997)	The health authority had acted unreasonably and their refusal to prescribe beta-interferon amounted to a blanket ban.
R v North West Lancashire Health Authority ex parte A and others (2000)	Health providers were free to prioritise types of treatment. While the health authority stated provision for gender reassignment surgery would be permitted in exceptional circumstances, their refusal amounted to a blanket ban.
AC v Berkshire West Primary Care Trust (2010)	PCTs have an absolute obligation to break even financially and have to balance clinical need and cost-effectiveness. It was neither unreasonable nor irrational to refuse to fund the treatment.
R v North and East Devon Health Authority ex parte Coughlan (2001)	The health authority's decision to close the residential home for severely disabled patients was wrong as it denied the patients their legitimate expectation. The decision to close the unit was 'an unjustified breach which amounted to an abuse of power'.

4.7.3 The exceptionality criteria

In *R v North West Lancashire Health Authority ex parte A* (2000), Auld said:

JUDGMENT

'it is proper for an authority to adopt a general policy for the exercise of such an administrative discretion, to allow for exceptions from it in "exceptional circumstances" and to leave those circumstances undefined.'

While there is a general acceptance of funding limitations, patients are able to argue that their case is so 'exceptional' in terms of likely benefit which the treatment would produce that their case should be funded. The exceptionality criteria require the provider to consider genuinely and transparently whether there is an overriding clinical need for the patient to be granted funding for treatment, and require each patient to be treated on their own particular merits.

Lord Scarman in *Re Findlay* [1985] 1 AC 318 (HL) said:

JUDGMENT

'... in my view, a policy to place transsexualism low in an order of priorities of illnesses for treatment and to deny it treatment save in exceptional circumstances such as overriding clinical need is not in principle irrational, provided that the policy genuinely recognises the possibility of there being an overriding clinical need and requires each request for treatment to be considered on its individual merits.'

CASE EXAMPLE

R v (Ann Marie Rogers) v Swindon PCT [2006] EWCA Civ 392

The patient suffered from stage 1, HER-2 positive breast cancer and underwent a mastectomy and related surgery. Following some personal research, she asked to be treated with Herceptin, which was at that time only licensed by NICE for stage 2 breast cancer. Her consultant supported her request. Trials for the use of Herceptin in stage 1, HER-2 breast cancer had shown some positive and encouraging results but there were also some concerns and research was incomplete. Therefore, Herceptin was still unlicensed for the treatment of stage 1 breast cancer and had not yet been endorsed by NICE. In turn, NICE would not give the endorsement if the drug has not been endorsed by the European Medicines Agency.

Nevertheless, the Secretary of State for Health's guidance was clear and unequivocal, stating that 'I want to make it clear that PCTs should not refuse to fund Herceptin solely on the grounds of cost'. Swindon PCT could fund Herceptin even though it was unlicensed in circumstances where 'a patient has a special healthcare problem that presents an exceptional need for treatment', but each case would be considered on its merits and given the cost of the treatment (approximately £25,000 per year) would have regard to funds. The Trust refused Ms Rogers' request for treatment based on 'exceptional need' on the grounds that she was a typical stage 1, HER2-positive patient and there was nothing exceptional about her particular case, despite her consultant's support and the guidance from the Secretary of State. The PCT denied that funding was an issue and Ms Rogers challenged the decision on the grounds that it was irrational.

At first instance, her case was dismissed but the Court of Appeal took a different approach. The primary question was whether the policy was rational and in deciding this the court opined that where there was no difference in the clinical need of different patients and since the question of funding was not an issue, the PCT were not at liberty to treat one patient who fulfils the clinical requirements differently from another. The Court of Appeal allowed the application for judicial review and referred it back to the PCT for reconsideration.

The interesting aspect of this case is that the PCTs refusal to fund Herceptin was not based upon cost considerations, as the Secretary of State's guidance was that PCTs should not refuse to fund Herceptin based upon lack of resources. Had this not been the case and the PCT argued that they had insufficient resources to fund Herceptin, the result may well have been different as indicated by the Court of Appeal:

JUDGMENT

'If that policy had involved a balance of financial considerations ... we do not think that such a policy would have been irrational.'

In reality this case is more about transparency of decision-making and the failure of this particular PCT to make a rational funding decision, as illustrated Sir Anthony Clarke MR who said:

JUDGMENT

'... once the PCT decided (as it did) that it would fund Herceptin for some patients and that cost was irrelevant, the only reasonable approach was to focus on the patient's clinical needs and fund patient's clinical needs and fund patients within the eligible group who were properly prescribed Herceptin.'

A similar case arose only a year later.

CASE EXAMPLE

R (Otley) v Barking and Dagenham NHS Trust [2007] EWHC 1927 (Admin)

The applicant suffered from cancer and secondary tumours had been discovered on her liver. Research had led her to become aware of Avastin which was licensed and prescribed in other countries but not yet in the UK. Her oncologist prescribed anti-cancer drugs that included Avastin, for which, as it was not available on the NHS, she paid privately. She responded positively and the oncologist applied for a further five prescriptions. However, a panel from the Trust decided that the patient's life would not be prolonged significantly to make it cost-effective. In response it was argued that the drug should be funded in exceptional circumstances but the Trust responded that her circumstances did not fit the exceptionality criteria and refused to fund the treatment. She applied for judicial review of the Trust's refusal.

Mitting J held that while the Trust's exceptionality policy was lawful, the application of the policy in this particular case to deny the patient the funding was both irrational and unlawful. Put simply, Avastin, together with other drugs, produced positive results and a chance at prolonged survival for the patient, and there were no alternative treatments that could produce the same benefits for her. The cost of the drug was not prohibitive and would not impact on funding other treatments for other patients.

Mitting J found that

JUDGMENT

'on any fair minded view of the exceptionality criteria identified in the critical analysis document, her case was exceptional.'

Only a year later the courts were obliged to hear a further and similar case concerning a Trust's refusal to fund drug treatment.

CASE EXAMPLE

R (Murphy) v Salford PCT [2008] EWHC 1908 (Admin)

The applicant had been refused renal cancer treating drugs, which had been recommended by her oncologist. The drugs were expensive and could extend her life, although could not cure her condition. The PCT's policy was that drugs which were refused in the ordinary course of events could be made available if the exceptionality criteria were satisfied. The PCT refused to grant the funding for the drugs and she applied by way of judicial review, having set out seven reasons why her case should be treated as exceptional.

The application for judicial review was granted and the case remitted back to the PCT for reconsideration. While each of the reasons she presented should be considered individually, all the circumstances of her case had to be considered jointly in order for a clear picture of her 'exceptionality' to become clear. Logically, if each of her factors were to be considered separately, while correct procedure, it becomes significantly easier for a unit provider to dismiss each separate factor as unexceptional.

CASE EXAMPLE

R (Ross) v West Sussex PCT [2008] 106 BMLR 1

Here the applicant and patient, Mr Ross, had applied for exceptional funding under the PCT's policy for Lenalidomide. The drug had been recommended by his consultant but was not available within that area on the NHS. He had been diagnosed as suffering from multiple myeloma and while he had initially responded well to previous treatment, he had now grown intolerant. It was recognised that without this drug his life expectancy was compromised, but it was refused on the grounds that it was neither cost-effective nor exceptional within the meaning of the Trust's policy. He applied for judicial review of the Trust's decision.

The High Court held the PCT's decision was unlawful and irrational, and ordered the PCT to fund the treatment while the PCT reconsidered its position. The court held that the PCT's exceptionality policy was unlawful because it called on a patient to show that his condition was unique. The PCT's policy meant that a patient was not 'exceptional' if his condition had characteristics similar to those of other patients.

In contrast to cases of resource allocation where the courts have steered purposefully away from any involvement, the above cases demonstrate the court's willingness to adjudicate on the lawfulness or irrationality of health providers' decisions not to fund expensive cancer drugs. While courts have sent cases back to panels for reconsideration, it does not necessarily follow that they will come to a different decision, just that they have reconsidered the case either with increased transparency or 'in the round'. Far from satisfactory, the exceptionality criteria exist as the only other avenue for a patient to pursue when denied life-saving or quality of life-enhancing drugs in an otherwise quagmire of scarcity of resources.

KEY FACTS

Key facts on the exceptionality criteria

Cases	Judgment
R v North West Lancashire Health Authority ex parte A (2000)	Recognised the correctness of being able to allow departure from a general policy and allow exceptional circumstances.
R (Ann Marie Rogers) v Swindon PCT (2006) and the Secretary of State	Court of Appeal referred the case back to the PCT for reconsideration on the grounds that the decision was irrational.

R (Otley) v Barking and Dagenham NHS Trust (2007)	The application of the exceptionality criteria to this particular patient was both irrational and unlawful. Case remitted back to the PCT for reconsideration.
R (Murphy) v Salford PCT (2008)	Case remitted back to the PCT for reconsideration.
R (Ross) v West Sussex PCT (2008)	The Trust exceptionality policy was both irrational and unlawful; case remitted back to the PCT for reconsideration.

4.7.4 The role of HRA 1998 in resource allocation

The HRA 1988 incorporated the ECHR into domestic law. It took effect in October 2000, making courts obliged to consider the application of human rights when deciding the lawfulness of actions of public bodies. It was initially thought that HRA 1998 would have a profound effect on medical law. In reality, it has not. While the statutory provisions provided that the judiciary can act creatively, they have been unwilling to do so and, as Alasdair Maclean submits, the real issue is more likely 'judicial concern regarding resource allocation and clinical integrity and a desire to avoid a flood of dubious claims underlying the court's caution' ('Crossing the Rubicon on the Human Rights Ferry', *Modern Law Review*, Vol. 64, No. 5, pages 775–94).

HRA 1998, Art 2

Article 2 states that 'everyone's right to life shall be protected by law'. A patient who believes they are denied treatment may argue their right to life, protected under Art 2, has been violated.

Article 2 imposes upon the State not only the obligation to ensure that a person's life is protected but also, further to the case of *Osman v United Kingdom* (1998), an obligation 'to take appropriate steps to safeguard life'. While one may consider whether this could extend to the allocation of resources, the court clarified that the obligation 'must be interpreted in a way that does not impose an impossible or disproportionate burden on the authorities'. Hence it is highly unlikely that any patient's claim that a refusal to fund treatment breaches their human rights under Art 2 will meet with any success.

Remarkably, there has been significant (albeit limited) success in enforcing Art 2. See Chapter 3, page 101 for an outline of *Savage v South Essex Partnership NHS Trust* (2008) in which there was an 'operational obligation' on the Trust imposed by Art 2. In contrast, the more recent case *Rabone v Pennine Care NHS Trust* (2010), examined on page 102, Chapter 3 held that there was no 'operational obligation' imposed by Art 2.

Article 3 prohibits 'inhuman and degrading treatment' and Art 8 (subject to the exceptions in Art 8(2)) protects the 'right to respect for private and family life'. Both of these Articles were tested in *R v North West Lancashire Health Authority, ex parte A and others* (2000) (see page 129 above) in which the applicants tried to argue their right to respect for a person's private and family life had been breached (Art 8) and that the denial of gender reassignment surgery amounted to inhuman and degrading treatment, under Art 3. Further, they argued that the refusal amounted to discrimination against them under Art 14.

The Court of Appeal took a restrictive approach, entertaining the claim for only the briefest moment. Referring first to Art 8, they rejected the suggestion that a positive obligation to fund treatment could be imposed, stating that 'such an interference could hardly be founded on a refusal to fund medical treatment'.

As far as Art 3 was concerned, there was a speedy dismissal that there could be any effect on allocation of resources. Buxton J stated:

JUDGMENT

'it has never been applied to merely policy decisions on the allocations of resources ... that is clear not only from the terms of Art 3 itself ... but also from the explanation of the reach of Art 3 that has been given by the Convention organs'.

Finally, with reference to Art 14, the applicants were not refused surgery on the grounds of their sexuality but on grounds of allocation of resources.

The more recent case below illustrates the court's insistence that Art 8 cannot be invoked to impose a positive obligation on unit providers to allocate resources for specific medical treatment.

CASE EXAMPLE

R (on the application of Condliff) v North Staffordshire Primary Care Trust [2011] EWCA CN 910

Mr Condliff appealed against his PCT refusal to fund weight-loss surgery. He was diabetic, had other medical conditions and was morbidly obese with a body mass index (BMI) over 40. The PCT policy for weight loss surgery was a BMI over 50, thus Mr Condliff was not entitled to the surgery. However, the PCT did operate a policy whereby a patient with exceptional reasons could still be eligible for surgery. He argued that the grounds of his case were exceptional but the Trust's exceptionality criteria specifically excluded 'social factors'. The Trust justified this on the grounds that decision-making should be made on clinical factors alone in order to avoid discrimination. He argued that as his condition had deteriorated further, the exceptionality criteria should apply. He further argued that excluding social factors from the exceptionality criteria was a breach of Art 8, and consequently his right to a private and family life was violated.

His application for judicial review was unsuccessful. Article 8 was not engaged when a public authority had to consider allocation of its own resources. Social factors and Art 8 factors were not interchangeable and could be two very different things. The court showed its reluctance to allow Art 8 to operate within the confines of this case. It did not interfere with a patient's Art 8 rights if funding was refused and there was no obligation on the public authority to provide the funding.

Wacksman J in the High Court said:

JUDGMENT

'when a PCT makes a policy decision about where to allocate its limited medical resources, assuming it does so on a rational basis, the Art 8 rights of any particular person who may be denied treatment as a result of a decision which applies that policy need not be considered by reason of some positive duty.'

As no positive obligation was imposed, there was no breach of Article 8 because of the exclusion of the social factors.

There is a strange irony about this case in that had Mr Condliff been more obese, he would have been eligible for the weight loss surgery in the first instance. In order to be eligible, all he needed to do was increase his weight, which in itself would have put his health at considerable risk! As his BMI was over 40 and he was suffering from other conditions, he would clearly have benefited from the surgery and subsequently, would probably be less of a burden on NHS resources. The Court of Appeal upheld the lower court's decision.

To date, it is clear that the courts will not entertain the provisions of HRA 1998 when considering resource allocation. While it is probably only a matter of time until the courts relent, the consequences of a decision in favour of a claimant would be to open the floodgates for all those patients who have been denied treatment due to lack of resources. If this occurs, it will be a decision any government who controls the NHS purse strings will find very difficult to bear.

4.7.5 The effect of European Union law

CASE EXAMPLE

R (on the application of Watts) v Bedford PCT and another [2003] EWHC 2184 (Admin)

The patient was a 72-year-old woman who was suffering from osteoarthritis in both hips and required a hip replacement for which she was placed on the NHS waiting list. The waiting period was 12 months and while her case was not medically urgent, she was in a great deal of pain. The waiting period was not itself an unreasonable one. She required authorisation from her PCT to be treated abroad under a scheme which allows patients to be treated in another member state of the EU. Her application was refused as the PCT argued that the waiting period was not one of 'undue delay'. Doctors in France had recommended surgery more urgently than doctors in the UK. She was then reassessed in the UK and placed on a three- to four-month waiting list. However, reluctant to delay any longer, she underwent surgery in France and claimed the cost of the surgery, nearly £4,000, back from the PCT. The PCT refused to pay the cost. She challenged the refusal and argued that Art 49 of the EC Treaty supported her claim. Article 49 states as follows:

ARTICLE

'Restrictions on the freedom to provide services within the Community shall be prohibited in respect of nationals of Member States who are established in a State of the Community other than that of the person for whom the services are intended.'

The Article, binding on domestic courts, prohibits member states of the European Union from restricting available services to their citizens. For example, a dental patient from Lithuania is perfectly within his rights to seek and obtain services from a dentist in Malta. Under Art 50(d) services referred to include professional services, of which medical services are recognised.

The issue which the courts had to consider was whether the waiting list meant that the patient would be unduly delayed. On appeal by the Secretary of State from the court of first instance, the Court of Appeal sought guidance from the European Court of Justice (ECJ) on a point as to whether the NHS's refusal to authorise treatment abroad would adversely affect its method of prioritising patient care through waiting lists.

In response the ECJ explained that prior authorisation is required before embarking on treatment abroad, if a patient wishes to ensure that costs incurred are refunded. However, when the NHS is considering whether to authorise payment, it must objectively consider the patient's condition and should not regard administration of waiting lists as the guiding factor. Whether a delay was 'undue' or not was dependent on the patient's medical condition.

ACTIVITY

Self-test questions

Ensure that your answers are supported by case law where appropriate.

- What are QALYs? Why are they relevant?
- Explain three criticisms of QALYs.
- What is the Secretary of State's duty in s 3 of the National Health Service Act 1977?
- How was this tested by the courts?

- What approach have the courts consistently taken where cases of judicial review are taken following decisions of healthcare rationing?
- Consider how successful a patient might be in relying on the exceptionality criteria. Refer to three cases.

ACTIVITY

Quick quiz

True or false?

1. In *R v Cambridge Health Authority ex parte B* (1995), Lord Bingham MR said, 'Difficult and agonising judgments have to be made as to how a limited budget is best allocated to the maximum advantage of a maximum number of patients. This is not a judgment that the court can make.'
2. Resource allocation is concerned with the effectiveness of the drug rather than the cost of the drug.

SUMMARY

- Section 1(1) of the National Health Service Act 1977 refers to 'promotion' of the health service.
- Section 1(2) expresses that the services provided are done so 'free of charge'.
- Section 3 explains the Secretary of State's duty to provide services 'as he considers necessary to meet all reasonable requirements'.
- The interpretation of s 3 was challenged in *R v Sec of State ex parte Hinks* (1980) where it was expressed not to impose a positive duty. A similar approach was taken in *R v North and East Devon Health Authority ex parte Coughlan* (2001).
- Judicial review exists as one of the only avenues in which to challenge a hospital's refusal of drugs or services on grounds of resource allocation.
- The courts remain steadfast in their refusal to become involved with executive decisions of allocation of resources.
- The courts will intervene where it is apparent that the *Wednesbury* criteria have been breached.
- The court will closely consider the exceptionality criteria where unit providers will consider exceptional circumstances as an exception from the general policy of funding limitations.
- There has been little impact of human rights legislation on resource allocation.
- A patient can by virtue of European Union law elect to be treated in a member state.

Further reading

Harris, J. (1987) 'QALYfing the Value of Life', *Journal of Medical Ethics*, 13, pages 117–123.
Harris, J. (2005) 'The Age-Indifference Principle and Equality', *Cambridge Quarterly of Healthcare Ethics*, 14, 93–9.
Newdrick, C. (2007) 'Low-priority treatment and exceptional care review', *Medical Law Review*, 15 (2), 236–44.
Syrett, K. (2008) 'NICE and judicial review: enforcing "accountability for reasonableness" through the courts?' *Medical Law Review*, 16 (1), 127–40.

5

Confidentiality

AIMS AND OBJECTIVES

After reading this chapter you should be able to:

- Understand the ethical basis for the role of confidentiality and be able to appreciate the role of professional guidance
- Appreciate the development of the law of privacy in England and Wales
- Appreciate the common law recognition of the significance of confidentiality of health records
- Understand the exceptions which exist to the principle that medical records remain confidential
- Evaluate the significance of legislative measures
- Comment critically on the common law and fully appreciate the judicial approach to the preservation of the tenet of confidentiality.

5.1 The ethical basis for the notion of patient confidentiality

Doctors are under an obligation to keep their patients' communications and details private and confidential. In this respect, the medical profession does not differ significantly from the legal profession who are under a similar duty to respect their clients' confidences.

The importance of this principle cannot be overstated, as a patient must be able to trust his doctor, that whatever he tells him will remain private. The duty of confidentiality represents both deontological and consequentialist ideals. Not only are doctors duty bound to keep a patient's confidence but the exercise of the duty also serves the greater good. If a patient feels that he cannot trust his doctor, he is less likely to seek medical advice. Trust and confidence in his doctor are essential for his care and treatment, not only for his personal health but also as far as wider concerns of public health issues are concerned.

The historical basis of this fundamental principle can be traced back to The Hippocratic Oath, some 2,400 years ago:

QUOTATION

'Whatever, in connection with my professional practice, or not in connection with it, I see or hear in the life of men, which ought not to be spoken of abroad, I will not divulge, as reckoning that all such should be kept secret.'

The ancient code did not, however, convey an absolute obligation as reflected in the use of the word 'ought', leaving room for discretionary disclosure. The Declaration of Geneva (amended at Sydney 1968, Venice 1983 and Stockholm 1994) removed the element of professional judgment altogether and replaced it with an absolute duty which extends even beyond the patient's death.

QUOTATION

'I will respect the secrets which are confided in me, even after the patient has died'.

Thus, the doctor is never free to divulge any information about the patient, even if he considers it to be in the patient's best interests or others closely related to him. Decisions of the courts and information tribunals have readily endorsed this crucial philosophical tenet, as demonstrated in *Bluck v Information Commissioner* [2007] 98 BMLR 1 and *Lewis v Secretary of State for Health and another* [2008] All ER 90 (see pages 167 and 165 for fuller examination of these cases).

5.2 Modern medicine and professional guidance

It needs no explanation to state that modern medicine presents a far different and more complex picture from the days of the Hippocratic Oath, or even from the Declaration of Geneva. Patient care is more diverse. On occasions different medical professionals are involved with one patient's care and treatment, all of whom may require access to a patient's medical records. Confidentiality must be preserved along every step of the way.

The British Medical Association

The British Medical Association (BMA) considers confidentiality to be vital to medical treatment:

QUOTATION

'Frank and open exchange between health professionals and patients is the ideal and patients need to feel that their privacy will be respected before they can enter into such an exchange.'

(BMA (2004) Confidentiality as part of a bigger picture)

The basic principle is largely unremarkable; doctors recognise and respect the need for confidentiality of their patient's medical details and records. Only if a patient truly trusts a doctor can he be sufficiently comfortable to trust the doctor with information which he considers to be most personal and private. While the concept of patient confidentiality is largely uncontroversial, its practice may be more troublesome as we later explore.

The Department of Health

The Department of Health Code of Practice (November 2003) reiterates these fundamental principles, stating that within the NHS:

QUOTATION

'A duty of confidence arises when a person discloses information to another (for example from patient to clinician) in circumstances where it is reasonable to expect that the information will be held in confidence.'

The Code of Practice continues by emphasising that the guidelines apply to *all* employees within the NHS. The reference to all employees is essential since an employee of the NHS who is not a medical professional may quite reasonably come across patient-sensitive information. Hence they are under the same duty of confidentiality as any clinician. In order to achieve its aims of securing a 'first class confidential service' it seeks to ensure that 'all patient information is processed fairly, lawfully and transparently', in order that the public:

QUOTATION

'understand the reasons for processing personal information ... give their consent for the disclosure and use of their personal information ... gain trust in the way the NHS handles information ... understand their rights to access information held about them.'

The General Medical Council

The General Medical Council (GMC), much like the other professional bodies, has also issued guidelines in relation to confidentiality. The guidance which came into effect in October 2009 states:

QUOTATION

'Confidentiality is central to trust between doctors and patients. Without assurances about confidentiality, patients may be reluctant to seek medical attention or to give doctors the information they need in order to provide good care. But appropriate information-sharing is essential to the efficient provision of safe, effective care, both for the individual patient and for the wider community of patients.'

The Nursing and Midwifery Council

The Nursing and Midwifery Council guidance 2004 provides the following

QUOTATION

'the common law of confidentiality reflects that people have a right to expect that information given to a nurse or midwife is only used for the purpose for which it was given and will not be disclosed without permission.'

Their caveat to breaching confidentiality is similar to other professional bodies, in that disclosure of a patient's information can be disclosed without their consent:

- by order of the court
- in order to prevent and support detection, investigation and punishment of serious crime
- to prevent abuse or serious harm to others.

The ethical approach of the professional bodies is not dissimilar; confidentiality is regarded as the bedrock of trust between clinician and patient, and effective medical treatment cannot operate without confidentiality. Given the ancient origins of the Hippocratic Oath it is no surprise that the ethical guidance is as consistent and stringent as it appears.

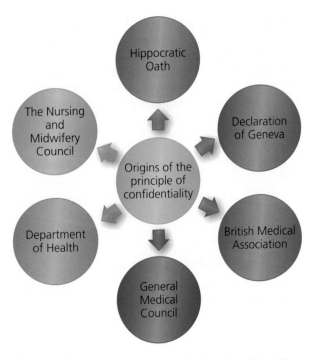

Figure 5.1 The origins of the ethical principles of confidentiality

5.3 Legal considerations

There is an equitable common law duty of confidence. The duty is not an absolute one. Any information that is obtained in confidence can only be disclosed if:

- the patient provides her consent, or
- if it is in the public interest for the information to be disclosed, or
- if disclosure is required by statute.

5.3.1 Introduction

It poses little difficulty to establish an equitable common law duty imposed upon those in the medical profession to ensure that the confidence of patients is respected.

An early example of the equitable duty of confidence (albeit in a non-medical case) can be seen in *Fraser v Evans* [1969] 1 QB 341 which emphasises the principle that a party is restrained from divulging confidential information to another.

Lord Denning MR stated:

JUDGMENT

'The jurisdiction is based not so much on property or on contract as on the duty to be of good faith. No person is permitted to divulge to the world information which he has received in confidence, unless he has just cause or excuse for doing so. Even if he comes by it innocently, nevertheless once he gets to know that it was originally given in confidence, he can be restrained from breaking that confidence.'

The principle was reiterated in *Hunter v Mann* [1974] QB 767, *per* Boreham J:

JUDGMENT

'in common with other professional men, for instance a priest and there are of course others, the doctor is under a duty not to disclose, without the consent of his patient, information which he, the doctor has gained in his professional capacity, save . . . in very exceptional circumstances.'

The principle has been repeated frequently, for example in the case of *W v Egdell* [1990] 1 All ER 835, where the court confirmed the existence of the equitable common law duty between a patient and his psychiatrist.

Per Bingham LJ referring to the psychiatrist's duty:

JUDGMENT

'Nor could he, without a breach of the law as well as professional etiquette, discuss the case ... unless he took appropriate steps to conceal the identity of *W*. It is not in issue here that a duty of confidence existed.'

5.3.2 The absence of a tort of privacy

In the United Kingdom, unlike other countries such as the USA, there is no cause of action in tort that can clearly be identified as an invasion of privacy. Even the recent case of *Wainwright v Home Office* [2004] AC 406 confirmed as much, where two prison visitors who were strip-searched unsuccessfully claimed that their privacy had been **breached**. The development of the law in the UK has however been significantly assisted by HRA 1998, which came into effect in October 2000.

It has been the role of common law to provide protection for those who were victims of the wrongful use of private information, which has slowly become known as breach of confidence. In other words, the courts could establish a breach of confidence arising out of a confidential relationship, such as a doctor/patient relationship.

There is often no express contractual relationship in medical law save for private medical treatment. Where there may be a contractual relationship between the parties, the case of *Saltman Engineering Co, Ltd and others v Campbell Engineering Co Ltd* (1948) 64 RPC 203 held that even where there is no express term in the contract, the subject matter should be kept confidential. Here, it was held that

breach
the infringement of a legal obligation

JUDGMENT

'there was an implied term of the contract that the drawings entrusted to the defendants for the purposes of such contract should be treated as confidential'.

The Court of Appeal stated as follows:

JUDGMENT

'if two parties make a contract, under which one of them obtains for the purpose of the contract, or in connection with it, some confidential matter, then, even though the contract is silent on the matter of confidence, the law will imply an obligation to treat such confidential matter in a confidential way.'

More recent case law suggests that it is not necessary to establish any basis of a contractual relationship in order to prove that the duty of confidence existed.

CASE EXAMPLE

Attorney-General v Guardian Newspapers Ltd (No. 2) [1990] 1 AC 109

A MI5 operative, Peter Wright, wrote a book called *Spycatcher* in which he recorded his memoirs of his work in the British security services in breach of the Official Secrets Act 1911. Following an unsuccessful application for an injunction by the Attorney-General, the book was subsequently published in several countries.

The question (for our purposes) for the House of Lords was twofold:

1. Were the *Observer* and the *Guardian* newspapers in breach of confidentiality in June 1986 when they reported on the injunction proceedings?
2. Was the *Sunday Times* newspaper in breach of confidentiality when it published its first intended serialisation of *Spycatcher* in July 1987?

The House of Lords upheld the Attorney-General's appeal. With reference to the first question above, the *Observer* and the *Guardian* newspapers were not in breach of confidentiality because they contained no information that was damaging. With reference to the second question, the *Sunday Times* was in breach of confidentiality because the duty could arise either in contract or in equity, and the significance of the duty meant that the newspaper, a third party, could not disclose confidential information to others.

For our purposes and for the study of medical law and ethics, the courts referred to the general principles of the equitable duty of confidence. The Law Lords' observations were particularly helpful.

Lord Bingham:

JUDGMENT

'... the duty of confidence does not depend on any contract, express or implied between the parties.'

Lord Griffiths explained that although the terms of a contract may impose a duty of confidence, any remedy is not dependent upon the contract and amounts to an equitable remedy. He referred to Megarry J who identified the three elements to found the duty of confidence in the case of *Coco v A. N. Clark (Engineering) Ltd* [1969] RPC 41 at 47:

JUDGMENT

'three elements are normally required if, apart from contract, a case of breach of confidence is to succeed. First, the information itself, in the words of Lord Greene MR in the *Saltman* case (1948) on page 215 must "have the necessary quality of confidence about it". Secondly, that information must have been imparted in circumstances importing an obligation of confidence. Thirdly, there must be an unauthorised use of that information to the detriment of the party communicating it.'

However, even this was seen as too limiting, and was developed by Lord Goff who stated that a duty of confidence exists where a person receives information that he knows or ought to know is both fairly and reasonably considered as confidential information. This principle should pose no difficulty for medical professionals as a doctor or those employed by the NHS know or ought to know from both their relationship with the patient and their own professional guidance that there is a duty of patient confidentiality. Lord Goff's statement:

JUDGMENT

'a duty of confidence arises where confidential information comes to the knowledge of a person (the confidant) in circumstances where he has notice, or is held to have agreed that the information is confidential with the effect that it would be just in all the circumstances that he should be protected from disclosing the information to others.'

Lord Goff set down three limiting principles:

■ The principle of confidentiality only applies to information that is confidential. Once the information enters the public domain, as a general rule, the confidentiality no longer exists.

- The duty of confidentiality applies neither to useless nor trivial information.
- It is in the public interest that confidences should be preserved and protected but on occasions, public interest may be outweighed by other public interests which favour disclosure.

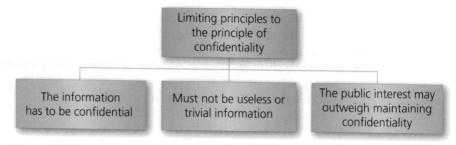

Figure 5.2 Limiting principles to the principle of confidentiality

5.3.3 The emergence of a new tort of privacy

The case of *Campbell v MGN* [2004] 2 AC 457 provided the courts with an enviable opportunity to extend and redefine the law.

CASE EXAMPLE

Campbell v MGN [2004] 2 AC 457

The famous model Naomi Campbell was photographed leaving a meeting of Narcotics Anonymous. The photographs were published by the *Daily Mirror* newspaper together with an article that described her battle with drugs. She had been no stranger to publicity, and given the nature of her occupation had often courted and welcomed publicity. She sued for breach of confidence, arguing that the photographs represented confidential information which could not be disclosed.

The House of Lords by a majority of 3:2 held that Mirror Groups Newspapers was liable. Both the taking of the photographs and the accompanying article were private and confidential, and were in breach of confidence.

During their consideration the House referred to the case of *A v B plc* [2003] QB 195, wherein the court had referred to a passage by Glesson CJ from *Australian Broadcasting Corporation v Lenah Game Meats Pty Ltd* [2001] 1 ALR 185. Glesson CJ had set down a test for determining whether the claimant has a reasonable expectation of privacy:

JUDGMENT

'certain kinds of information about a person, such as information relating to health ... may be easy to identify as private ... The requirement that disclosure or observation of information or conduct would be highly offensive to a reasonable person of ordinary sensibilities is in many circumstances a useful practical test of what is private.'

It was this test that was considered by Lord Hope in *Campbell v MGN*. Lord Hope observed:

JUDGMENT

'there will be a reasonable expectation of privacy where the information is obviously or can be easily identified as private'.

Lord Nicholls (dissenting) said:

JUDGMENT

'Essentially the touchstone of private life is whether in respect of the disclosed fa   the person in question had a reasonable expectation of privacy.'

In this case it posed no difficulty. The information could clearly be identified as private a. hence, in situations where privacy is easy to determine, there is no need to consider whethe the act is highly offensive. Whether disclosure of material can be regarded as 'highly offensive' is a subjective test: that is, it is judged according to the mind of the person affected by the disclosure. The courts clearly support the view that any reference to medical information is where a person could have a reasonable expectation of privacy.

Therefore, there is a reasonable expectation that information that is private or personal, such as medical records, will be protected.

5.3.4 Consideration of human rights

In *Campbell v MGN* (2004) the House of Lords had to decide whether there was a public interest, such as freedom of the press under Art 10, HRA 1998 which justified the breach. As Lord Hope stated:

JUDGMENT

'the right to privacy had to be balanced against the right of the media to impart information to the public. And the right of the media to impart information to the public has to be balanced in its turn against the respect that must be given to private life.'

It was simply a balancing act. In this case, the court concluded that there was little public interest in the story, and Campbell's right to a private life prevailed.

5.3.5 Comment on disclosure of private information

However, in *Campbell v MGN* (2004), Lady Hale stated:

JUDGMENT

'Not every statement about a person's health will carry the badge of confidentiality or risk of doing harm to that person's physical or moral integrity. The privacy interest in the fact that a public figure has a cold or a broken leg is unlikely to be strong enough to restrict the press's freedom to report it. What harm could it possibly do?'

This view is contrary to the BMA guidance which states that, subject to limited exceptions (which we will consider slightly later):

QUOTATION

'There should be no use or disclosure of any confidential patient identifiable information gained in the course of professional work for any purpose other than the clinical care of the patient to whom it relates'.

Press interest is not an exception to the cardinal rule that confidential information should remain confidential, but what the courts seem to be suggesting is that disclosing information to the press that a famous footballer has a broken leg and will be unable to play for several months does not bear the weight of the breach of confidentiality as if it was disclosed that the same footballer was HIV-positive.

5.3.6 Comment on disclosure of human rights

As stated above, a balancing act between Art 8 and Art 10 HRA 1998 will be required. It is highly likely that medical information will fall comfortably within the protection of Art 8, and it would be hard to justify how disclosure could be justified under Art 10. When balancing the two rights, Lady Hale in *Campbell v MGN* (2004) said:

▪ The interference or restriction with the Article right must meet a pressing social need.
▪ It must be proportionate to the legitimate aim pursued (the interference must be no more than is necessary to protect the other right).
▪ The reasons given for the interference must be both relevant and sufficient.

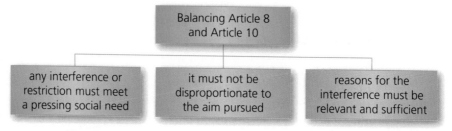

Figure 5.3 Balancing Arts 8 and 10, HRA 1998

5.3.7 A developing tort of misuse of private information

CASE EXAMPLE

Murray v Express Newspapers plc [2008] EMLR 12

The 19-month-old son of author J. K. Rowling was photographed with a long-range lens without his parents' consent. A photograph was later published in *The Sunday Express*.
The court rejected the notion that everyday acts could not attract a reasonable level of privacy. Taking the photograph was contrary to reasonable expectations.

JUDGMENT

'[The] question of whether there is a reasonable expectation of privacy is a broad one, which takes account of all the circumstances of the case. They include the attributes of the claimant, the nature of the activity in which the claimant was engaged, the place at which it was happening, the nature and purpose of the intrusion, the absence of consent and whether it was known or could be inferred, the effect on the claimant and the circumstances in which and the purposes for which the information came into the hands of the publisher.'

In summary, in determining whether there was a reasonable expectation of privacy, the following had to be taken into account:

• the attributes of the claimant
• the nature of the activity in which he was engaged
• where the activity was taking place
• the nature and purpose of the intrusion

- the absence of express consent or implied consent
- the effect on the claimant
- the circumstances in which and the purpose for which the information came into the hands of the publisher.

The court then had to consider striking the balance between the child's right to respect for his private life by virtue of Art 8, HRA 1998 and the rights of the publisher to freedom of expression under Art 10, HRA 1998. The court concluded that the approach was in line with the reasoning in *Campbell v MGN* (2004) and also the European judgment of *Von Hannover v Germany* (2004) 40 EHRR 1. The court held that reasonable expectation rested on the circumstances of the case and, particularly in this case as the complainant was a child, held that his right to a private and family life had been breached.

CASE EXAMPLE

McKennitt v Ash [2006] EWCA Civ 1174

The claimant, a Canadian folk singer, had obtained an injunction against the publication of the defendant's book. The defendant was a former friend and business associate of Ms McKennitt and was privy to personal and sensitive information about the claimant. One particular aspect that the claimant did not wish to be published was information relating to her health and diet. Lord Justice Buxton expressed the inviolable precept of confidentiality of medical material in the following terms:

JUDGMENT

'A person's health is in any event a private matter, as the *Campbell* case demonstrated. It is doubly private when information about it is imparted in the context of a relationship of confidence.'

He continued by stating that there is a reasonable expectation of privacy in relation to such matters, and that the question that needed to be addressed was as follows:

JUDGMENT

'First, is the information private in the sense that it is in principle protected by Art 8? If "no" that is the end of the case. If "yes", the second question arises: in all the circumstances, must the interest of the owner of the private information yield to the freedom of expression conferred on the publisher by Art 10?'

The second question above was not relevant to address as the medical information was both private and confidential.

The case confirms that the primary consideration is whether there has been a misuse of private information, rather than whether the information is true. The real legacy of this case lies in the fact that unless there are special circumstances that justify publishing private information Art 8, the right to a private and family life, prevails over Art 10 and freedom of expression.

5.3.8 Conclusion

Does the common law offer the patient any more protection than the professional guidelines issued by the governing bodies of the medical profession? Perhaps the reality of the matter is that a public figure would be able to seek an injunction from the courts to restrain material about their health being disclosed to the public. It is very unlikely that the courts will deny such an injunction given the precedents that have now been established, particularly in light of the most recent relevant case of *McKennitt v Ash* (2006). But what if the medical information has already been disclosed in a *Campbell*-style situation? In this situation, awarding damages is the only remedy and in these circumstances, where a person's private and personal medical information has been disclosed, damages are woefully inadequate. It is not the damages the claimant desires, but the confidentiality. Perhaps, the more effective remedy for the complainant is through the medical professionals' disciplinary body, in order to highlight the seriousness of the breach of confidence.

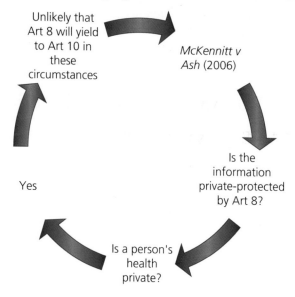

Figure 5.4 Misuse of private information

KEY FACTS

Key facts on confidentiality and privacy case law

Case	Judgment
Saltman Engineering Ltd v Campbell Engineering Ltd (1948)	There does not need to be an express term in the contract for material to be kept confidential.
Fraser v Evans (1969)	Emphasises the principle that a person cannot divulge another's confidential information.
Hunter v Mann (1974)	Refers to the doctor's duty not to disclose confidential information, save in limited circumstances.
W v Egdell (1990)	Equitable doctrine of confidentiality referred to between doctor and psychiatrist.
Attorney-General v Guardian Newspapers (1990)	The duty of confidence does not rely on any express or implied contractual term. There must be an unauthorised use of confidential material, the disclosure of which is detrimental to the person to whom the confidence is owed.
Wainwright v Home Office (2004)	Establishes no common law tort of privacy.
Campbell v MGN (2004)	There was a reasonable expectation of privacy.
McKennitt v Ash (2006)	Medical information was both private and confidential and was protected by Art 8.
Murray v Express Newspapers (2008)	There was a reasonable expectation of privacy which had been breached in this child's case. Art 8 has been violated.

ACTIVITY

Self-test questions

Ensure that your answers are supported by case law where appropriate.

- What is the ethical basis for the concept of confidentiality?
- Why is confidentiality important in a doctor–patient relationship?
- Is there a tort of privacy in England and Wales?
- Is a contractual relationship required in order to prove that a duty of confidence exists?
- When is a reasonable expectation of privacy established?
- Which factors need to be taken into account?

5.4 Exceptions to the confidentiality rule

5.4.1 Express consent

It would be misleading if one was to describe the granting of consent to disclosure as a specific exception to the rule of confidentiality as no duty of confidentiality exists if a patient consents to disclosure of their medical records. The express consent of the patient removes the doctor's duty of confidentiality.

CASE EXAMPLE

C v C [1946] 1 All ER 562

The parties were divorcing and the petitioner sought disclosure of information relating to venereal disease from the respondent's doctor. The respondent consented. The doctor refused but indicated that he would disclose the information if he was *subpoenaed* by the court.

In order to avoid the cost and unnecessary court attendance in future cases, the court indicated that in circumstances where a patient consents, the doctor cannot refuse to disclose medical records.

5.4.2 Implied consent

Although consent may not have been given expressly, it may have been impliedly granted. It is important for patients to recognise when this may occur and therefore when they have impliedly consented to disclosure of their medical records. The General Medical Council's guidance, *Confidentiality 2009*, para 25 states as follows:

QUOTATION

'Most patients understand and accept that information must be shared within the healthcare team in order to provide their care. You should make sure information is readily available to patients explaining that, unless they object, personal information about them will be shared within the healthcare staff, including administrative and other staff who support the provision of their care.'

The approach is entirely logical; if a patient attends their GP, who then refers the patient to a specialist, it would be both time-consuming and burdensome if the GP was to be required to seek the patient's express consent on each and every occasion.

5.4.3 The use of anonymous medical information

There is no breach of confidentiality where a patient cannot be identified from information that is disclosed.

CASE EXAMPLE

R v Department of Health ex p Source Informatics Ltd [2001] QB 424

Source Informatics was an American company which wanted to obtain information on doctors' prescribing habits in order that they could sell the information to drug companies for marketing purposes. The information to be disclosed was anonymous in the sense that the patients were not identified, although the area in which they lived would be disclosed by way of postcode. However, a Department of Health policy document warned GPs against disclosure as it would, even if data was made anonymous, breach patient confidentiality. Source Informatics sought to challenge this decision by way of judicial review.

There was no proprietary right in the prescription forms themselves from which the information was derived. Even though the patient had not expressly consented to disclosure there was no breach of confidentiality.

In the Court of Appeal, Simon Brown LJ held that the basis of the decision on whether to disclose confidential information which has been made anonymous was one of 'fairness' and this in turn was to be assessed according to the 'conscience of the confidant'. He therefore addressed the question:

JUDGMENT

'one asks, therefore, on the facts of the case: would a reasonable pharmacist's conscience be troubled by the proposed use to be made of patient's prescriptions?'

This subjective question was to be guided by the protection of the patient's privacy and in this case the patient's privacy was not infringed and the pharmacists had not breached their duty of confidentiality. However, this decision does not suggest that all data once made anonymous loses its confidentiality.

The difficulty with this decision is immediately ascertainable. The primary consideration is the fairness of disclosure rather than the overriding principle of ensuring that the patient's confidentiality is respected. It therefore suggests that all that a doctor needs to consider is whether it would be *fair* to disclose the material. Fairness is a particularly subjective term to use, and in these circumstances entirely contrary not only to the ethical position but also the professional guidance and common law.

The use of anonymised data suggests that if a person is not readily identifiable, they cannot be upset or offended by the use of such material. That does not necessarily follow as data could relate to, for example, the prevalence of certain conditions within a particular postcode or an age group or an ethnic grouping. It would not stretch the imagination too far to suggest that it would indeed be possible to identify a particular individual, which was the specific concern in *H (a healthcare worker) v Associated Newspapers Limited and N (A Health Authority)* [2002] EWCA Civ 195 (see later).

Nevertheless, the GMC in their professional guidance *Confidentiality, Protecting and Providing Information* (2000) does not reflect the suggested tone of this decision; indeed neither does subsequent case law. The guidance emphatically states that even where a patient does not object to data or information being disclosed, it is still incumbent upon the clinician to ensure that there is a likely benefit to the public before disclosure is made. If there is 'little or no evident' public benefit, disclosure should not be made without the patient's consent. If it is impractical to seek consent or where the patient lacks capacity, then the doctor must weigh the likely benefit to the public against the possible harm that may be caused to a patient. While this is still a subjective assessment, the guidance strongly supports the principle that the patient's confidentiality is the primary concern despite the judgment in *R v Department of Health ex p Source Informatics Ltd* (2001).

5.4.4 Public interest

This area poses real problems and immeasurable difficulties. Picture the situation where the patient 'confides' in the doctor that he is guilty of some violent crime, for example rape or murder, and the doctor honestly and genuinely feels that he should warn the authorities in case the patient reoffends. Does he break his patient's confidence, or is he bound to respect the patient's confidentiality as professional guidelines suggest?

Unsurprisingly, the law suggests that, if it is in the public interest that the information is disclosed, the doctor or medical professional will not be breaching the confidentiality of the patient.

CASE EXAMPLE

W v Egdell [1990] 1 All ER 835

W was detained in a secure hospital having been convicted of manslaughter. The defendant, a psychiatrist, was asked to prepare a report for the patient's legal representatives as W was seeking a transfer to another unit. The report was prepared but the hearing did not proceed. The defendant, aware that his report would not come to light when the patient was next routinely reviewed, sent a copy to the medical director of the hospital and urged a copy to be sent to the Home Office. The defendant was concerned that decisions about W's possible release could be made without taking the unfavourable contents of his report into account. W brought an action under the equitable doctrine of breach of confidence and also brought an action for breach of contract.

There was no question about the existence of the duty of confidence but 'the breadth of that duty' was carefully considered. The court referred to the *Spycatcher* (1990) case in the House of Lords where Lord Goff accepted that:

JUDGMENT

'the broad general principle ... that a duty of confidence arises when confidential information comes to the knowledge of a person ... in circumstances where he has notice, or is held to have agreed, that the information is confidential, with the effect that it would be just in all the circumstances that he should be precluded from disclosing the information to others.'

However, he added, there are limiting circumstances. There are circumstances where the public interest outweighs the principles that confidences should be preserved and protected. It was the court's duty to weigh up:

JUDGMENT

'the public interest in maintaining confidence against a countervailing public interest favouring disclosure ...'

The court held that the defendant had not breached the equitable obligation of the duty of confidence and found support in the GMC guidelines. Rule 81 sets out the exceptions to the duty of confidentiality and reflects the reality that the duty of confidence is not as absolute as it first appears. Rule 81 states:

QUOTATION

> 'Rarely, disclosure may be justified on the ground that it is in the public interest which, in certain circumstances, such as, for example, investigation by the police of a grave or very serious crime, could override the doctor's duty to maintain his patient's confidence.'

Let us consider what the situation may be if the patient tells the doctor that when he leaves the surgery/hospital he is going to harm his wife or girlfriend. What is the doctor's duty then? It may seem an obvious answer bearing in mind the guidance given in the case of *W v Egdell* (1990), as the medical professional would feel within the boundaries of both common law and professional guidance to alert the police. Is this enough? Should he warn the wife/girlfriend as well? Where does his responsibility end? This was precisely the situation that arose in the case of *Tarasoff* (1976) below.

CASE EXAMPLE

Tarasoff v The Regents of the University of California (1976) 17 Cal 3d 358

The defendant began a romantic attachment with the victim who was uninterested in him. He became mentally ill and sought mental health counselling at the University of California. He confided in his doctor and told him of his intention to kill Tatiana Tarasoff. The psychologist reported him to the university's police who briefly detained him but released him when he promised not to harm Tatiana. A few months later he killed Tatiana and her parents sued the university for failing to warn of the potential risk of harm.

The California Supreme Court considered the importance of confidential communications but held that the public health policy interest in protecting the public from a known risk of harm outweighed the duty of confidentiality. The case was settled out of court but the effect of the case is that, following the opinion of the California Supreme Court, those who are involved in the treatment of psychiatric patients have a *duty* to warn the authorities if a patient is a particular threat. Other US states such as Illinois have followed this judgment. Illinois law now states that a medical professional involved in a special relationship (doctor–patient) *must* warn third parties (relevant authorities and the victim) if the threat of harm to an identified victim is reasonably foreseeable.

Response of domestic law

The decision of *Tarasoff* (1976), while morally supportable, places an undue burden on the medical professional, and the extent to which the warning to the victim should take place is worthy of a lengthy discussion in itself. Domestic UK law has not to date encountered a similar case to *Tarasoff*, although the case of *W v Egdell* (1990) above has come close. However, tort law in England and Wales has more recently established that a health authority cannot be held liable for the actions of a third party.

CASE EXAMPLE

Palmer v Tees Health Authority [1999] EWCA Civ 1533

The claimant was a patient who had been diagnosed as having a personality disorder and had been abused as a child. When he was admitted to hospital he admitted he had sexual feelings towards young children. After he was discharged from hospital and while he was still an out-patient, he sexually assaulted and killed a young girl who lived in the same street. The mother sued the health authority, alleging a breach of duty of care for failing to diagnose the patient and failing to eliminate the risk that he posed.

The case was struck out and did not proceed to trial. It was not reasonably foreseeable that the patient would kill the victim; therefore there was insufficient proximity between the parties and the ultimate victim to establish a duty of care and accordingly there could be no course of action where the victim was not identifiable at risk.

If the facts had been a little different and the patient had clearly identified his potential victim then the courts may have found themselves in a *Tarasoff* situation, having to determine whether the medical professionals owed a duty of care to breach confidentiality. The GMC guidance referred to above states that disclosure can only be justified on the grounds of public interest where there is disclosure of information relating to 'a grave or very serious crime'. It is clear that it is not in the public interest to breach a patient's confidentiality relating to for example a theft or a burglary. *The Lancet* (vol. 374, 9707, page 2041) reports that doctors in the UK are now obliged to advise the police when they treat a patient whom they suspect has been involved in a serious gun or knife crime. Guidance from the GMC which came into force in October 2009 now makes the reporting of such serious crimes obligatory.

KEY FACTS

Key facts on cases considering the confidentiality rule

Case	Judgment
C v C (1946)	Express consent to disclosure of medical records adequate for doctor to disclose without breaching confidentiality.
R v Department of Health ex p Source Informatics Ltd (2001)	Anonymised data would not breach confidentiality if it was disclosed.
Tarasoff v The Regents of the University of California (1976)	Protecting the public outweighed the duty of confidentiality.
W v Egdell (1990)	No breach of the equitable duty of confidence.
Palmer v Tees Health Authority (1999)	Insufficient proximity between the parties to establish a duty of care.

5.4.5 Child protection

The area of child protection represents a further area where doctors are not always bound by confidentiality. Where a child is at risk of serious harm, public policy will prevail over the duty of confidentiality. However, it is a matter for the clinician as to whether he considers the harm to be sufficiently serious to inform the police or appropriate authorities. Guidance from the GMC document entitled *Confidentiality* (2009) states that if a doctor believes that a minor may be a victim of neglect or physical, sexual or emotional abuse, information *must* be disclosed to the appropriate authority if the medical professional believes it is in the patient's best interests or it is necessary to protect that person from serious harm.

5.4.6 The issue of confidentiality and HIV infection

ACTIVITY

Applying the law

Alan attends his GP. Alan tells him that he has recently discovered he is HIV-positive. The GP knows that his partner Brigit is pregnant and that he is also involved in more than one extra-marital relationship. What should the GP do? While Alan is entitled to have his confidentiality respected and not to be disclosed without his consent, there is a wider picture, to be considered.

There is a need to balance conflicting interests. Alan needs to have his confidentiality respected, not only as this is his right, but also because of the social stigma that is often associated with patients who are HIV-positive. Alan is likely to be concerned about potential discrimination and repercussions should his employers or friends find out. These real difficulties need to be balanced against the medical risk of HIV being transmitted as a result of sexual relations with Alan and, for Brigit, there is also a possible adverse effect on the unborn child. Furthermore there is also the risk to the women with whom Alan is having extra-marital relations.

The GP counsels Alan to inform his respective partners but Alan returns to the GP a while later and tells the GP that he has not informed any of his partners and is not going to as he is, firstly, embarrassed and, secondly, his partner Brigit will more than likely discover that he has been involved in other relationships. What steps should the GP now take?

Although the GMC had guidance on serious communicable disease, this has since been withdrawn and the guidance is now contained in the more generic *Confidentiality* (2009). This states that the GP could inform Alan's partners if he believes that Alan has not done so and cannot be persuaded to do so, in order:

QUOTATION

'to protect individuals or society from risks of serious harm, such as serious communicable disease.'

The guidance advises the GP to tell Alan that he is going to make contact with those concerned, if 'it is safe and practicable to do so'. It is of course possible that Alan resents what he may perceive to be the GP's interference. It continues:

QUOTATION

'you must be prepared to justify a decision to disclose personal information without consent ... You must not disclose information to anyone, including relatives who have not been, and are not, at risk of infection.'

Provided the GP can justify his actions he is permitted, rather than obliged, to disclose Alan's medical condition to his partner. He may also tell other women with whom Alan has been involved in a relationship. There is an obligation not to disclose the information to others who may not be directly at risk. The onus on the GP is significant and burdensome – what decision should he make? He needs to balance the harm he will cause by telling the parties with the harm he may cause by not telling them.

- If he tells Alan he is going to inform other parties, then he will risk losing Alan's trust and confidence. This is a significant problem for Alan's ongoing treatment of his HIV status.
- If his tells the women with whom Alan is having a relationship then he is protecting them from a potentially fatal condition but conversely he also may destroy their relationship.
- If he tells Brigit then the same principle above applies, but the fact that Brigit is pregnant may present a more compelling reason to tell her.

It is a matter for the clinician who has to be able to justify a delicate balancing act between public interest demands and the patient's confidentiality, with the hopeful expectation that his decision will benefit the public more than it will harm the patient concerned.

The conflicting issue of confidentiality towards HIV-positive patients and protecting society from the risk of serious harm may also become relevant when considering the Public Health (Control of Disease) Act 1984, amendments to which came into force in April 2010. Local authorities have been granted more extensive powers to prevent and control against the spread of infectious diseases, which could prevent significant harm to human health. While it appears that the legislation is largely directed towards the spread of contagious and/or infectious diseases around schools, there is a real concern that HIV patients could fall into this category. The effect of this is that if a medical professional was of the opinion that an HIV patient presented 'a serious and imminent risk to public health', he could report the patient to the local authority who could then apply to the Magistrate's Court for an order that he be detained for treatment.

While this could be a draconian interpretation on legislation, it is intended to deal with genuine fears such as the spread of measles in schools. The risk that this presents to the breach of confidentiality is real and alarming. Even more worrying is the potential conflict with *The NHS Trust and Primary Care Trusts (Sexually Transmitted Diseases) Directions (2000)*. This states that all NHS and PCTs shall take all necessary steps to ensure that no disclosure of any material, relating to a person who is being examined or treated for any sexually transmitted disease, should be made to anyone other than a medical practitioner involved in the treatment of the patient.

Thus far we have considered the limited situation where there is a relationship between a doctor and a patient. We have already seen in tort law, in the case of *Palmer v Tees Health Authority* (1999), that there was no common law duty to warn of the risk, although this was largely due to the victim being unidentified and the lack of reasonable foreseeability. It is worth considering the possible common law duty if Alan did transmit HIV to Brigit (however unlikely this may be) and she began an action in negligence for a failure to warn of the risks.

The case of *Goodwill v BPAS* [1996] 1 WLR 1397 may bear some relevance. The case concerned a failed vasectomy, and the partner of the patient sued the hospital for breach of duty of care. She was not the partner of the patient at the time of the operation, but a future partner to whom the court said that no duty of care was owed. If however she was the current partner then it is possible she would be owed a duty of care as it would be reasonable foreseeable that she would be affected; she could be readily identified and the relationship would be sufficiently proximate.

Accordingly, although there is no common law precedent in England and Wales, it is possible that if Brigit contracted HIV from the GP's failure to warn her, the court could impose such a duty. If the court took this approach, it would be in line with some parts of the USA where there is a general common law duty to inform, as illustrated in the American case of *Reisner v Regents of the University of California* (1995) 37 Cal Pptr 2d 518.

5.4.7 The public interest, freedom of the press and confidentiality

CASE EXAMPLE

X v Y [1988] 2 All ER 648

Two doctors working at a hospital had been diagnosed with HIV and the information had been disclosed to the newspapers. The health authority sought an injunction to restrain the newspapers from publishing the names of the doctors. The newspapers accepted that they had received the information in breach of confidentiality, but argued in favour of disclosure on the basis that matters such as whether HIV patient/doctors were at risk of infecting their patients were of public interest.

The court rejected this rather sensationalist media-based argument and held that medical records should remain confidential and that a person's expectation concerning confidentiality should be fulfilled. The judgment simply reflects the absolute duty of confidentiality save for where consent is given or where it is in the public interest. It was not in the public interest to be able to identify which doctor had been diagnosed with HIV as the risk of transmission was so insignificant.

JUDGMENT

'the public in general and patients in particular are entitled to expect hospital records to be confidential and it is not for any individual to take it upon himself ... to breach that confidence whether induced by a journalist or otherwise.'

Rose J stated:

JUDGMENT

'... in my judgment those public interests are substantially outweighed when measured against the public interests in relation to loyalty and confidentiality both generally and with particular reference to AIDS patients' hospital records.'

CASE EXAMPLE

H (a healthcare worker) v Associated Newspapers Limited and N (A Health Authority) [2002] EWCA Civ 195

The fact that the risk of transmission of HIV is very small was relevant in this case. Here the claimant, a healthcare worker, had tested positive for HIV. The health authority wished to notify all his patients so that they could be tested for HIV if they so wished. He claimed that this would be unlawful since the risk was so small that his breach of confidentiality could not be justified. In the meantime the *Daily Mail* newspaper wished to publish the story including information about the identity of the health authority and the specialty in which he worked. The health worker sought an injunction restraining the newspaper from publishing any material that could directly or indirectly lead to his identity being disclosed.

On the hearing of the injunction, the court upheld the health worker's right to confidentiality. The court had considered disclosing his area of specialism but H argued that if this was disclosed then it would become easier to identify him, especially if the name of the health authority was also disclosed. The argument was accepted but the court ordered that the information regarding his specialty be disclosed as the court accepted there was a genuine cause for debate among the public about dentists who were HIV-positive.

An interesting aspect about this case and one that distinguishes it from *X v Y* (1988) is that HRA 1998 came into force in 2000 and thus became relevant here. It was necessary to balance the healthcare worker's right to respect for his private life (Art 8) against the press freedom of expression (Art 10). It was one that the courts considered seriously and reflected in the court's decision to allow disclosure of his specialism. The court refused to accept that any harm could be done by allowing this disclosure, particularly in light of the health authority not being named. The court did remark that any inconvenience or expenditure would not restrain freedom of expression, stating that 'such consequences are the price which has to be paid, from time to time, for freedom of expression in a democratic society'.

5.4.8 Human rights in action

We have already touched upon the role of HRA 1998. Patient confidentiality complements the provision of Art 8 which provides for the 'right to respect for private and family life'. This right is qualified by Art 8(2) which provides that there shall be no interference with this right unless it:

ARTICLE

'is necessary in a democratic society in the interests of national security, public safety or the economic wellbeing of the country, for the prevention of crime, for the protection of health and morals, or for the protection of the rights and freedom of others.'

The cases below demonstrate the approach which the European Court of Human Rights hase taken when considering issues of medical confidentiality.

CASE EXAMPLE

MS v Sweden [1997] 45 BMLR 133 (ECHR)

The appellant had injured her back and was unable to return to work for a considerable time. Several years later she made an application for compensation. It transpired that her medical records had been disclosed at the request of the Social Insurance Office. Her claim for compensation was rejected. She complained to the European Commission of Human Rights, alleging that the unauthorised disclosure of her records amounted to an unjustified interference with her right to respect for private life under Art 8.

The court agreed that the disclosure of her records by the clinic to the Social Insurance Office amounted to an interference with Art 8. She had not expressly consented to the disclosure and there was no implied consent as her records had been disclosed for entirely different reasons, unconnected to her treatment. However, the court held that the interference could be justified under Art 8(2) as the disclosed information was necessary for assessing her initial claim. The court further explained that the interference sought to pursue the legitimate aim of protecting the economy by ensuring that compensation should only be paid in the correct circumstances. Since the staff to whom the information was disclosed were under their own duty of confidentiality, there was no breach of Art 8.

CASE EXAMPLE

Z v Finland (1998) *25 EHRR 371*

The applicant Z was married to X, who was HIV-positive. It was alleged that he had had sexual intercourse with a number of women despite being aware of his condition. The prosecution, in attempting to prove that he knew he had HIV and either knowingly or recklessly had sexual intercourse with women, obtained Z's medical files (who was also HIV-positive). The doctor was ordered to give evidence as to Z's condition in an attempt to prove X's knowledge. X was convicted and the press identified Z in their reports. Z appealed arguing that Art 8 had been breached.

- The doctor could be called to give evidence about her medical condition without her consent as the case was concerned with allegations of a most serious criminal nature. The interference was subject to strict limitations and Art 8 had not been breached.
- The seizing of the medical records was sufficiently important to outweigh the appellant's right to confidentiality and the hearing was heard in private. Again, Art 8 was not violated.
- The case papers were to remain confidential for ten years. The court held that to make it accessible would be a further infringement of her right to confidentiality. Furthermore, the court had violated her right under Art 8 when it permitted publication of her identity.

KEY FACTS

Key facts on cases of disclosure

Case	Principle
X v Y (1988)	Disclosure of the doctor's condition was not in the public interest.
H (a healthcare worker) v Associated Newspapers Limited and N (a health authority) (2002)	Limited disclosure would not breach the health worker's right to confidentiality. Balancing act between Art 8 (the right to a private life) and Art 10 (freedom of expression).
MS v Sweden (1997)	Article 8 was not breached by the disclosure of her medical records. The records were necessary to assess her claim and the interference was justified under Art 8(2).
Z v Finland (1998)	Article 8 was not breached as the importance of disclosure of the medical records outweighed her right to confidentiality.

5.5 Statutory provisions

There are some statutes which positively require disclosure of confidential information.

5.5.1 The National Health Service Act 2006

Section 251, National Health Service Act 2006 replaces s 60, Health and Social Care Act 2001, although there is very little, if any, change in the wording. It applies only in England and Wales, with no equivalent provision in Scotland or Northern Ireland. This extraordinary provision permits disclosure of confidential medical information for research purposes without a patient's consent. It states as follows:

SECTION

'the Secretary of State may by regulations make such provision for and in connection with requiring or regulating the processing of prescribed patient information for medical purposes as he considers necessary or expedient –

a) In the interests of improving patient care, or

b) In the public interest.'

With approval of the then newly introduced Patient Information Advisory Group (PIAG), medical information which identifies patients and where consent is considered impractical can be used without consent of the patient, provided the PIAG is satisfied that the disclosure is in the interests of patients or the public.

The PIAG's role is to 'assess applications by medical and research institutions to use non-anonymised information about patients without their consent' and to ensure that there are no alternatives to the use of this information.

More recent legislation, the Health and Social Care Act 2008, established the National Information Governance Board for Health and Adult Social Care (NIGB) for England which will absorb the functions of the PIAG. A new committee will be formed to hear applications for s 251 approval, more suitably known as the Ethics and Confidentiality Committee.

5.5.2 The Data Protection Act 1998

The Data Protection Act 1998 (DPA) is the most significant piece of legislation that governs the storage and usage of our personal data, originally enacted to absorb the Data Protection Directive 95/46/EC. It covers information that is held either on computer systems (or other electronic device) or in manual hard form. It does not include verbal communications which have not been physically recorded. The DPA 1998 now needs to be read in light of the more recent Freedom of Information Act 2000 which was drafted to include elements of the Data Protection Act 1998 concerning the storage of personal information in hospitals and GP surgeries.

The Data Protection principles are contained within Sched 1, Part 1 of the Act and state as follows:

SECTION

'(1) Personal data shall be processed fairly and lawfully and, in particular shall not be processed unless

a) at least one of the conditions in Schedule 2 is met and

b) in the case of sensitive personal data, at least one of the conditions in Schedule 3 is also met.'

Medical records are considered to be personal data.

SECTION

'(2) Personal data shall be obtained only for one or more specified and lawful purposes, and shall not be further processed in any manner compatible with that purpose or those purposes.

(3) Personal data shall be adequate, relevant and not excessive in relation to the purpose or purposes for which they are processed.

(4) Personal data shall be accurate, and where necessary, kept up to date.

(5) Personal data processed for any purpose or purposes shall not be kept longer than is necessary for that purpose or those purposes.

(6) Personal data shall be processed in accordance with the rights of data subjects under this Act.

(7) Appropriate technical and organisational measures shall be taken against unauthorised or unlawful processing of personal data and against accidental loss or destruction of, or damage to, personal data.

(8) Personal data shall not be transferred to a country ~~~~~~~~~~~~~~~~~~~~~~ Economic Area unless that country or territory ensures an adequate level of protection for the rights and freedoms of data subjects in relation to the processing of personal data.'

The eight principles which describe how data must be handled are presented in Figure 5.5.

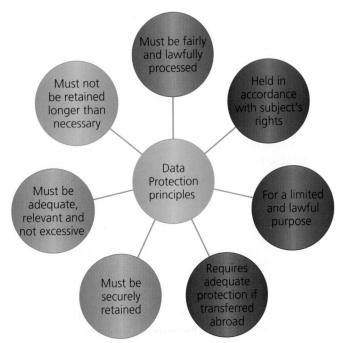

Figure 5.5 The eight principles of handling data

By virtue of s 68(2), a health record is defined as one which:

SECTION

's68(2) a) consists of information relating to the physical or mental health or condition of an individual and

b) has been made by or on behalf of a health professional in connection with the care of that individual.'

Schedule 3 refers to conditions that are relevant for the purposes of the first principle:

SECTION

'1) The data subject has given his explicit consent to the information being used.

2) (1)The processing is necessary for the purposes of exercising or performing any right or obligation which is conferred or imposed by law on the data controller in connection with employment.

3) The processing is necessary –

a) in order to protect the vital interests of the data subjects or another person, in a case where –

i) consent cannot be given by or on behalf of the data subject; or

ii) the data controller cannot reasonably be expected to obtain the consent of the data subject; or

b) in order to protect the vital interests of another person in a case where consent by or on behalf of the data subject has been unreasonably withheld.'

Furthermore, para 8 allows processing if it is necessary for medical purposes and is undertaken either by a medical professional or a person who although not a medical professional would still owe that duty of care.

Where the term medical purpose is referred to, this includes medical diagnosis, research and preventative medicine, providing care and treatment, and managing healthcare services.

It is the data controller's responsibility to ensure that all statutory obligations are complied with. A data controller is defined as a person who 'determines the purposes for which and the manner in which any personal data are, or are to be processed'.

Remedies

The importance of this legislation in protecting personal data is enforced by the penalties that can be enforced. Section 55(1) makes it a criminal offence to breach its provisions. Section 55 states:

SECTION

'a person must not knowingly or recklessly, without the consent of the data controller

a) obtain or disclose personal data or the information contained in personal data, or

b) procure the disclosure to another person of the information contained in personal data.'

In these circumstances under s 55(A) a financial penalty payable to the Data Protection Commissioner can be imposed, which can in turn be enforced through the civil courts in cases of non-compliance.

Compensation can also be payable to the person who has suffered distress or damage as a result of breach of the DPA 1998. Mere distress by itself is not enough. If a patient seeks compensation for medical data that was wrongly disclosed, it is insufficient to rely on distress and the patient has to prove damage caused as a direct result. However, if the defendant can demonstrate that he had taken such care in all the circumstances as was reasonably required, under s 13(3), the defendant may have an effective defence.

While this legislation aims to protect and effectively restricts the dissemination of personal data, s 28 in Part IV of the Act exempts personal data from the DPA principles if it is necessary for 'safeguarding national security'. Furthermore, under s 30(1) the Secretary of State can exempt information relating to the data subject's physical or mental health.

5.5.3 The Coroners and Justice Act 2009

The Coroners and Justice Act 2009 makes some minor amendments to the DPA 1998, although it would appear to affect data held by healthcare professionals only minimally.

Section 173 introduces Part 8 which provides the Information Commissioner with greater powers and allows him to investigate whether a public authority is complying with data protection principles. The objective of this section is to ensure that personal and sensitive data remains secure, although this does not appear to be particularly troublesome in the healthcare professions.

Section 174 requires the Information Commissioner to establish a Data Sharing Code which complies with best practice, while s 175, only partly in force at the time of writing, increases the powers of the Information Commissioner.

The highly contentious clause 152 has been withdrawn: this would have provided government departments with power to enable information-sharing which would have had significant implications for the confidentiality of a patient's medical records.

5.5.4 A patient's rights to access their own medical records

Patients have a right to access their own medical information, and legislation has provided the avenue to exercise this right.

The Access to Medical Records Act which was amended in 1990 has been largely repealed and replaced by DPA 1998. The only remaining part of any relevance is disclosure of medical records relating to a deceased person.

The three main relevant Acts are:

- **Data Protection Act 1998** which permits a patient to be able to access their own medical records. An authorised representative can exercise this right on behalf of the individual who is seeking access.
- **Access to Health Records Act 1990** which allows access to the health records of a patient who has deceased.
- **Medical Records Act 1988** which allows a patient under s 1 to access medical reports which have been prepared by a medical professional for insurance or employment purposes. The Act also allows an individual the right to refuse consent to disclosure of a medical report to an employer or insurance company.

The Data Protection Act 1998

We have already seen how DPA 1998 regulates the processing and disclosure of medical information of patients and contains eight guiding principles relating to disclosure. The DPA 1998 provides individuals (referred to as data subjects) with the right to access their own personal data. This includes access to medical records. Medical records are not limited to the written word and, according to the Department of Health's *Guidance for Access to Health Records Request* (2010), can include laboratory reports, radiographs, monitoring reports, imaging records and even videos and tape recordings of all telephone conversations.

Data controllers are people or organisations who are entitled to hold these records. They can be the NHS, a GP's practice or members of any private professional's practice who are obliged to comply with patients' rights. These rights which are known as 'access rights' are contained within ss 7, 8 and 9 of the Act.

Section 7 states that an individual is entitled

SECTION

'a) to be informed by any data controller whether personal data of which that individual is the data subject are being processed by or on behalf of that data controller'

The data controller must then provide a description of

SECTION

'(b) (i) the personal data of which that individual is the data subject,
     (ii) the purposes for which they are being or are to be processed, and
     (iii) the recipients or classes of recipients to whom they are or may be disclosed'

The data controller is not obliged to disclose any information about the data subject until he is satisfied as to the data subject's identity and the appropriate fee has been paid.

Section 4 states that if the data which the data subject requests refers to another individual, the data controller cannot release this information until:

- s 4(a) that other person has consented or
- s 4(b) it is reasonable to comply with the request of the data subject without first obtaining the other individual's consent.

With reference to s 4(b), s 6 sets out whether it is reasonable to proceed to disclosure without the consent of the identified individual. The following factors need to be taken into account:

SECTION

'(a) any duty of confidentiality owed to the other individual,
 (b) any steps taken by the data controller with a view to seeking the consent of the other individual,
 (c) whether the other individual is capable of giving consent, and
 (d) any express refusal of consent by the other individual'

The obligation contained in s 7(1)(c)(i), that is, 'the information constituting any personal data of which that individual is the data subject', must be supplied with unless:

SECTION

'(a) the supply of such a copy is not possible or would involve disproportionate effort, or
 (b) the data subject agrees otherwise;'

The implications of the above provision could be that if the data subject's medical records are particularly extensive, the data controller could refuse to process them on the grounds that the effort would be disproportionate to any potential gain. However, where an access request has been met, a further request does not need to be met until a reasonable period of time has elapsed. A request should be complied with by 21 days although, if this is not possible, the applicant should be informed.

The Data Protection (Subject Access) (Fees and Miscellaneous Provisions) Regulations 2000 set out the cost of copying the medical records, which even if held in electronic form must not exceed £50. Complying with a data subject's request should not be done with profit in mind.

More importantly, the Data Protection (Subject Access Modification) (Health) Order 2000 sets out limitations to the data controller's obligation to comply with a patient's right to access to their medical records.

Section 5 states that personal data can be exempt from s 7 if disclosure:

SECTION

'would be likely to cause serious harm to the physical or mental health or condition of the data subject or any other person'.

Furthermore, if access would relate to a third party, disclosure need not be made unless:

- the third party is a health professional who has either contributed to the health records or has been involved in the care of the patient, or
- the third party, who may not be a health professional, consents to the disclosure of that information, or
- it is reasonable to proceed with disclosure without that person's consent.

As we can see from above, there is no absolute right to a data subject's medical records.

CASE EXAMPLE

R v Mid-Glamorgan Family Health Service Authority ex parte Martin [1995] 1 WLR 110

The applicant had been a patient at a number of different hospitals and sought access to all of his medical records. The records were not subject to the statutory provisions of right of access under DPA 1998 or the Access to Health Records Act 1990 due to the period in which they were made. The hospitals were reluctant to disclose the records directly to the applicant as it was felt that they might harm the applicant since he had a history of mental illness. The hospital was content to disclose them to the applicant's legal adviser.

Sir Roger Parker LJ rejected the proposition that at common law a medical professional had an absolute property in a patient's medical records. On the other hand, he equally rejected the idea that a patient had an absolute right of access to his medical records. The reasons why a patient may want his medical records were so diverse that the court was unable and unprepared to specify the exact nature of the duty to disclose or restrict access to a patient's medical records.

The court held there was no common duty of access and a health authority as the owner of the records could refuse disclosure if it considered it was in the best interests of the patient.

A more recent example of this principle can be seen in the case below.

CASE EXAMPLE

Roberts v Nottinghamshire Healthcare NHS Trust [2008] EWHC 1934 (QB)

The claimant suffered from mental illness and was an in-patient at Rampton, a high-security psychiatric hospital. He had made an application under DPA 1998 for access to a report prepared by a psychologist on behalf of the defendants for use in a Mental Health Review Tribunal. Disclosure to the claimant's solicitors had already been refused and the defendants relied on DPA 1998 together with the Subject Access Modification to justify non-disclosure. The defendants relied on the argument that it would not be in the patient's interests to read the report as it could be harmful to his health.

The court accepted that the report was not to be disclosed to the patient. It considered the possibility of limited disclosure to the patient's representatives, but recognised the potential difficulty if their client asked to see the report. That would cause the solicitors to be professionally embarrassed and they would be obliged to withdraw. Furthermore, there was no statutory authority for part-disclosure and accordingly the application for judicial review failed.

Disclosure of medical records and patient access to their records reflects the fourth principle of accurate and up-to-date medical records clearly expressed in DPA 1998. To this end, a patient may seek to amend their medical records if the patient feels they are inaccurate. In the first place, the patient should discuss the proposed amendment with the healthcare professional and, if they are both agreeable, the amendment can be made to the records, with the original still visible. If the medical professional does not agree to the proposed amendment, the patient can enter a statement on the records to express their disagreement.

The Access to Health Records Act 1990

This statutory provision allows a limited group of people to be able to access a deceased's medical records.

Personal representatives are able to access a deceased person's medical records without any reservation. Section 3(1)(f) states that access is permissible 'where the patient has died' to 'the patient's personal representative and any person who may have a claim arising out of the patient's death'.

The latter group referred to, that is, those who may have a claim arising out the patient's death, will have to justify their claim before they may have access to a deceased patient's data. In a similar manner to the DPA 1998, disclosure should be made promptly and it is the data controller's responsibility to ensure that any person who does not have an automatic right to disclosure is able to clearly identify that they can properly seek access to the medical records of the deceased.

Interestingly enough, the Department of Health's *Guidance for Access to Health Records Request* (February 2010) indicates that access to a deceased person's medical records can be made in the absence of a statutory provision if it is considered that it is in the public interest to do so.

However, the public interest must be weighed against the breach of confidentiality which would inevitably occur, not only to the deceased patient but also the effect on the health service as a whole. Moreover, close consideration would be made to the effect on living individuals who could be affected by such disclosure and the damage that may be caused to the deceased's reputation. Recognition is made that the significance of confidentiality towards a deceased's medical records would diminish with time, a point we return to later.

The sensitively drafted guidance clearly expresses that those who wish disclosure of a deceased's records must have a:

QUOTATION

'legitimate purpose, generally a strong public interest justification and ... a legitimate relationship with the deceased patient'.

It is also recognised that reasons for disclosure could include a need or desire for relatives to understand more about the deceased's medical condition, particularly with genetic considerations in mind.

The courts have had to consider carefully the issue regarding access to a deceased person's medical records, and balance the public interest and the deceased's right to continuing confidentiality even after his death.

CASE EXAMPLE

Lewis v Secretary of State for Health and another [2008] All ER 90

In 2007, some workers at the nuclear industry at Sellafield in Cumbria who had died between 1962 and 1991 had had tissues removed for analysis. It later transpired that tissues from other workers at nuclear installations had also been taken for analysis. As the circumstances of why this took place were unclear, an investigation was ordered and a request was made to the claimant medical practitioner for disclosure of the medical records and documents. He was concerned that to do so might breach his own duty of confidentiality, and also the other doctors that were consulted when the other patients were alive. The question arose as to whether confidentiality survived the patient's death. The Secretary of State argued that disclosure should be made under the Health Service (Control of Patient Information) Regulations 2002. The claimant questioned whether the statutory provision granted sufficient authority, but it was for the courts to consider having balanced the competing interests.

In these circumstances, the duty of confidence did not survive the death of the patient. The statutory argument was rejected. The court relied on its inherent jurisdiction to hold that on this occasion the public interest to disclose the medical records outweighed maintaining the patient's confidentiality after death. The court also emphasised that safeguards should be in place to ensure that no information became public.

The GMC's guidance in *Confidentiality* (2009) is specific about the duty of confidentiality that is owed to a deceased patient. Paragraph 70 explains that where a patient has asked for information to be kept confidential, this request must be adhered to. In the absence of such a statement, there are a number of factors to be considered before information should be disclosed. These include:

- whether disclosure would be likely to cause distress to, or be a benefit to, the patient's partner or family
- whether the disclosure would disclose information about the patient's family or anyone else
- whether the information is already in the public domain or can be anonymised
- the purpose for the disclosure.

However, a deceased's records can be disclosed in the following circumstances:

- to help a coroner or similar officer with an inquest or fatal accident
- when required by law
- when authorised under s 251, NHS Act 2006
- when justified in the public interest
- when a parent asks for information about the circumstances and cause of a child's death.

Discussion point

Whether confidentiality is preserved once a patient has died has become the subject of recent interest from a historical perspective. Dr Raus Straus explores in his article 'To protect or to publish: confidentiality and the fate of the mentally ill victims of Nazi euthanasia' (2009) Journal of Medical Ethics, 35, pages 361–4) whether the identity of mentally ill patients who were murdered by the Nazi atrocities under the guise of euthanasia can be released. The question is whether Yad Vashem, the remarkable educational institution dedicated to preserving the memories of the victims of the Holocaust, can for these purposes and for public interest publish the names of the victims.

One of the difficulties would be that families who previously had not known the fate of their loved ones, would not only discover the manner in which they died but also that they suffered from mental illness. It is possible that a relative may not wish it made public knowledge that his or her grandparent suffered from mental illness.

This most unusual situation required a delicate balance to be made between disclosure in the public interest and preserving the confidentiality of a patient approximately 60 years after their death. The decision was so difficult to resolve and the confidentiality of the victims considered so vitally important to preserve that a decision was made to allow the names of the victims to be stored in a locked database but only to be assessed by committed researchers or family members.

KEY FACTS

Key facts on cases regarding a patient's rights to see his medical records

Case	Principle
R v Mid-Glamorgan Family Health Service Authority ex parte Martin (1995)	Disclosure of medical records could be refused if non-disclosure considered to be in the best interests of the patient.
Roberts v Nottinghamshire Healthcare NHS Trust (2008)	Disclosure to the patient of his records was refused on the grounds that it could harm his health and was therefore not in his best interests.
Lewis v Secretary of State for Health and another (2008)	Public interest in disclosure of medical records outweighed patient confidentiality.

5.5.5 Freedom of Information Act 2000

The Freedom of Information Act 2000 provided a general right of access to information held by public authorities. There are certain statutory exemptions; these include where the disclosure of the information could cause harm to an individual and where the information is given in confidence. Where there is a refusal to disclose, an application can be made to the Information Tribunal (formerly the Data Protection Tribunal).

CASE EXAMPLE

Bluck v Information Commissioner [2007] 98 BMLR 1

The complainant sought disclosure of her deceased daughter's medical records. Karen Davies died at Epsom General Hospital in 1998; the Trust had admitted liability and damages had already been settled. The complainant wished to know the circumstances surrounding the patient's death. The hospital acknowledged that they were in possession of some of the records but refused disclosure stating that the information was confidential. They relied upon s 41, Freedom of Information Act 2000, arguing that a duty of confidence survived death and that said duty was owed to the deceased. Section 41 states as follows:

SECTION

's41(1) Information is exempt information if —
  (a) it was obtained by the public authority from any other person (including another public authority), and
  (b) the disclosure of the information to the public (otherwise than under this Act) by the public authority holding it would constitute a breach of confidence actionable by that or any other person.
(2) The duty to confirm or deny does not arise if, or to the extent that, the confirmation or denial that would have to be given to comply with s 1(1)(a) would (apart from this Act) constitute an actionable breach of confidence.'

The Information Commissioner agreed with the hospital's refusal to disclose her medical records. The exemption from disclosure in s 41 was absolute and was not subject to a public interest test. Section 42 which applies to information which would be covered by legal professional privilege could be disclosed if there was some public interest element in doing so. However, this had to be balanced against the public interest of maintaining confidentiality between lawyers and client. On balance the tribunal came to the decision that the exemption under s 41 was valid and s 42 applied to some of the information.

This interesting case, being before an Information Tribunal, is not binding upon the court but was followed in *Lewis v Secretary of State for Health* (2008) above.

KEY FACTS

Key facts on disclosure under Freedom of Information Act 2000

Case	Judgment
Bluck v Information Commissioner (2007)	Exemption from disclosure of medical records pursuant to the Freedom of Information Act was valid.
	The duty of confidentiality survived the patient's death and medical records could not be disclosed.

5.5.6 Criminal offences

Police and Criminal Evidence Act 1984

Even where a crime can be considered serious, there is no statutory provision that requires the automatic release of confidential information. However, under Part 2, ss 8 and 9 of this Act, if there is a reasonable suspicion that an indictable offence has been committed, an application can be made to the court for disclosure of material. Section 12 confirms this can relate to documents and other records relating to a person's physical and mental health.

Misuse of Drugs (Notification of and Supply of Addicts Regulations) 1973

Any doctor who considers or has reasonable grounds to suspect that a person is addicted to a notifiable drug, for example cocaine, morphine or pethidine, shall notify the Chief Medical Officer within seven days, furnishing and thereby disclosing the patient's personal details.

Prevention of Terrorism (Temporary Provisions) Act 2000

Under these provisions, enacted to provide greater powers with which to fight terrorism, a person is under a duty to report his belief or suspicion that another is involved in terrorism or terrorist-related acts if such information comes to his attention through his trade, profession, business or employment. While it is a defence for that person failing to disclose to rely on reasonable excuse to justify his failure to disclose, reasonable excuse does not extend to the duty of confidentiality.

Road Traffic Act 1988

Section 172 provides that any person called upon must provide to the police information which can assist them in identifying a person alleged to have committed a road traffic offence. The information simply relates to identifying the person, and it is unlikely that any further information could be disclosed without an order from the court. Failure to comply is in itself a criminal offence.

CASE EXAMPLE

Hunter v Mann [1974] 2 WLR 742

A car was involved in an accident after it had been reported missing. That evening Dr Hunter treated a man and a girl who had been involved in the accident, advising them to admit their involvement to the police. He did not ask their consent to disclose the information himself. Section 168(2) of the Road Traffic Act 1972 states that 'any other person' shall if required as aforesaid give any information which it is 'in his power to give and may lead to the identification of the driver'. Dr Hunter was charged with failing to comply with this section. He argued that, although he did not have absolute privilege not to disclose information, the section did not apply as he was acting under the duty of confidentiality.

The court accepted that a doctor should never disclose confidential information unless there is a clear justification for doing so. However, applying the literal meaning of the words 'any other person' would include a doctor and accordingly his conviction was upheld.

5.5.7 Human Fertilisation and Embryology Act 1990 (HFE Act)

By virtue of s 31, HFE Act 1990, the Human Fertilisation and Embryology Authority is permitted to keep a register which contains details of all individuals who receive treatment or services provided by the Act. Section 33A creates an obligation on those who hold information not to disclosure.

5.5.8 Public health concerns

NHS (Venereal Disease) Regulations 1974, the NHS Trusts (Venereal Diseases) Directions 1991 and NHS Trusts and Primary Care Trusts (Sexually Transmitted Diseases) Directions 2000

The statutory provisions state that all information relating to a patient being treated or examined with and for a sexually transmitted disease shall not be disclosed unless for the purpose of contacting those people with whom the patient may have had sexual relations. This can be done without the patient's consent if the patient has not informed them and cannot be persuaded to do so. If it is practicable, the identity of the patient is not disclosed.

Public Health (Control of Disease) Act 1984 and Public Health (Infectious Diseases) Regulations 1988

Doctors in England and Wales are under a statutory duty to notify and disclose patient details to the local authority officer (a public health officer) if they are aware or have cause to suspect that a patient is suffering from a notifiable disease.

This includes diseases such as cholera, food poisoning and measles but excludes HIV and AIDs. This exclusion is essential as patients with HIV and AIDs must not feel that, if they seek medical help, their condition will be reported. This would undoubtedly deter many patients from seeking help. Furthermore, if people who are HIV-positive and suffer from AIDs treat their conditions responsibly, they pose virtually no risk to others.

Abortion Regulations 1991

By virtue of Reg 4, a medical professional who carries out a termination of pregnancy is obliged to notify the Chief Medical Officer. Under Sched 2 he must provide details of the woman's name and address, date of birth, marital status and her history of pregnancy and history. However, more recent provisions require her NHS number rather than her name and address, a simple step to help preserve her anonymity. Regulation 5 ensures that abortion information is kept confidential.

Births and Deaths Registrations Act 1953

Medical staff have a duty to inform the district medical officer of a baby's birth.

Section 22 requires a doctor who has attended a patient during his last illness to sign a death certificate and forward it to the Registrar of Births and Deaths.

Section 11 requires all stillbirths to be registered.

Key facts on disclosure under Road Traffic Acts

Case	Principle
Hunter v Mann (1974)	S 168, Road Traffic Act 1972 applied to a doctor and he was under a duty to disclose relevant information.

5.5.9 Duties of a doctor to the Driving and Vehicle Agency (DVA)

If a doctor considers that his patient is suffering from such a medical condition that he considers that patient should not be driving, he should persuade that patient to report it to the DVA.

If the patient lacks capacity to understand the advice he is being given, the doctor should advise the DVA himself. The doctor can also discuss the matter with the patient's family with the patient's consent. A doctor may disclose personal information if he decides that such disclosure is in the public interest without the patient's consent, and can still disclose in exceptional circumstances where the patient has withheld consent. The circumstance within which this operates is where the doctor considers that the benefit to an individual or to society as a whole justifies intrusion into a patient's confidential information. Therefore careful consideration must be given to the circumstances as they appear and, if necessary, the doctor should take such steps as he considers he can justify.

5.6 Children and the role of confidentiality

While a doctor must ensure that he maintains his patient's confidence, it is axiomatic that this is impossible where the treatment of young children is concerned. Parents are involved with the decision-making process of their child's treatment and there is an obvious need to ensure that they are kept informed at every conceivable stage. When considering a young child, the duty of confidentiality must be owed to the child's parents as well as to the patient.

We have already seen in the case of *Gillick* (1986) that where a child reaches an age of sufficient maturity and understanding, he or she has a right to keep their medical information from their parents. It follows that provided a child has achieved the status of having capacity to consent, their medical records will also be kept confidential from their parents.

Some 20 years after the case of *Gillick* (1986) established such ground-breaking principles, the case below sought a fresh challenge to such a prized status.

CASE EXAMPLE

R (Axon) v Secretary of Health [2008] EWHC 372 (Admin)

By way of judicial review Mrs Axon challenged the 2004 Department of Health guidance document, arguing that it was unlawful and had misrepresented the law in *Gillick* (1986).

Firstly, she maintained that the duty of confidence of medical professionals that was owed to a child when consulted on matters such as contraception, sexually transmitted infections and abortions was subject to parental knowledge unless doing so 'would or might prejudice the child's physical or mental health so that it is in the child's best interests not to do so'.

Secondly, Mrs Axon argued that the *Gillick* decision needed to be read in light of Art 8, ECHR, which conveyed a right to a private and family life, which she maintained included the right to be advised of treatment to a child aged under 16 on matters involving contraception, sexually transmitted infections and abortions. An obligation to keep confidences did not, she maintained, include those between parent and child.

The application for judicial review was rejected. The DOH guidance was not unlawful as it embodied the *Gillick* guidelines.

In rejecting the first argument the court stated that *Gillick* was to be applied in all cases involving advice and treatment to children concerning contraception, sexually transmitted infections and abortion.

In relation to Mrs Axon's reliance on Art 8, the court rejected this argument, stating that *Gillick* had already decided that the duty of confidence between health professional and child should be preserved. Silber J could not see any justification for reliance on Art 8; a parent could not maintain authority over medical advice given in relation to sexual matters where a child had capacity and an adequate understanding so as to be '*Gillick* competent'.

While the duty of confidentiality is not absolute, confidentiality in this sense would be subject to the health professional's clinical opinion as to whether a child under 16's physical or mental health may be called into question. However, if a child under 16 is deemed to have capacity to consent to treatment then a child should be entitled to have such confidences respected and maintained. Failure to do so would make a mockery of a child having capacity to consent and renders the *Gillick* decision worthless. If Mrs Axon succeeded, it would reverse a child's willingness to have faith and trust in their doctor and the ability to consult them on such important yet personal and sensitive matters.

The position of adults who lack capacity is similar to that of children, as was established in the earlier case below.

CASE EXAMPLE

R (on the application of S) v Plymouth City Council [2002] EWCA 388

The mother of an incapacitated patient wished to have access to the medical records of her child as part of an ongoing dispute with the local authority concerning her son's guardianship order. Although the local authority agreed to disclose some medical records, they refused to disclose them either to her solicitors or herself directly.
Hale LJ held in the Court of Appeal that:

JUDGMENT

'both at common law and under the Human Rights Act, a balance must be struck between the public and private interests in maintaining the confidentiality of information and the public and private interests in permitting, indeed requiring, its disclosure for certain purposes'.

In a difficult balancing exercise and on the facts of this case, the court allowed disclosure, stating:

JUDGMENT

'there is a clear distinction between disclosure to the media with a view to publication to all and sundry and disclosure in confidence to those with a proper interest in having the information in question'.

The principle reflected in the case is mirrored in guidance from professional bodies. In recognising that a duty of confidentiality is owed to patients who may lack capacity, there is also recognition that there may be occasions where medical information may need to be disclosed. If a person who lacks capacity refuses disclosure, every effort should be made to have an appropriate adult at a consultation.

In order to assess the patient's best interests, it may be necessary to share personal information with the patient's relatives, friends or carers or a person entrusted to represent the patient's interests. Even so, disclosure must be relevant and pertinent to the reasoning behind the current disclosure.

KEY FACTS

Key facts on disclosure where patient is a child or adult who lacks capacity

Case	Judgment
R (Axon) v Secretary of Health (2008)	A '*Gillick* competent' minor had a right of confidentiality and this could not be overridden by Art 8 in order to allow her parents to access medical information.
R (on the application of S) v Plymouth City Council (2002)	On occasions, where patients lack capacity, it may be necessary to permit a breach of confidentiality in order to determine a patient's best interests.

ACTIVITY

Self-test questions

Ensure that all your answers are supported by case law or appropriate authority.

- If a patient cannot be identified from disclosed information, can there be a breach of confidentiality?
- Provide examples of where confidentiality can be breached in cases of public interest.
- If a doctor is diagnosed with HIV, can his status be disclosed to his patients?
- What effect has HRA 1998 had on confidentiality?
- Explain how a patient can access their own medical records.
- Can a deceased's medical records be disclosed?
- Describe four situations where there is a statutory duty to disclose medical records.

SUMMARY

- The notion of confidentiality is a fundamental and historical principle of the relationship between doctor and patient. Without the principle of confidentiality, a patient may be reluctant to confide in their doctor – a situation which could have a direct effect on the patient's treatment.
- Although there is no tort of privacy recognised in the UK, there has been a development of the tort of misuse of private information, within which a patient's medical records doubtless falls.
- However, there are some occasions where either the public interest or statutory provisions indicate that confidentiality can or should be breached. These are however retained within close perimeters in order that the sacred principle maintains intact.

SAMPLE ESSAY QUESTION

Critically evaluate the view that while health professionals are obliged to maintain confidentiality, there may be circumstances where the interest in maintaining confidentiality is outweighed in the public interest and disclosure is then justified.

This essay-style question is straightforward, requiring you to explain how a duty of confidentiality arises and then critically evaluate occasions on which breaching a patient's confidentiality is permitted. It is largely dependent on the time you are allowed for writing an answer as to how much of the material below you would have the time to include. Therefore, this answer is all-inclusive but it is not expected you would include *all* of the material below in a 45-minute essay.

- It is advisable to progress through the essay logically and to begin with discussing the origins of the duty of confidentiality; the Hippocratic Oath and the Declaration of Geneva would be a good place to start.
- Refer to the professional guidelines – demonstrate a knowledge of their statements on confidentiality.

- The common law has demonstrated that there is no right to privacy – *Wainwright v Home Office* (2004) is an excellent example of this and so is *Hunter v Mann* (1974), but it is also necessary to be able to discuss the development of the new tort of misuse of private information through cases such as *Campbell v MGN* (2004) and *McKennitt v Ash* (2006). While there is no difficulty in proving that medical information amounts to confidential information, these dicta may have some very useful reference to health records, and these are the types of references that should be included.
- It is worthwhile making reference to HRA 1998, Arts 8 and 10, and how a right to a private and family life will always triumph over the press's freedom of expression as far as confidentiality of medical records is concerned.

- The question now requires you to critically evaluate the occasions on which public interest allows disclosure.
- *R v Department of Health ex parte Source Informatics Ltd* (2001) – anonymous confidential information could be disclosed if the clinician considered it was fair to do so. This was to be judged according to the conscience of the confidant.
- You may wish to be critical about this judgment, as the element of fairness as a tool for assessment is not comparable with respect for the overriding principle of confidentiality. The GMC guideline *Confidentiality* (2009) confirms that anonymous data should still only be disclosed if there is a likely benefit to the public.
- Clinicians deal with real-life problems and sometimes the public interest may outweigh confidentiality, but it can be a difficult balancing exercise.
- Discuss the case of *W v Egdell* (1990) and the breadth of the duty that was discussed when making reference to the *Spycatcher* case (1990).
- The case of *Tarasoff* (1976) represents a good illustrative example even though it is not binding on UK jurisdiction, and reference to *Palmer v Tees* (1999) would illustrate how no duty of care can be imposed if it is not reasonably foreseeable.
- Public interest is also an issue where a patient may be HIV-positive, and this should form part of a discussion. Reference should be made to GMC guidelines, other statutory provisions and also common law, *X v Y* (1988) and *H (a healthcare worker) v Associated Newspapers Limited and N* (2002) as all these areas highlight the public interest argument.

- There are also a number of statutory provisions that require disclosure to be made, and several of these should be mentioned as they focus on the public interest element. Among these are child protection, the National Health Service Act 2006, DPA 1998, statutes governing public health concerns, statutes governing criminal offences and the Road Traffic Act 1988.
- Statutory provisions should be highlighted, discussed and reference made clearly to where the public interest arises.

- An appropriate conclusion should be drawn, perhaps suggesting that while the tenet of confidentiality is paramount, there are exceptions as it is not an absolute duty. In concluding, mention should be made of the professional guidelines; while disclosure can be made, it is still within very strict parameters.

Further reading

Department of Health (February 2011) *Guidance for Access to Health Records Requests.*
General Medical Council (October 2009) *Confidentiality Guidance for doctors.*
McLean, A. and Mackey, C. (2007) 'Is there a law of privacy in the UK? A consideration of recent developments', *European Intellectual Property Review*, 29(9) pages 389–95.

6

Ethical theories

AIMS AND OBJECTIVES

After reading this chapter you should be able to:

- Understand the role of ethical theories in context of the study of bioethics
- Be able to demonstrate an appreciation of different ethical theories
- Demonstrate an ability to apply the theories to ethical dilemmas.

6.1 Introduction

Medical ethics is the term used to describe traditional dilemmas within the doctor–patient relationship, such as the question of confidentiality or a patient's consent. It is the study of moral dilemmas as they are applied to the field of medicine. There is an overlap between medical ethics and bioethics, the latter being the more modern and progressive term that reflects twenty-first century issues. The term 'bioethics' comes from the Greek words '*bios*' meaning life and '*ethos*' meaning behaviour. The remarkable advances in medical technology over recent years mean that the dilemmas faced by society are much more complex than more traditional dilemmas that can occur in the doctor–patient relationship. For example, whether a person should be allowed to sell their kidney is not a question that can be resolved in a doctor–patient relationship as it has profound effects on the whole of society. This is precisely the type of dilemma that needs to be considered. Other issues we will consider throughout this book include the following:

- Is it ethically permissible to turn off a patient's life support machine?
- If a minor child can consent to medical treatment, why can they not refuse treatment?
- Can an adult refuse treatment even if it will lead to their death?
- Can a person seek another's help to end their own life?
- Is abortion of a child with disabilities ethically permissible?

How do we start to approach these complex issues? One often instinctively knows whether something is ethically permissible without any recourse to ethical theories. We may have a 'gut instinct' response to whether something is ethically acceptable or not, but caution should be used when relying on instinct alone. It is important to be able to substantiate a view by support and explanation to a theory. One cannot simply say 'selling a kidney is wrong because I feel strongly about it'; it is necessary to provide an explanation of why it is wrong.

Challenge your own beliefs in the following chapter. If you feel strongly that an act is ethically permissible or not, there is nothing wrong with maintaining this view, provided you can support it by reference to an ethical principle and, most importantly, provided you can see the opposing argument as well. You can then reject the argument if you feel so inclined and explain why you reject it. One can either take a secular approach or a more theological approach and it is important to note that many modern medical technologies such as pre-implantation genetic diagnosis are with some limited exceptions supported by religious groups. Abortion however probably remains one of the most controversial areas where religious views can still dominate.

We begin by considering the more secular and dominant theories.

6.2 The secular perspective

 ### 6.2.1 Consequentialism and utilitarianism

QUOTATION
....

'A consequentialist is someone who thinks that what determines the moral quality of an action are its consequences.' (Hare (2010))

Consequentialism allows us to decide whether an act is ethically or morally permissible according to its consequences (hence the term consequentialism). The more favourable the consequence, the more the act should be encouraged. If the act allows favourable or good consequences then it should be encouraged, but if it allows bad consequences then it should be discouraged. In order to determine the value of an act, one must weigh up the alternatives of each of the actions and decide which has the best consequence. On a superficial level, this is an attractive theory as it addresses issues on a basic level – what will give me greater pleasure, a visit to the cinema or a trip to the theatre? What will give the patient the greatest pleasure, having a kidney transplant or not? Obviously, assuming the kidney is not rejected by the patient, the favourable consequences are that he receives a transplant.

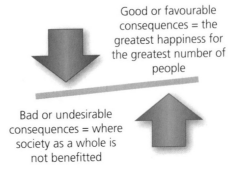

Good or favourable consequences = the greatest happiness for the greatest number of people

Bad or undesirable consequences = where society as a whole is not benefitted

Figure 6.1 Balancing favourable or undesirable consequences

One form of consequentialism is utilitarianism, which has been 'regarded by many as underpinning modern ethical medicine' (Mason and Laurie (2010), page 6).

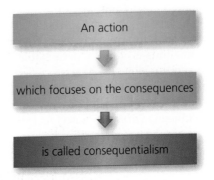

An action

which focuses on the consequences

is called consequentialism

Figure 6.2 What is consequentialism?

Act-utilitarianism

Act-utilitarianism is concerned with the moral value of an act, and this is judged by assessing its utility. Its objective is that the consequences of any action should be only favourable so that a person experiences pleasure. A good consequence is one that results in pleasure, not pain. Happiness and pleasure are the ultimate goals, and what does not make a person happy or pleasurable should not be adopted or pursued. The moral value of an action is judged only by its potential outcome: the consequences of the act.

Historically, the most significant proponents of utilitarianism and the development of the wider notion of consequentialism are John Stuart Mill (1806–73) and Jeremy Bentham (1748–1832). The Bentham principle can be defined as the moral act which emits 'the greatest good for the greatest number of people'. In 1789 Bentham wrote *The Principle of Morals and Legislation*, and in Chapter 4 he described a formulaic approach or 'felicific calculus' to be applied in order to determine the greatest happiness to the greatest number of people. This approach has been described as 'Bentham's way of becoming the Newton of the moral world' (Wesley C. Mitchell (June 1918) *Political Science Quarterly*, Vol. 33, No. 2, pages 161–83).

In Chapter 1 of *The Principle of Morals and Legislation*, Bentham said:

QUOTATION

'Nature has placed mankind under the governance of two sovereign masters, pain and pleasure. It is for them alone to point out what we ought to do, as well as to determine what we shall do. On the one hand the standard of right and wrong, on the other the chain of causes and effects, are fastened to their throne.'

Therefore, in order to determine whether an action is morally acceptable, the various pleasures and the pain that may be derived from it should be determined according to their:

propinquity
close or proximate

fecundity
the ability to produce further pleasures

- Intensity – how strong is the pleasure?
- Duration – how long will the pleasure last?
- Certainty – how certain is it that there will be pleasure?
- **Propinquity** – how soon will the pleasure happen?
- **Fecundity** – the probability that the pleasure to be derived from the action will reoccur.
- Purity – the probability that pleasure will not be followed by pain.
- Extent – the extent to which people will be affected.

The 'felicific calculus' was to be applied to a multitude of utility areas such as economics and criminal justice. We will refer to its application to modern day medical ethics shortly.

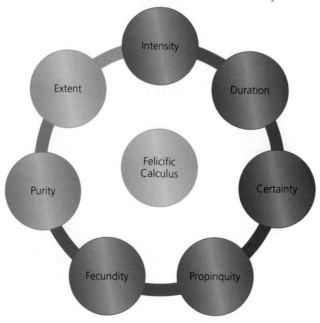

Figure 6.3 The components of felicific calculus

Discussion point

If we attempt to apply act-utilitarianism in practice, there are possibilities of unsavoury outcomes, the consequences of which invade our social values and principles of justice. For example, an often-quoted scenario (see Herring (2011) or Pattinson (2009)) is of a doctor presented with several ill patients, all of whom are waiting urgent transplants without which they will surely die. If, however, the doctor was to kill one healthy visitor then all three patients would survive. A utilitarian may be satisfied by this approach as it would cause the greatest happiness to the greatest number of people. Imagine also that all three of the patients have partners, dependent children, valuable jobs and the healthy visitor has no family at all and few friends. From a consequentialist point of view, the three patients' survival would outweigh one person's death, as the greatest happiness would be derived from all those family members and friends that would celebrate the transplant.

In order to combat this clear injustice and almost radical application, rule-utilitarianism seeks to provide a balance.

Rule-utilitarianism

This principle suggests that a set of rules is adopted to assist with what creates the best possible outcome. As an alternative to considering the potential consequences of an action, the rule-utilitarian considers the rules of the action in order to determine how right or correct the act would be. Once the correct rule is applied, the consequences of the outcome with the rule are considered. The rule with the best consequences is the one that should be morally adopted. The difference between the two concepts is that act-utilitarianism considers the most favourable outcome by actions, and rule-utilitarianism considers the outcome by an application of rules.

Rule-utilitarianism can be self-contradictory. If we adopt the rule that one should not kill, on the face of it we should be content with such a fundamental principle. However, if we consider the rule a little further, we start to challenge ourselves. As a society we largely consider it acceptable to kill another with whom we are lawfully at war, and indeed it is not unlawful to do so, but as a rule-utilitarian it would not be ethically permissible to do so even though it would cause happiness to the greatest number of people. Another such example is the act of self-defence: if a person may not kill then it follows it would not be ethically permissible to kill another in self-defence even though it is legally permissible to do so.

In order to remedy the significant defect that appears in rule-utilitarian, John Stuart Mill introduced the idea of **weak rule-utilitarianism** which states that although rules are relied upon in order to determine what benefits society to the greatest extent, the rule need not be followed if it creates the greatest happiness *not* to follow that rule. Weak rule-utilitarianism offers the greater opportunity of justice as opposed to **strong rule-utilitarianism** which imposes an absolute position: rules are there for the benefit of society and should not be broken under any circumstances.

6.2.2 Criticisms of consequentialism and utilitarianism

Utilitarianism is concerned with trying to achieve the greatest happiness for the greatness number of people. However, in order to achieve this ultimate goal, the risk of overlooking a person's right for the good of society is unavoidable. One of the difficulties with applying wholly utilitarian principles is that it ignores the principles of justice (disregarding the need of one person in favour of the greater good of many) and autonomy (as utilitarianism implies that all persons must act in a similar way and accordingly denies a person self-determination and free will).

Since an act is morally acceptable according to its perceived consequences, one insurmountable difficulty is that it is impossible to predict the consequences of a given action with any degree of accuracy. For example, will the kidney transplant be successful, and how long will the success last? Since it is not possible to predict the accurate consequences of an action, it is not possible to judge the value of one consequence over another.

6.2.3 Deontology

Deontology contrasts with utilitarianism in the sense that while utilitarianism is concerned with the consequences of an action, deontology's primary concern is whether an action is intrinsically wrong. For example, murder is wrong not because of the consequences of the act, that is, the pain as opposed to pleasure caused to the friends and family, but because the act itself is intrinsically wrong. Deontology's principle revolves around whether an act is deemed to be good or bad, and the role of a person's duty in everyday life. A doctor has a duty to diagnose and treat his patient to the best of his skill and ability, and it is this duty that is his primary concern rather than the consequences of his action.

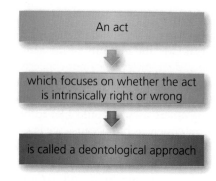

Figure 6.4 What is deontology?

ACTIVITY

We can illustrate the deontological principle by considering the following example. A woman gets dressed to go out for the evening and she asked her husband whether she looks nice in her new dress. The utilitarian replies 'Yes' even if she does not look nice because by answering affirmatively he is conveying pleasure, not pain and creating happiness for the greatest number of people – his wife because she feels as if she looks nice, even if it is not true, and himself because he has made her feel happy! On the contrary, a deontologist addresses the same question differently. He has a duty to tell the truth and he knows inherently that lying is not right. The deontologist will tell the truth, regardless of the consequences and his wife's feelings. Which is the better approach?

Immanuel Kant

Immanuel Kant (1724–1804) is the most significant and well-known deontologist. He argued that the most important approach is doing the right action combined with the will or motive of the person involved in making that decision. In order to do what is morally right, people should act from a sense of duty, not from a consideration of the possible consequences.

Thus, rights-based or duty-based theories are associated with Immanuel Kant and deontology. In his *Groundwork of the Metaphysic of Morals* (1785) the Categorical Imperative set out his formulae for guiding moral principles. They are as follows:

QUOTATION

'Act only according to that maxim whereby you can at the same time will that it should become a universal law.

Act in such a way that you treat humanity, whether in your own person or in the person of any other, never merely as a means to an end, but always at the same time as an end.

Therefore, every rational being must so act as if he were through his maxim always a legislating member in the universal kingdom of ends.'

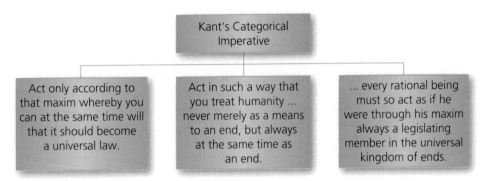

Figure 6.5 Kant's Categorical Imperative

With reference to the first of the Categorical Imperatives, referred to as the Formulae of the Universal Law, the morality of the action must not be dependent on the individual person. Since deontology does not concern itself with the individual, the maxim must have universal application and broadly reflects the accepted principle that one should only do to others as they would expect others to do unto them. More simply put, we should treat others as we would like to be treated, not through any consideration of potential consequences but because we have a duty to do so.

There is a link between the two rules, the latter of which is probably regarded as one of the most important maxims; we should never act in a way which treats ourselves or others merely as a means to an end. By applying the Formulae of the End in Itself, we maintain an ultimate respect for the way we treat others which is, after all, a laudable concept. With this in mind, deontology is an attractive moral theory.

Discussion point

The moral superiority of deontology over utilitarianism can be seen in the following example. Utilitarianism is often considered to be the moral principle that was used to justify the Nazi's deplorable experiments in the Second World War (such as experiments on twins, sterilisation experiments, mustard gas and freezing experiments) which were allegedly carried out in the name of science. They argued that scientific experimentation would benefit mankind as a whole, but from a deontologist's point of view these acts were morally wrong and deontologists could quite rightly never justify such inhumane actions. The victims of the atrocities were treated solely as a means to an end – a principle rejected by deontologists. The perpetrators were tried at Nuremberg, and the Nuremberg Code of Medical Ethics is the basis of many countries' code of medical ethics today.

Let us revert to the earlier example on page 178 where a doctor has three seriously ill patients – a consequentialist may be able to justify the killing of the healthy visitor in order to save three seriously ill lives, but a deontologist could not. One cannot kill the visitor for the simple reason that it is wrong; one cannot use a person simply as a means to an end; killing one person to save three is not morally right and therefore cannot be condoned.

Discussion point

President George Bush disclosed in recent media reports that torture methods of 'water boarding' had been used in the USA with the result that alleged terrorist suspects divulged terrorist targets in the USA, Europe and the UK. How would a utilitarian view this statement? It is likely that a utilitarian point of view would find this acceptable even though Art 3 of the European Convention on Human Rights (ECHR) does not permit torture or degrading treatment. Utilitarianisms would consider this act to be acceptable as it would cause the greatest happiness to the greatest number of people, because more lives would be saved by extracting this information. Deontologists however would find this is unacceptable, as they do not believe it is ever right to use a person as a means to an end and this act, which many would describe as torture, would never be morally right.

However, deontology can be criticised for the lack of flexibility projected by its theory. If there is a dispute between consequentialists it can be resolved through a discussion of what is the best possible outcome or consequence. A deontologist cannot resolve a dispute because there is no dispute to resolve. An act is right or wrong based upon the concept of duties and obligations.

6.2.4 Ethical principles applied

In this section we attempt to apply utilitarianism and deontology to some essential principles that we have explored in this book so far, or will encounter shortly.

Informed consent

We have already considered the legal importance of informed consent in Chapter 2, from which we understood that it is essential to obtain a patient's consent prior to treatment, and in order to do so it is essential to provide the patient with sufficient information in order that he or she can make an informed decision.

The interaction of both consequentialism and deontology can be seen in the ethical justification for informed consent.

From a consequentialist view, it is more beneficial to treat a patient who has been fully informed about the treatment she is to undertake, together with all the potential risks involved in the treatment process. A patient is more likely to be willing to follow recommended treatment if she is involved in the process rather than having the process imposed upon her. Modern medicine is less about deference to a doctor's opinion of the appropriate treatment to follow and more about the forging of a relationship where the doctor is best placed to advise, but the patient may be better placed to consider what treatment is more appropriate for them, given their lifestyle, available time, potential side effects, their personal priorities or life goals.

The difficulty with the consequentialist approach is with its actual application. How does the patient know what is the best approach? Has the patient truly understood everything she has been told, or does she simply believe she understands? This does not mean that the average patient is incapable of understanding what she is being advised, simply that understanding what she is being told is not the same as having a clear and focused appreciation of the advice and the consequences of treatment. If a patient seeks medical help to the extent that informed consent is being sought, it is unlikely to push credulity too far to suggest that the patient may be feeling vulnerable, scared or apprehensive and may not actually comprehend what is in her best interests.

Furthermore, what does 'good' mean? What is 'good' for me is a difficult question to address, and who determines what is good for me does not present any easy answers. When consequentialism refers to the greatest happiness for the greatest number of people, it becomes difficult to apply to medical issues.

From a deontology perspective, the rights-based approach would be that informed consent is necessary because it reflects the patient's own autonomy; a patient has the right to understand what treatment he may undergo, and only by being fully informed is he able to express his own self-determination and reflect bodily integrity. The doctor informs the patient of the treatment and associated risks, not necessarily because he appreciates the importance of informed consent but because he has a duty to do so.

Confidentiality

In Chapter 5 we explored the principle of confidentiality and the importance of the clinician's role in maintaining that duty. This reflects clear consequentialist ideas – if a doctor ensures that (subject to any exceptions) he maintains his patient's confidence, the patient is more likely to trust the doctor with personal and possibly sensitive material. Take for example the patient who has a sexually transmitted disease. If he can trust his doctor, he will confide in him, he will seek advice, diagnosis and treatment. Conversely, if he does not feel that his confidence will be respected, he is less likely to seek help. Perhaps he feels embarrassed and does not want his neighbours, friends or family to discover his condition. If confidentiality is maintained then the consequentialist principle is intact – the greatest happiness for the greatest number of people will be secured as the patient will be treated and the risk of the spread of disease is eliminated.

On the contrary, if his confidence is not respected, the repercussions for public health could be significant. As a principle, consequentialism is adequately demonstrated in the notion of confidentiality.

Discussion point

We know that a doctor has a duty to maintain his patient's confidences. What if the patient tells the doctor that he has aspirations of shooting passengers on the rush-hour train after work? This patient poses a serious threat to society and the doctor would be justified in breaching the patient's duty of confidence and reporting the patient to the police. However, there is a difficult conflict here for the deontologist who is not concerned with consequences. He owes a duty of confidentiality, but on occasions he may have to weigh this duty against the public interest. This would require him to consider the consequences of the breach of the duty which deontology does not represent. The conflict to resolve two competing duties is difficult as one must take precedence over the other, but a deontologist would consider that all duties bear an equal weight. A consequentialist would have little difficulty with this scenario: the greatest happiness is caused by protecting the public interest and, thus, the duty of confidence is broken.

KEY FACTS

Key facts on utilitarianism and deontology

Utilitarianism	Deontology
The moral quality of an act is determined by its consequences.	The moral quality of an act is determined by rights or duties.
Jeremy Bentham and the felicific calculus.	Immanuel Kant and the Categorical Imperative.
The morality of an act is determined by application of intensity, duration, certainty, propinquity, fecundity, purity and extent.	Universal law. Not treating a person solely as a means to an end.
Criticism – focuses on the greater good and can therefore ignore justice and patient autonomy.	Criticism – bound by rules and duties and therefore little room for debate. While consistent, deontology can be inflexible.

ACTIVITY

Self-test questions

- Explain what is meant by consequentialism.
- What is the felicific calculus? Consider how it can be applied to an ethical dilemma.
- What is meant by deontology?
- Which do you consider is the most flexible approach?

6.2.5 Principlism

Arguably the most influential set of guidelines which can be applied to any situation in bioethics is principlism. The brainchild of Tom Beauchamp and James Childress, principlism is based on four principles which represent the overarching principles to be applied in modern medicine. Their application to modern medicine has made them overwhelmingly accepted, as the principles recognise that there is often *not* a finite answer to a clinical dilemma. The four principles are shown in Figure 6.6.

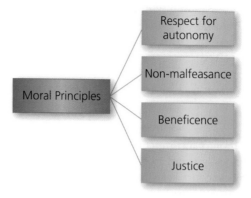

Figure 6.6 The principles of principlism

Respect for autonomy

The courts for some considerable time have recognised the importance of patient autonomy, although perhaps more readily in the USA than the UK. The fundamental nature of patient autonomy was recognised as long ago as 1914 when Cardozo J in *Schloendorff v New York Hospital* (1914) uttered the well-known dictum:

JUDGMENT

'every human being of adult years and sound mind has a right to determine what shall be done with his own body; and a surgeon who performs an operation without his patient's consent, commits an assault.'

According to Beauchamp and Childress, the principle of autonomy does not override any of the other four principles, although it is often thought of as having the predominant role. They define autonomy as:

QUOTATION

'at a minimum, self-rule that is free from both controlling interference by others and from limitations, such as inadequate understanding that prevent meaningful choice'.

(2008, page 58)

Autonomy remains one of the foremost guiding principles, and our choice to express our own free will is one of the most fundamental of all basic principles. We may not make the right decisions, we may make uninformed decisions but they are our autonomous decisions, a reflection of our own self-determination and an essential part of our lives.

To illustrate autonomy in practice, consider the case of *Re C (Adult: Refusal of Medical Treatment)* (1994) where C, a paranoid schizophrenic, was competent to refuse medical treatment to remove his gangrenous foot even though there was a high probability that he would die without the amputation. His decision to refuse the amputation was, many would say, entirely irrational, but it was his own autonomous decision and, in modern medicine, had to be respected.

An often-quoted example of autonomy in action is that of the Jehovah's Witness who after a serious accident requires a blood transfusion. He refuses all blood products, and understands and appreciates the consequences of his refusal. Should a patient be permitted to die when treatment could save him, or should his religious (or other) objections be adhered to? We might be incredulous at their decision that any person would rather give his life than refuse to adhere to their own religious scriptures, but it is the patient's right to choose and not for the doctor to impose his will upon the patient even if, by imposing his will, he can successfully treat the patient. What the patient is really saying is that you cannot violate my bodily integrity and if I do not consent, you cannot act. Beauchamp and Childress state that:

QUOTATION

'... such respect involves respectful action, not merely a respectful attitude. It also requires more than non-interference in others' personal affairs.'

(2008, page 63)

Even though a competent patient has a right to refuse medical treatment, we know that the opposite is not true, as in *R (on the application of Burke) v The General Medical Council* (2005) the court held that a patient cannot demand medical treatment, when he reaches a specified stage of an illness, if it is contrary to his best interests. In this case, autonomy has its limitations.

Lord Phillips said:

JUDGMENT

'autonomy and the right of self-determination do not entitle the patient to insist on receiving a particular medical treatment ... Insofar as a doctor has a legal obligation to provide treatment this cannot be founded upon the fact that the patient demands it.'

Why is it that a patient's autonomous decision to die is respected but a patient's autonomous decision for life-sustaining treatment will be denied? It can be difficult to see how autonomy is respected in one scenario but is replaced with paternalism in the other. The clearest indication given from the case is not an ethical one but a legal one, as the court indicated that it would be difficult to determine medical treatment at some time in the future and divorced from the facts. How the patient may wish to be treated at some time in the future is not necessarily the same as what the patient's best interests might be and, where there is potential for collision, the courts will not allow autonomy to be enforced for the future.

We have seen in Chapter 2 on consent that a young patient can only express their autonomy where they have the appropriate level and understanding or are '*Gillick* competent'. However, it is perhaps worth considering the case of *Re E (a minor) (wardship: medical treatment)* (1993) which we looked at on page 72. E was a Jehovah's Witness and shared his parents' belief about a refusal to share blood products. At 15 and a half years of age, he was sufficiently intelligent to understand most of his treatment and condition, but the courts took a paternalistic approach concluding that he would not understand the true manner of his death or the likely distress on his parents. In other words the court deemed that there were some aspects that were beyond his understanding. Ward J authorised the blood transfusion as he was motivated primarily by the welfare of the child, and in doing so outweighed autonomy with paternalism. While the court viewed the approach they took to be in the best interests of the child, the court was assisted by the fact that he was aged 15 and a half; once this patient was 18 years old he refused all further blood transfusions and subsequently died.

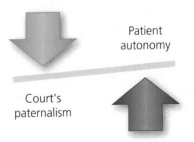

Figure 6.7 A balancing act

The case of *Gold v Haringey Health Authority* (1988) is another example of where a patient had been denied her autonomy. Here, Mrs Gold consented to a sterilisation procedure, but she alleged that she had neither been advised of the risk of spontaneous reversal nor that a male vasectomy was statistically more successful. She fell pregnant, gave birth and then sued the health authority arguing that as this was a non-therapeutic intervention, she should be told of *all* the risks, in order that she could make an autonomous decision. She failed in her action as the court determined there was no difference between therapeutic and non-therapeutic and the *Bolam* test (see Chapter 1) should be applied. The decision demonstrates that her autonomy was irrelevant even though there were bodies of professional opinion to support each view. The difficulty here is that she sought and consented to a procedure based upon an incomplete picture of the risks and benefits, which completely removed her autonomy to make her own decisions about a medical procedure and adversely affected her bodily integrity. As Margaret Brazier observes 'The judgment in *Gold* left patient autonomy woefully thin in substance' ((2003) *Medicine, patients and the* law, third edition. London: Penguin, page 106).

The case of *Airedale NHS Trust v Bland* (1993), which we consider in more detail in Chapter 11, contains significant judicial opinion of the importance and value of autonomy and self-determination. Lord Mustill confirmed the principle seen in *Re T* (1992) where a competent patient can determine his or her own future even if it may not be in their best interests:

JUDGMENT

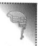

'If the patient is capable of making a decision on whether to permit treatment … his choice must be obeyed even if on any objective view it is contrary to his best interests.'

Lord Goff made a similar point, explaining that the:

JUDGMENT

'principle of self-determination requires that respect must be given to the wishes of the patient, so that if an adult patient of sound mind refuses, however unreasonably, to consent to treatment or care by which his life would or might be prolonged, the doctors responsible for his care must give effect to his wishes, even though they do not consider it to be in his best interests to do so.'

Such indication of the significance of autonomy can further be seen in the decision of *Re B (Adult: Refusal of Medical Treatment)* (2002) where Butler-Sloss J permitted the competent patient's request that her ventilator be switched off, allowing her to die, and stated:

JUDGMENT

'unless the gravity of the illness has affected the patient's capacity, a seriously disabled patient has the same rights as the fit person to respect for personal autonomy. There is a serious danger, exemplified in this case, of a benevolent paternalism which does not embrace recognition of the personal autonomy of the severely disabled patient.'

Hence, the natural inclination towards paternalism by the medical profession gives way to patient's autonomy. One difficulty with autonomy may be that if we respect a patient's desire to refuse medical treatment even where they know it might lead to their death, how can we really be sure that their decision is one freely made? By way of explanation, if a patient refuses medical treatment believing it to be their autonomous decision, are they not really distressed, frightened and vulnerable? Clearly, the court was at pains to address the point in *Re B* (2002) and the patient was emphatic in her wish for the ventilation on which she was entirely dependent to be switched off. In other situations, autonomy may be respected but the patient has died when they could have been saved. If we imagine for a moment that death was not quite so final and there was a short window of communication, how many patients would thank medical professionals for respecting their autonomy, and how many would ask, 'Why didn't you save me when you could, while I was confused, anxious and distressed?'?

Non-malfeasance

non-malfeasance
not harming one's patients

The principle of **non-malfeasance** imposes upon us a duty not to harm others. In medical ethics, the principle *Primum non nocere*, translated as 'above all do no harm' is particularly pertinent and one of the fundamental guiding principles in medical treatment. There is also evidence of non-malfeasance in the Hippocratic Oath as it states:

QUOTATION

'I will prescribe regimens for the good of my patients and according to my ability and my judgment and never do harm to anyone.'

The difficulty in the principle of non-malfeasance is well illustrated by the following American case.

CASE EXAMPLE

McFall v Shrimp (1978) 10 Pa D & C 3d 90

McFall was suffering from a serious illness and was advised that his condition would benefit from a bone marrow transplant from a donor. His cousin, Shrimp, initially volunteered, was tested and found to be a suitable match, but then withdrew his consent to proceed. While the donation of bone marrow is a purely altruistic act, an application was made to court to compel Shrimp to donate bone marrow.

McFall argued that a duty was imposed to help save a life where it is in one's power to do so. The court seeking some authority referred to the English courts, asking whether 'society (can) infringe upon one's absolute right to his bodily security'. The court observed that in English law there is no duty to assist a stranger, while in other countries there is 'a contrary view which has the individual existing to serve the society as a whole'. The defendant was being asked to forego his autonomy and, if the claimant succeeded, be compelled to give up part of his body (even though it would regenerate within a short period of time). Here was a conflict of ethical principles: would it harm the defendant more if his bodily integrity was violated and living tissue was forcibly extracted from him contrary to his wishes, or would this act be for the greater good, that is, saving McFall's life?

The court refused the application to force Shrimp to donate his bone marrow. They said:

JUDGMENT

'(Forcible) extraction of living body tissue causes revulsion to the judicial mind. Such would raise the specter of the swastika and the inquisition, reminiscent of the horrors this portends.'

The suggestion here is that the courts may have been reluctant to order the bone marrow donation to proceed for fear of the slippery slope and where it could lead. If this court ordered bone marrow to be donated, could another court order a kidney to be transplanted? The court concluded that there was no legal duty even though many would consider his refusal to be acceptable. McFall died shortly afterwards.

This case can also usefully demonstrate the conflicting principles of consequentialism and deontology. A consequentialist would observe that the greatest happiness would be caused to the greatest number of people if Shrimp donated bone marrow, as McFall may survive and this would create pleasure not pain, even though the duration of the pleasure is uncertain as one cannot guess how much longer he would live with the bone marrow transplant. In contrast, a deontologist would approach the scenario differently. Forcing a person to donate bone marrow is using a person solely as a means to an end and ignores that person's individuality. However, Kantian theorists refer to duties. Does Shrimp have a duty to donate bone marrow to save his cousin?

Reverting to the principle of non-malfeasance, it can be hard to define. While we must 'do no harm', how can this principle be reconciled with euthanasia? We accept that a doctor cannot harm a patient but it may be hard to pinpoint where the greater harm lies.

For example, Mildred is an elderly terminally ill patient who is in constant pain and suffering. She begs her doctor to end her pain and suffering and allow her to die in dignity. Is greater harm caused in allowing her to die and ending her suffering, or refusing her request and allowing her to remain alive to continue to suffer and ensure more pain and distress? If the doctor denies her euthanasia, which he invariably will as it is unlawful, he has also denied the patient her autonomy. Supporters of euthanasia would criticise this refusal of patient autonomy as Mildred's free will and self-determination is denied at the most important time of her life. Not ending her life may ironically be doing Mildred the greater harm.

Beneficence

While non-malfeasance requires us not to harm, **beneficence** imposes a positive obligation to act in a person's best interests. Although there is a distinct overlap between the two, there is often an attempt to keep them distinct from each other.

There is no statutory provision in the UK which legally requires one to positively assist another, save in the rarest of circumstances where a duty through a special relationship is imposed (see for example *R v Stone and Dobinson* [1977] QB 354), but it seems straightforward enough to state that medical professionals act in the best interests of their patients. In its nature, beneficence veers slightly more towards utilitarianism than deontology, even though deontologists still regard beneficence as a valuable principle. From an ethical perspective, the idea of doing more good than harm is a principle that guides the medical profession throughout. The healthcare profession is singularly one of the most beneficent professions, with its aim or objective as the healing of the patient at its core, and beneficence exists as one of its most predominant values.

It is sometimes difficult to determine with any precision what acting in a patient's best interests means. In the case of the Jehovah's Witness who refuses a blood transfusion when seriously injured, it could mean taking a paternalistic approach and ensuring that the patient receives the blood transfusion, albeit against his wishes but in order to save the patient's life. While this may achieve what was originally intended by the Hippocratic Oath, it is in direct conflict with the principle of autonomy, as the act of saving the patient is not in the best interests of the patient if that is not what the patient perceives them to be.

Since beneficence means doing good for patients, this principle encounters difficulty with the problems related to rationing of healthcare. A medical professional acts in his patient's best interests, but if the patient is denied expensive medicine as there are insufficient resources to fund treatment, the principle of beneficence simply cannot be met. This is turn affects the principle of justice.

Non-malfeasance	Beneficence
• A duty not to harm others.	• A positive duty to do good and act in the patient's best interests.

Figure 6.8 Definitions of non-malfeasance and beneficence

There is the potential for these two important principles to clash. An illustration of this can be seen in the unique case of *Re A (Conjoined Twins)* (2001). Here, Mary and Jodie were **conjoined**; Mary, being the parasitic twin, was largely dependent on Jodie's blood supply. If they were not separated, both twins would die but if they were separated, Mary, the weaker twin, would not be able to live without depending on her twin. How do we apply ethical principles? The principle of non-malfeasance tells medical professionals not to harm others, but the separation would led to Mary's certain death. It is not easy to reconcile the principle of beneficence as there is a duty to act positively and do 'good'. How can 'good' be done when Mary will die as a direct result of the separation? The answer lies in the 'best interests' application – the conjoined twins were separated as it was deemed to be in the best interests of Jodie. The case illustrates the difficulty of the application of ethical principles and how, in real dilemmas, they can often conflict.

conjoined
twins fused by one embryo failing to divide into two

Justice

R Gillon has observed that 'the idea that justice is a moral issue that doctors can properly ignore is clearly mistaken' (*BMJ*, Vol. 291, 20 July 1985). The idea of justice is of paramount importance in the application of medical ethics. Every patient should be treated equally regardless of their race, religion and social class. This much is easy to accept, but it is however a balancing act. Gillon demonstrates an example of the general practitioner who decides to spend 30 minutes with a bereaved mother and five minutes with a lonely elderly lady with a sore throat. Here, the patients are not being treated equally by a simple mathematical allocation of time, but maybe they are being treated equally in terms of need.

Justice implies fairness and equitable treatment. In the UK, a person is entitled to medical care provided free at source by the State. If a person does not receive the treatment recommended by his physician, and does not have an effective remedy, an injustice is automatically created.

It is clear that the demand for resources outstrips supply and there are insufficient resources to be able to fund all the treatment that every patient may desire. It is a complex balancing act as to who should get the limited resources.

In Chapter 4 we considered the example of two patients, Patient A and Patient B who, both suffering from the same condition, required the same drugs in order to cure their condition. Patient A was unemployed, a drug abuser and a petty criminal with no dependants. Patient B was a renowned heart surgeon, married with dependants. The question remains: which patient should receive the drugs? In a very simple application, it would appear that Patient B has the most to lose and, given that his contribution to society is immeasurable, a form of justice may suggest that he should be treated and Patient A should not. This is however the challenge for healthcare. The principle of distributive justice dictates that all citizens should be treated as equitably as possible, but where there are financial constraints imposed upon the providers, this simply is not possible. All patients should be treated equally regardless of their class and social utility.

There are harder issues to identify. Although it is straightforward to accept that patients should be treated equally, we often assume that patients walk into their doctors' clinic and adequately express their difficulties, or maybe present themselves at Accident and Emergency Departments and allow others to determine their medical complaint for them. However, there is also a proportion of the population who find it considerably more difficult to access healthcare, whether because of a lack of understanding of their own health, reasons of poverty or an inbuilt distrust or fear of the medical profession. These are the patients who often have complex social and health problems and whose access to healthcare is more difficult but who must be treated as equally as any other patient. Justice is therefore sometimes hard to identify.

6.2.6 The four principle approach in action

If we use the four principle approach as designed by Beauchamp and Childress and advocated by Gillon, it is possible to conclude that assisted suicide is morally ethical, despite a considerable body of opinion that is opposed to it.

If a patient suffers from a terminal condition, and is in continual relentless pain and suffering to an extent that he or she expresses a clear intended wish to die, if their desire is unhindered, uninfluenced and not subject to any element of duress and if the principle of autonomy is to be applied, their view should be respected. If a Jehovah's Witness's autonomous refusal to accept a blood transfusion, understanding and fully appreciating the consequences, is respected, then it is difficult to justify why the patient who wishes to end their life cannot be afforded the same respect for their self-determination. The answer lies in the effect which such decisions may have on society as a whole, as we will consider in more detail in Chapter 10.

The principle of non-malfeasance is an obligation not to inflict harm knowingly upon a person. Arguably, denying a person the right to determine how they end their life when faced with such adversity does impose considerable harm upon them. The patient has had considerable opportunity through the progression of their illness to weigh up the harm that would be caused by ending their life and the benefits that could be achieved as a result. The harm could be the emotional effect which their death would have on their loved ones or the potentially serious legal implications involved in assisting a suicide. The benefit would be the objective of the assisted suicide: that their life would be ended; they would be relieved from their lifetime of suffering; and be allowed the dignified death which they desire. The benefits from the patient's perspective are likely to outweigh the potential harm that could be caused, although many patients are naturally concerned about legal repercussions on their loved ones to assist.

Beneficence conveys the positive obligation to act in a way that is best for the patient. As we have already explained, UK law does not impose such an obligation; it is axiomatic that we should behave in this way. While a doctor may consider that a patient suffering from an incurable condition may benefit from palliative care, this is not in the patient's interests if this is not what the patient desires.

Justice is harder to apply. It is fair, just and equitable that a person's autonomy should be respected and that a person should be allowed to choose when to end their own life. Perhaps it is unfair and unjust to deny a person the right to assist their loved one to end their life, and inequitable that the State should interfere with a person's life to the extent that they are denied this right. Perhaps one might agree that the State's fear of the unknown consequences of permitting assisted suicide should not outweigh such a fundamental right.

KEY FACTS

Key facts on principlism

Respect for autonomy	Non-malfeasance	Beneficence	Justice
Respecting a patient's free will and self-determination.	Acting in a way so as not to harm the patient.	Acting positively to do good.	Fair and equitable treatment.
Case examples include *Re T* (1992) and *Airedale NHS Trust v Bland* (1993). Many cases can illustrate patient autonomy.	Case examples: *McFall v Shrimp* (1978) *Re A (conjoined Twins)* (2001).	Potential conflict of all principles. *Re A (conjoined Twins)* (2001).	Consider examples from resource allocation as illustrative of lack of equal justice.

6.2.7 Paternalism

Historically, the approach of the medical professional was paternalistic. Paternalism is the flip side of autonomy. The doctor acting in the patient's best interest would treat and the patient would comply. The effect of such an approach was that the patient may not have been sufficiently or adequately informed; alternatives may not have been discussed with the patient; and the patient's informed consent would not have been relevant to obtain. This approach is now seen as unethical.

Beauchamp and Childress define paternalism as:

QUOTATION

'the intentional overriding of one person's known preference or actions by another person, where the person who overrides justifies the action by the goal of beneficence or avoiding harm to the person whose will is overridden'. (2008)

Since the development of the doctrine of informed consent in the USA and the more recent case of *Chester v Afshar* (2004) suggesting the evolution of informed consent here in the UK , paternalism has often given way to a more patient-centred approach, as Lord Steyn indicated: 'in modern law paternalism no longer rules'. This view is fundamental to modern medicine which insists 'that due respect is given to the autonomy and dignity of each patient'.

Nevertheless paternalism still exists in the medical profession. We have already seen in the judicial approach to children and their capacity to consent that the courts will err on the side of protecting the children and ordering treatment in situations where the child has already made an autonomous decision to reject medical treatment.

As demonstrated in *Re T* (1992) where the patient has capacity to consent, autonomy is respected and the patient is free to determine his own destiny. If a patient lacks capacity it follows that it must be right for the courts to determine what is in the patient's best interest. However, as autonomy has increased in significance over recent years, there is a natural conflict with the principle of beneficence as it does not follow that a patient's expression of autonomy is necessarily the most beneficent approach.

Autonomy and older children

The judicial approach to decisions of children under the age of 18 is that by virtue of s 8, Family Law (Reform) Act 1969, a child can consent to treatment in the same way as an adult. However, where a child refuses medical treatment, the court will reject a child's autonomy and act paternalistically. The courts have consistently rejected a minor's attempt to refuse medical treatment. The judiciary may be sympathetic to an adolescent's attempts at autonomy but still regard them as children who have yet to mature and experience life. Many adolescents would consider this patronising as they are given the right to be treated as an adult including the right to make unwise decisions, but that right cannot be exercised if it does not concur with the adult's view. If an adolescent's autonomy is not to be respected then clear reasons should be given why.

Ward J recalls in *Re E* (1993):

JUDGMENT

'those of us who have passed beyond callow youth can all remember convictions we have loudly proclaimed which we now find somewhat embarrassing'.

Despite the common sense approach that is being demonstrated, there is little value of affording the older child autonomy if that autonomy can easily be overruled as Brazier and Bridge argue:

QUOTATION

'If society is not prepared to allow adolescents to court unfavourable outcomes in judgments relating to medical treatment, we should say so openly.' (1996)

Autonomy and childbirth

In cases concerning childbirth, the courts have displayed a particularly paternalistic view and demonstrated a readiness to declare a woman temporarily incompetent in order for a Caesarean section to be performed. However, in *St George's Healthcare NHS Trust v S, R v Collins and others* (1998) the appeal courts held that the Mental Health Act 1983 had been wrongly relied upon and her autonomy should have been respected.

Despite this dictum, subsequent case law is still willing to take a paternalistic approach and reject a woman's competency where she puts her baby at risk in labour. In doing so, the courts apply a more common sense and practical approach, and act to prevent avoidable harm. In this respect it may be an admirable principle to act in the best interests of the patient but it violates a woman's autonomous decision.

Is paternalism wrong? The Hippocratic Oath imposes an obligation upon a doctor to act 'for the benefit of my patients'. Thus historically it is his obligation to adopt paternalism and act in his patient's best interests. Even with the development of autonomy, some may argue that too much decision-making is left to the patient and, since the patient may not know what is best for them from a clinical perspective, they simply wish to be treated and leave the decision-making to those who are learned in the art of medicine.

6.2.8 Virtue ethics

Virtue ethics is a character-based moral theory which emphasises the character and virtue in the action. Instead of considering the duty of the individual as deontology does, or the consequences of the action as utilitarianism does, virtue ethicists place the value on the virtue of the action to be taken.

Virtue ethics derives largely from ancient Greek philosophers Aristotle and Plato who said that an action is only morally right or acceptable if a virtuous person would adopt it. It is associated with the Greek term *'eudaimonia'* which despite being translated in a number of ways means 'human flourishing'. A virtue ethicist does not ask 'what is my duty?' or 'where can the greatest happiness be achieved?', but 'what would a virtuous person do in this situation?'.

One of the criticisms of virtue ethics is perhaps the lack of boundaries and its complete subjectivity. Who is to define what a virtuous person is? If I believe a person is virtuous because they donate blood, does another person believe the same? Perhaps the other person will only consider them to be truly virtuous if they donate bone marrow (being infinitely more intrusive). We would probably all agree that a virtuous person does good things to another person and abides by our laws but, even so, one person may put the virtue of compassion, understanding or empathy on a different scale of importance. Where does the virtue of truth-telling or respect fit into this? Virtue ethics does not allow us to appreciate the utility of an action rather than the person taking the action.

If virtue ethics is applied to the principle of informed consent above, it focuses on the question, 'what would a virtuous person do in these circumstances?'. The answer may well be that a virtuous doctor would advise the patient of the risks of the procedure in order that they may fully consent, but this ignores entirely the legal obligation or duty which the doctor is under as illustrated in the case of *Sidaway v Board of Governors of the Bethlem Royal Hospital and the Maudsley Hospital* (1985). The principle of informed consent is not about a doctor's virtuous nature, but about the patient being able to provide true consent to a medical procedure. Thus, the focus should be on the patient and not on the doctor's well-meaning.

Virtue ethics could be described by critics as being self-centred. Morality should not be about oneself; we should not judge whether an action is morally right or wrong according to how it makes *us* feel and whether it makes *us* happier. Intrinsically there seems to be something wrong with acting compassionately because of any potential benefit for ourselves; we should act compassionately out of respect or regard for the other person, regardless of how it makes us feel.

Virtue ethics, a theory of ethics guided by actions, is considered flexible and able to adapt to a given situation. It is critical of deontology and consequentialism as they are bound by either rules or principles, lacking the individuality of being able to respond to a specific situation. Conversely, one of the strengths of both deontology and consequentialism is the inflexibility of their theory. As they are both bound by rules, there is clarity as to how one should act, creating consistency through direction.

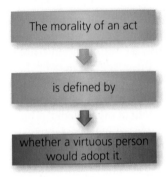

Figure 6.9 Virtue ethics

6.2.9 Casuistry

With its ancient origins in Rome and Greece, the term 'casuistry' is derived from '*casus conscientitae*' or cases of conscience. Casuistry is a historical method of applying ethics based upon a practical approach. The Roman philosopher Marcus Cicero (1061–43 BC) wrote in *On Duty* that 'different circumstances should be carefully scrutinised in every instance'.

Casuistry progressed with the Christian confessors, the Penitentials in around the sixth century AD, who explained that 'not all persons were to be weighed in one and the same balance'. This largely had theological application whereby the clergy were attempting to treat like cases alike in terms of penitence through confession.

Casuistry differs from other ethical principles in the sense that, while other principles may consider the morality of an action by determining whether an act is right or wrong, casuistry considers each case distinctly but, much like the doctrine of judicial precedent, uses previous cases to determine whether like cases should be treated alike. The circumstances of the case are essential to the method of casuistry. It therefore follows that the more similarly one case resembles another, the more likely it is to follow the previous application.

The Jesuits built upon ancient casuistry to the height of its popularity around 1556–1656 until its decline shortly thereafter. The Jesuits were of particular significance as they were not only powerful within the Church but wielded considered influence within the Roman State; hence casuistry enjoyed a high profile during this period. Thus, casuistry extended into secular society as a flexible approach to problem-solving.

One of the most significant critics of casuistry was Blaise Pascal, a French seventeenth century philosopher, who with considerable support argued that there was no moral support to the principle of casuistry, and created a number of possibilities or probabilities to a situation that could be subjectively applied. Nevertheless, modern casuistry had retained a degree of support, and supporters of casuistry such as Albert Jonsen have regarded it as a practical and useful approach in modern medical ethics. Jonsen argues that 'no ethical problem is completely unprecedented' and will often have some similarity to previous cases. Consequently, the ethical reasoning can be described as reasoning by analogy.

Critics of casuistry consider the analogous approach to be faultworthy as, even if two cases are similar on the facts, there are often inherent differences in them, sufficient to justify them being treated differently. Furthermore, the reliance on the similarity of judicial precedent is misguided. Judicial precedent treats legal cases alike if they are similar on the facts, and such decisions are binding on future decisions. This can only occur as there is some authoritative basis for this to occur, that is, the hierarchy of the courts and the expertise of the judicial system. Thus it is false to treat like clinical cases alike as there is no similar structure of authoritative decision-making in bioethics, and no hierarchy of arbiters to which to adhere. Bioethics is often subjective, dealing with real issues and cannot be treated with the clinical objectiveness of legal decision-making.

Sokol (2008) has observed that the 'four quadrants' approach accurately represents the casuistry approach. The approach outlined in Jonsen's *Clinical Ethics* (2010) (written also with Siegler and Winslade) and used in the USA and in the United Kingdom has true value.

The 'four quadrants' refer to four areas to be considered when a patient presents clear ethical dilemmas: medical or clinical indications, patient's wishes, quality of life and 'contextual features'. The four quadrants approach is in Sokol's view compatible with the four principles of Beauchamp and Childress, but:

QUOTATION

'in the domain of clinical ethics and practical decision-making, it presents a considerable advantage over the other'.

as it presents a practical method for considering real-life dilemmas. Sokol recognises that the approach:

QUOTATION

'cannot single-handedly resolve moral dilemmas ... it is a kind of a moral stethoscope, increasing the clinician/ethicist's ability to see what is morally relevant while revealing at the bedside, the moral dynamics of the case.'

While casuistry has been widely criticised, there is a justifiable role for the method in modern medical ethics.

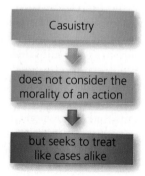

Figure 6.10 What defines casuistry

6.2.10 Feminist ethics

While the development of feminist perspectives in bioethics has been slowly emerging for several decades, it is in the last 'fifteen years (that) feminist approaches in bioethics emerged as a distinct and recognizable constituency' (Rawlinson (2008)).

While feminism bioethics is not necessarily an approach to bioethics that applies only to women, it is an area of bioethics where there is one specific perspective towards an aspect of bioethics. That is not to suggest that the vision is blinkered; on the contrary, feminist bioethics closely considers other principles and methods but the role of feminism is of primary importance. Feminism is concerned with issues of justice, equality and oppression.

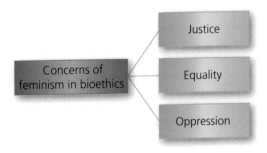

Figure 6.11 Feminist ethics

Feminism bioethics is concerned with oppression and how medical practices often act to oppress women, whether or not that is the desired intention. Sherwin said:

QUOTATION

'Questions about dominance and oppression are essential dimensions of feminist ethical analysis'. (Wolf (1996))

Karem Lebacqz expressed the universal view that 'all feminists agree that women are oppressed and this oppression is wrong' (1995).

Feminism and assisted reproduction

It is argued that women felt oppressed when new reproductive techniques were introduced, and in a mostly male-dominated environment felt treated as pawns in medical experimentation and that their natural desire for children was a conduit for exploitation. Petersen argues that assisted reproduction should be rejected because it 'socially coerces' women 'into desiring to have children by their patriarchal society in which they live' and they are directly harmed as a result (2004).

While **in-vitro fertilisation** (IVF) offered women the opportunity to bear children, it was also a path to succumb to the social and often economic pressure to be able to have biologically-related offspring. Once medical advances established that infertility was not necessarily a woman's condition, social pressure intensified. Donchin observes that 'infertile women are urged to fulfil their "full reproductive potential" regardless of the economic, psychological or bodily cost' (1996). The procedure of IVF is intrusive, often painful and can be harmful to a woman's health. Moreover, more than one cycle is often needed in order to achieve success. Since multiple pregnancies are also a complication of IVF, women argue that oppression continues when faced with this potential scenario.

While IVF is available on the NHS, it is subject to strict criteria and guidance set down by NICE in 2004, entitled *Clinical Guidelines Fertility: assessment and treatment for people with fertility problems*. IVF is more readily available privately; thus, one might argue that it is only those women who can afford it who can truly access it. There are a significant number of women who due to their social class do not have the financial security to access such technology and are oppressed due to the lack of distributive justice in assisted reproduction. A report entitled *Holding back the IVF revolution? A report into the NHS IVF provision in the UK today* (June 2011) highlights the inconsistency in the number of cycles of IVF offered on the NHS according to location of the PCT, together with the considerable variance of lower and upper age limits. Such imbalance in access to assisted reproduction creates an injustice to women where IVF is less available.

As medical technology continues to progress, human embryonic stem cell research has caused widespread feminist consternation. While the focus of stem cell research has largely been the moral status of the embryos together with the associated arguments of personhood, the effect of stem cell research on women has not received equal coverage. Embryo experimentation is only possible if eggs are obtained from the women's bodies and, in order to obtain eggs, it is necessary to stimulate the ovaries artificially by

in-vitro fertilisation

a form of assisted reproduction where eggs or ova are removed from a woman's ovary. In laboratory conditions, the eggs are then fertilised with male sperm and returned to the woman's uterus.

hormone treatment. Much like IVF, there are risks associated with such a procedure. Such acts can be contrary to one of the most significant ethical theories as deontologists would argue that women are being treated as a commodity and a person should never be treated solely as a means to an end.

Women may choose to donate their eggs as an altruistic act but others may seek payment for the embryos. Here, it can be argued that women are being exploited as it is likely to be the poorest women in the population, often those of an ethnic minority, who have the greatest financial need and who are likely to endure the inconvenience and possible repercussions on their health. Exploitation of a person because of their sex, social class and racial grouping is morally wrong. It is these women, the ones who have the most to lose, who will be unable to gain from any technologies that may be developed as a direct result of embryonic stem cell research as they will undoubtedly be costly. Such women from a poorer social class or ethnic minority are unlikely to be able to afford such benefits privately, and rationing may render them unobtainable on the NHS.

Women as carers

Feminism in bioethics seeks to redress the balance between the inequalities of the sexes. Historically, medicine was concerned with the doctor–patient relationship, the former of which was predominately male. More recently, while there are considerably more female doctors, women still represent by far the greater percentage of patients within the NHS. Partly this is due to reproduction itself, but women are also the primary carers of children and are considerably more likely to be caring for elderly relatives than are men.

The caring relationship predominately carried out by women is often overlooked but it is invaluable to the working of the NHS. Herring highlights that work traditionally regarded as in the domain of women is often overlooked in the 'male gaze' and, if care work is described as 'voluntary' and 'informal', it is marginalised as 'unimportant' (2007). Thus while the doctor achieves a degree of recognition, the inequality of the sexes is perpetuated as the carer, the one whom the patient has come to rely on and who undoubtedly has created a close bond, is all but unrecognisable.

Women as sexual commodities

On a more global scale, the inequality between the sexes has a profound effect on the wellbeing of both children and women, both of whom are the most socially disadvantaged. Statistics from the Child and Woman Abuse Studies Unit (Hughes *et al*, 1999) reflect some alarming figures. In Indonesia, prostitutes number 650,000, of whom 30 per cent are children; India has 10 million prostitutes of which 160,000 are Nepalese women being held in Indian brothels, and in the Philippines 400,000 women are involved in prostitution, a quarter of whom are children. These appalling figures show oppression of women on an almost incomprehensive scale. They come from the poorest economic background with little access to healthcare services and oppressed by male dominance. The rate of child pregnancy is high and is the direct cause of deaths of many women worldwide.

Female genital mutilation (FGM)

The World Health Organisation statistics (February 2010) state there are between 100–140 million girls and women worldwide living with the effects of FGM. The effect of such a practice on women is notable; there is an increased risk of severe bleeding, difficulty urinating and significant childbirth complications. Women are at a greater risk of having a Caesarean section (even if they can access healthcare) and statistics show there is a greater risk of newborn deaths among women who have had female genital mutilation. Here in the UK, it is estimated that at least 20,000 young girls (many of them in London) are at risk of FGM. Legislation to help protect such abuses, more often than not without informed consent, has been in place since 1983 with the enactment of the Female Circumcision Act, although the Female Genital Mutilation Act 2003 extended its provisions and now makes it a criminal offence to take a child out of the country for the purposes of FGM.

Key facts on paternalism, virtue ethics, casuistry and feminist ethics

Paternalism	Virtue ethics	Casuistry	Feminist ethics
Originates in the Hippocratic Oath.	Originates from Aristotle and Plato.	Originates in ancient Rome and Greece.	More recent origins.
Overrides a patient's autonomy. Largely rejected in modern-day medical practice.	Considers an act to be morally acceptable if there is some virtue in the act.	Referred to as cases of conscience. The aim is to treat like cases alike.	Symbolism by justice, equality and oppression.
Still prevalent in denying a minor the right to refuse medical treatment.	Criticised for being self-centred with the focus on the virtue of the actor rather than the patient.	Does have some application in medical practice today.	Continuing evidence of oppression of women and lack of equality on a global scale.

6.3 The religious perspective

6.3.1 Introduction

Thus far, we have considered a number of theories that help us try to apply ethical principles to medical issues. There are, however, other theories that need to be taken into account. The role that religious belief plays in medical ethics is still questionable. Should religious belief have any role in decisions regarding medical ethics at all? Even though society in the UK is regarded as largely secular, there are many who hold spirituality close to them even though they may not be overt in the practice of their religion. Many turn to religious belief when their lives become suddenly disrupted by illness and, even if a person is not religious, it is likely there is an element of spirituality within them. Even before modern medicine, those who were suffering from disease or illness sought help, not from the physician but from their deities whom it was felt could heal them directly.

There has been considerable progression of thought since this ancient period and there are few who would prefer to place faith in divine rather than medical intervention. Society has changed significantly; here in the UK we now live in a diverse, multi-cultural society which is largely secular, but there is still the belief prevalent in many religions that life originates from God and it is only for God to determine when it ends. There is a surprisingly cohesive approach between the main religions among many topics as the discussion below on abortion demonstrates. Among the main religions of the world there is a consensus of opinion for one another and respect for the sanctity of life.

However, the difficulty that arises when applying religious belief to ethical dilemmas is that religious belief is not flexible. It is impossible for a secular ethicist to persuade a Jehovah's Witness to accept a blood transfusion or a staunch Catholic to accept an abortion. Religious doctrine of any religion is contained within sacred texts and is the fundamental essence of that person's life. No amount of secular persuasion is likely to persuade a person with deep-rooted beliefs.

6.3.2 Doctors and religion

Should a medical professional's own religious belief be permitted to influence the decision-making process?

The GMC guidance entitled *Personal belief and Medical Practice* (March 2008) states that a doctor must respect a patient's personal beliefs as they may contribute to the patient's wellbeing and ability to cope with their illness. Their belief however may mean that they may ask for treatment which a doctor does not consider to be in their best interests, or refuse treatment which a doctor considers to be in their best interests. The guidance states that doctors should avoid being judgmental about others' personal beliefs and must ensure that they do not inflict their own beliefs upon patients.

However, if a doctor is asked to perform a procedure where he has a conscientious objection, such as abortion, he can refer that patient to another doctor. The case of *Janaway v Salford Area Health Authority* [1989] 1 AC 537 confirms that if one is called on to 'participate' in an abortion, one has the right to refuse. This right is also enshrined in statute, which applies in England, Wales and Scotland (but not Northern Ireland) as s 4(1), Abortion Act 1967 allows a doctor to refuse to participate in an abortion if he conscientiously objects.

In the next two sections we discuss religions' approaches to abortion and new medical technologies.

6.3.3 Abortion and religion

In this section we will be comparing and contrasting the principles of Christianity, Hinduism, Islam, Judaism and Buddhism in relation to their approaches to abortion – a controversial topic not only in ethics but also in religious dogma. It should be noted that the views given below do not necessarily represent all the views within each religion, especially where that view is a more conservative or liberal view.

Christianity

In Catholicism, abortion is regarded as a grave sin since the soul enters the body at conception and is therefore a person, simply waiting *in utero* to be fully formed. Its rejection of abortion and its unceasing condemnation are rooted in authorities from the early Church; for example, Letter of Barnabas 19 in 74 AD states 'Thou shalt not slay the child by procuring abortion; nor, again, shalt thou destroy it after it is born', and the First Text, The Didache Apostolorum in 90 AD said 'You shall not kill by abortion the fruit of the womb'.

The Catholic Church has a deontological approach to abortion as, since one may not use another as a means to an end, Catholicism forbids the termination of one life in order that another is preserved. Pious XII stated in 1951 that abortion at any period amounted to 'a grave and unlawful attack upon the inviolability of human life'.

More recently, in 1995, Pope John Paul ll referred to abortion as 'a grave moral disorder'. In confirming that the Church's position on abortion was 'unchanged and unchangeable' the Pope stated there are no 'circumstances' that would make 'licit an act which is intrinsically illicit' (*Evangelium Vitae* (*The Gospel Of Life*), paragraph 62).

The Catholic Church is unremitting in its condemnation of abortion, which extends to where the foetus is suffering from disability or deformity. Even in these circumstances the foetus cannot be terminated as the Church states that killing the foetus is contrary to the wishes of God.

While the Anglican Church encourages subjective contemplation, it directs followers to the Church of England direction and the statement of the General Synod 2005 which states:

QUOTATION

'The Church of England combines strong objection to abortion with a recognition that there can be – strictly limited – conditions under which it may be morally preferable to any available alternative.'

The objection to abortion lies in the understanding that God has given the foetus life created in the image of God, and it should not be destroyed. Hence, the foetus is a human being from the moment of conception and has every right a person is entitled to, which includes the right to life.

The Anglican Church argues the law in England and Wales which legalises abortion is too liberal and considers the number of abortions to be 'unacceptably high'. However, the Church of England does recognise that there are circumstances where the life of the mother would be threatened if the pregnancy were to continue and in these circumstances the termination of a pregnancy can be justified but should be carried out as soon as is possible. In order to avoid terminations of pregnancy after 24 weeks' gestation, the direction given by the Church of England is that this should only occur in situations where there is 'severe foetal handicap', although there is little guidance as to precisely what this entails.

Hinduism

Ancient Hindu texts, in common with other ancient religions, condemn abortion as tantamount to murder. The Institutes of Vishnu (translated by Julius Jolly (1880) *Sacred Book of the East, Volume 7*. Oxford: The Clarendon Press, paragraph 1, page 133) states that 'killing an embryo is tantamount to killing a Brahmin (Priest)'. No allowance is made for the health of the foetus or the mother. More modern writings recognise that abortion is more commonplace and is prevalent in contemporary India, particularly among female foetuses.

Islam

Islamic law considers life to be sacred, much like other religions. As a general rule, Islam forbids abortions; however, Sharia law permits abortion where there is a risk that the foetus will threaten the mother's life. The justification for this is the balance of the two evils, and in these circumstances the unborn foetus can be sacrificed for the life of the mother. Islamic law does not allow abortion for economic reasons or in order to reduce the size of a family.

Abortion after the four-month period is not permitted, save in circumstances to save the mother's life, as by that stage ensoulment will have taken place. After the soul is said to enter the body, any abortion will be considered analogous to murder.

If it transpires that the foetus suffers from severe abnormality, the traditional approach is that the foetus cannot be aborted. However, more recently, Islamic guidance has modified its approach and has begun to consider the effects which severe abnormality of the foetus would have on the mother and the family. It therefore appears that if the abnormality puts the mother's life at risk, the foetus can be aborted.

It therefore follows that abortions under Islamic or Sharia law can be performed if:

i. the pregnancy is under four months (before ensoulment)
ii. the foetus is suffering from severe abnormality
iii. the severe abnormality causes the mother or the foetus itself extreme hardship which causes the mother's life to be endangered
iv. both the mother and the father consent to the termination of the pregnancy.

Judaism

Halacha or Jewish law states that a foetus should not in principle be harmed. However, if there is a direct threat to the mother either in childbirth or the continuation of the pregnancy, then abortion is permitted. Before birth, while the foetus is considered to be alive, only the mother is a person; the foetus has not yet achieved this status and, where it threatens the mother's life, 'her life comes before the life of the foetus' and abortion is permitted. In this respect, the mother's life will always come first and, while great respect is afforded to the foetus, the foetus's potential as a person is irrelevant and is disregarded. Once the foetus is largely delivered, the mother and the baby's life are deemed to be equal in value.

Halacha does not in principle consider one life to be less valuable than another. It is therefore the majority opinion of most Orthodox Jews that abortion is not permitted in cases of foetus abnormality or disability. However, there is a contrary, minority view that does permit termination of pregnancy within the first three months in cases of abnormality which would cause the baby to suffer if the pregnancy was allowed to continue. This view would also allow a foetus to be aborted up to the six-month period, if it is discovered that it was suffering from Tay-Sachs. Given that babies with Tay-Sachs suffer considerably and their lifespan is severely curtailed, Jewish couples are encouraged to be tested for Tay-Sachs to establish whether they are carriers of the defective gene.

Since Halacha does not recognise an embryo as a potential person prior to 40 days, then it follows that abortion prior to 40 days is permitted in some circumstances. Furthermore, if an embryo prior to this period is not clearly recognised, then it follows that pre-implantation diagnosis is permitted within Orthodox Judaism.

Buddhism

There is no single Buddhist view on abortion. The first Precept of Buddhism is not to kill any living being; therefore aborting a baby is clearly against this principle. Life for Buddhists begins at conception, and traditional Buddhists regard abortion as deliberately destroying a life. Both the intention to abort and the action are against the principles of Buddhism.

However, modern Buddhists are divided about the morality of abortion, and it is possible for them to argue that abortion is permissible, for example in cases where not performing an abortion causes a child to be born who will suffer greatly because of medical conditions. Buddhism stresses the individual's personal responsibility for everything that they do and the consequences thereof; the decision to abort would be highly personal, requiring substantial examination of the ethical issues for that individual.

6.3.4 Assisted reproductive techniques and religion

Developments in medical technology now allow patients to receive assistance with reproduction (IVF), embryo screening or pre-implantation genetic diagnosis (PGD) to help eliminate foetal abnormality by screening embryos prior to implantation. Here, we take a brief look at different religious approaches to modern medical technology.

Christianity

There is no clear consensus within the different branches of Christianity to PGD. The one consistent element within Christianity is the belief in Jesus as the son of God together with his teachings and revelations. The process of PGD involves selection of an embryo; those which are not wanted are discarded. The destruction of the embryo would amount to infanticide of the embryo which violates Christian ethics which state that human life begins at conception and therefore any destruction of any embryo is tantamount to murder.

Islam

Islam is broadly accepting of a procedure which would allow a couple to conceive a child free from genetic material which could present a significant risk to the child. This acceptance is in line with Islamic thinking and can be distinguished from other technologies such as sperm donation which 'fractures links of family genetic lineage and this is analogous to adultery and condemned' (Serour and Dickens (2001)). However, while the importance of PGD is recognised, Islam is reluctant to approve its use for sex selection of embryos or for the purposes of establishing a desirable family unit. Nevertheless, the emphasis on the need of a son in a Muslim family might allow the use of PGD where the family unit already had daughters and multiple pregnancies are not in the mother's best interests.

Judaism

Halacha or Jewish law considers the use of pre-implantation genetic diagnosis positively. This advance in medical technology is perhaps particularly relevant for a community which has prevalence to Tay-Sachs disease, especially those Jews whose ancestry is Eastern European (Ashkenazi). In such circumstances it is permissible to perform pre-implantation genetic screening in order to determine which zygotes are carriers of Tay-Sachs and then implant only those which are healthy. What is the implication of the discarded zygotes? There is little significance in Judaism of the disposal of embryos, as an embryo must achieve implantation in the woman's womb before it is truly recognised. Therefore, prior to the 40-day period the embryo is considered to be simply fluid.

ACTIVITY

Self-test questions

- What is principlism?
- Why is the principle of autonomy important?
- Does autonomy override other principles?
- Do principles ever conflict? Illustrate with examples.
- What is virtue ethics? Is there a role for this theory in modern medical ethics?
- Is casuistry relevant in modern-day bioethics?

SUMMARY

■ The ethical dilemmas that bioethics pose can be resolved with consideration of a number of ethical theories. The most common (utilitarianism, deontology and the four principles) allow us to apply different approaches. Ethical theories are an invaluable tool and should not be used in isolation to each other, but the use of each theory, where appropriate, allows us to weigh up the dilemmas that are often faced in modern medicine.

■ In contrast to a secular approach, ethical dilemmas are sometimes also resolved by the use of religious guidance or principles. These of course tend by their very nature to be less flexible as there is little room for debate or non-adherence. Nevertheless, we can observe that the majority of mainstream religions embrace medical techno-logical advances.

Further reading

Beauchamp, T. and Childress, J. (2008) *Principles of Biomedical Ethics*, sixth edition. Oxford: Oxford University Press.

Brazier, M. and Bridge, C. (1996) 'Coercion or caring: analysing adolescent autonomy', *Legal Studies*, 16 (1), pages 84–109.

Donchin (1996) 'Feminist Critiques of new fertility techniques', *Journal of Medical Philoso-phy*, 21, pages 476–97.

Hare, R. M. (2010) 'A Utilitarian Approach', in *A Companion to Bioethics*, edited by Kuhse, H. and Singer, P. Oxford: Blackwell.

Harris, J. (1985) *The Value of Life – An Introduction to Medical Ethics*. Oxford: Routledge.

Harris, J. (2001) *Bioethics*. Oxford: Oxford University Press.

Herring, J. (2007) 'Where are the Carers in Healthcare Law and Ethics?' *Legal Studies*, vol. 27, pages 51–73.

Jonsen, A., Siegler, M. and Winslade, W. (2010) *Clinical Ethics: A Practical Approach to Ethical Decisions in Clinical Medicine*, seventh edition. Lange Clinical Science.

Lebacqz, K. (1995) *Encyclopaedia of Bioethics*, edited by Reich, W. T. Basingstoke: Macmillan.

Mason, J. K. and Laurie, G. T. (2010) *Mason and McCall Smith's Law and Medical Ethics*, eighth edition. Oxford: Oxford University Press.

Pattinson, S. (2009) *Medical Law and Ethics*, second edition. London: Sweet and Maxwell.

Petersen, M. (2004) 'A woman's choice? – on women, assisted reproduction and social coercion', *Ethical Theory and Moral Practice*, 7.

Rawlinson, M. C. (2008) 'Introduction', *The International Journal of Feminist Approaches to Bioethics*, vol. 1, No. 1.

Serour, G. I. and Dickens, B. M. (2001) 'Assisted reproduction developments in the Islamic world', *International Journal of Gynaecology and Obstetrics*, vol. 74, pages 187–93.

Sherwin, S. (1996) *Feminism and Bioethics: Beyond Reproduction*, edited by Wolf, S. Oxford: Oxford University Press, pages 3–43.

Sokol, D. K. (2008) 'The "four quadrants" approach to clinical ethics case analysis; an application and review', *Journal of Medical Ethics*, 34, pages 513–16.

7

Assisted conception

AIMS AND OBJECTIVES

After reading this chapter you should be able to:

■ Understand the meaning and relevance of assisted conception
■ Demonstrate a clear understanding of the provisions of the Human Fertilisation and Embryology Act 2008
■ Understand both the legal provisions and the ethical arguments relating to pre-implantation genetic diagnosis
■ Demonstrate a clear understanding of the law and ethics of both therapeutic cloning and reproductive cloning
■ Appreciate the legal complexities and ethical issues surrounding surrogacy.

Introduction

In this chapter we explore the legal regulation and the ethical arguments concerned with assisted conception. The regulation of assisted conception is provided by the Human Fertilisation and Embryology (HFE) Acts 1990 and 2008, and constant reference to the Act is made throughout the chapter. Any form of assisted conception is required to be licensed by the Human Fertilisation and Embryology Authority (HFEA), and we consider not only the legal provisions but also the effects of assisted conception on the child born as a result.

Assisted conception is one of the most significant breakthroughs in medical technology. In 1978, Louise Brown was the world's first IVF baby to be born and, within four years of her birth, a Committee of Enquiry into Human Fertilisation and Embryology was tasked with recommending regulation for this fast-growing area of medicine. It is essential that the law matches pace with medical advances to ensure adequate regulation. The Warnock Report (named after the Chair and eminent philosopher, Baroness Warnock) reported in 1984. It was another six years until the Human Fertilisation and Embryology Act 1990 was passed.

It will become apparent in this chapter that assisted conception is an extensive yet intriguing and thought-provoking area. The reader must be aware that many provisions in the Human Fertilisation and Embryology Act are simply not addressed as entire books are devoted to this subject alone. This chapter provides a mere snapshot of the legal and ethical issues relating to infertility.

According to NICE, infertility is defined as 'failing to get pregnant after two years of regular unprotected sex'. If a couple are attempting to conceive, this can be extremely distressing and put an added stress upon their relationship. According to the HFEA, the concerns of infertility are, after pregnancy, the most common reason for young women to seek medical advice. While the casual observer may consider infertility to be uncommon, a significant 3.5 million people per year suffer from infertility in the UK. A small minority remain unable to conceive.

Part 1 will briefly investigate ownership of gametes (sperm in the case of a man and ova or eggs in the case of a woman) before examining some specific difficulties that have arisen relating to consent. These have largely been remedied by statutory amendments. Part 2 explores pre-implantation genetic diagnosis, which can be colloquially described as health screening for embryos. Part 3 will discuss cloning, a particularly fascinating area of extensive ethical debate, of which we can just scratch the surface. The final part of this chapter investigates surrogacy – the legal complexities and potential injustices.

7.1 Part 1: The ownership of gametes and issues of consent

7.1.1 Who owns the gametes?

An issue arose in the case of *Yearworth* (2009) as to who had legal ownership of gametes in a case of negligence.

CASE EXAMPLE

Yearworth v North Bristol NHS Trust [2009] EWCA 37

Five patients were diagnosed with cancer and after seeking advice from their hospital were advised to produce samples of sperm to be stored, in case chemotherapy treatment rendered them infertile. The sperm was stored in liquid nitrogen but fell below the required level, with the effect that the sperm thawed and they perished. The parties sued in negligence. While it was apparent there was a breach of duty of care as the storage unit failed to work as it should, there was no direct personal injury and, more importantly, there was no guidance from the law as to who owned the sperm. Was it the person whose sperm was in storage and was now of no use, or were the gametes owned by the hospital?

The Court of Appeal held that where a hospital had stored a sample of sperm on behalf of a patient who was undergoing chemotherapy, in case he became infertile after treatment, the sperm was the property of the person who produced it; thus there was loss or damage sufficient to establish negligence. The patient had produced the bodily product for the specific purpose that it be frozen in case it was required at a later stage. The storage of the sperm is regulated by the HFE Act 2008 and the patients consented to the storage as required by the Act and also in the way it could or could not be used. Accordingly, it appears to be correct to impose a duty on the hospital towards the patients which they subsequently breached, with the direct result of the loss of the patients' sperm causing them irrevocable loss.

7.1.2 Anonymity and gamete donation

Prior to 2005, s 31(5), HFE Act 1990 stated that neither the couple who received the donor gametes nor the offspring produced as a result were entitled to any information that would identify the donor. Anonymous donors were anonymous in the true sense of the word. The donor's identity was known to the licensed authority as the HFEA kept a register of those who had been born as a result of artificial donor insemination and those who had donated. Although the principle of anonymity was sacrosanct, there was certain information which could be disclosed. This related to the following situations:

- If the child born suffered a hereditary disorder, the donor could be contacted to restrict further donations
- There is a possibility that the child born from an anonymous donor could become involved in a relationship where he or she might be related to the person they were due to marry or bear a child with, with potentially disastrous consequences.

It was argued in the case detailed below that a child has a right to information about her genetic identity under Art 8, ECHR.

CASE EXAMPLE

R (on the application of Rose) v Secretary of State for Health [2002] EWHC 1593 (Admin)

The claimants were all born as a result of artificial insemination by donors and wished to be able to identify their biological parents. The Secretary of State responded by explaining that there was a consultation exercise in progress and failed to respond directly to the applications request. They sought judicial review of the decision arguing that Art 8 was engaged and their right to a private and family life included identification of their biological parent.

The court accepted that Art 8 was engaged and that it was important for children who were born as a result of gamete donation to be able to identify their biological father in the case of sperm donation or the biological mother in the case of egg donation. The court recognised the social and psychological importance of being able to identify clearly who they are as individuals.

The court, however, failed to address the conflicting right of a donor wishing to retain his anonymity. If a donor was assured anonymity and that assurance was not honoured, one might also conclude that the donor's rights under Art 8 had also been violated.

7.1.3 Human Fertilisation and Embryology Authority (Disclosure of Donor Information) Regulations 2004

As public attitudes changed and assisted conception became more commonplace, accessible and less stigmatised, the law acted in response. The UK was not swift in this respect. The first country to change their law regarding gametes' anonymity was Sweden in 1984, and thereafter offspring born could discover the identity of their biological father or mother. It is, however, worth stressing at this point, that the gametes' donor has no legal, parental or financial responsibility to the child born as a result.

As a number of countries followed suit. The UK introduced the Human Fertilisation and Embryology Authority (Disclosure of Donor Information) Regulations 2004. Reg 2(3) allows children who are born as a result of gamete donations from 1 April 2005 to discover the donor's identity, once they reach the age of 18.

The information to which they are entitled includes:

- the donor's full name and date of birth
- where he or she was born
- the appearance of the donor
- the last known postal address.

The provisions even allow information such as the donor's eye colour, ethnicity, occupation and religion to be disclosed.

7.1.4 Ethical issues of removing gamete anonymity

Applying the ethics

Discussion point

Sam and Vicky are the first- and second-born children of Michael and Katie. They are the direct product of their parents' gametes; they are biologically related. Michael becomes infertile but Michael and Katie have always wanted three children and, with the help of donor sperm, Katie is able to have her third child, Sophie.

It is often argued that we have a right to know our genetic heritage and this is particularly true in the case of gamete donation. Knowing our genetic links is important not only for fulfilling our true sense of identity but also for the purposes of identifying any genetic disease. For Sophie, this may be particularly important as she becomes an adult and seeks to have a family herself. The knowledge could be important for the purposes of preventative treatment of certain conditions and thus such knowledge is extremely relevant.

As we have already seen, it appears that the right to know one's biological parent is protected by Art 8, ECHR but this needs to be balanced with the donor's right of anonymity (which has now been removed), and also Michael and Katie's right *not* to tell their child of their genetic linkage.

Frith (2001) explores some of the reasons why parents may not wish to tell their child they were the product of gamete donation. They include the concern of what psychological and social effects the information would have on the child. Sophie could perhaps be teased at school at an early age when there is a natural lack of understanding and sensitivity among children in the playground. The fears of psychological damage also extend to the reaction of other members of the family which include not only the extended family but also perhaps the donor child's own siblings. If Sophie looks at her brother and sister, she will recognise that she is different to them, in the sense that she is not genetically linked to her parents in the same way that they are. She may suffer from lower self-esteem and a sense of not belonging.

Of course, this presupposes that Sophie has been told of her genetic background. There is no legal provision to compel parents to tell their children of their biological origins, and statistics suggest that the majority of parents do not tell their children if they are a product of gamete donation. Michael and Katie may not wish to tell Sophie of the genetic reality for fear that she will not consider her mother or father to be her 'real' parent, as such disclosure could affect the nature and the perception of their relationship.

Arguably, if Sophie was told from a very early age, then potentially difficult information could be explained sensitively and supportively, rather than embarking upon explaining to a child when they reach the more emotionally charged teenage years. Furthermore, this must be preferable to either allowing Sophie to find out accidentally, or suspecting she is not genetically linked to one of her parents or, perhaps worst of all, allowing her to enter into a prohibited relationship at some point in the future. If Sophie finds out in later childhood or early adulthood the true nature of her genetic parentage, her memories of her presumably contented childhood could be adversely affected as a result. However, it is probably worth bearing in mind that even where children are conceived through sexual intercourse, there is no real certainty about a child's paternity.

7.1.5 Embryos and the issue of consent

The HFE Act 1990 provides that a person's gametes cannot be used without their express consent.

Schedule 3, para 6(3) is expressed with precision and states that:

'An embryo the creation of which was brought about *in vitro* must not be used for any purpose unless there is an effective consent by each person whose gametes were used to bring about the creation of the embryo to the use for that purpose of the embryo and the embryo is used in accordance with those consents'.

The issue of consent became extremely controversial when two couples who had frozen embryos to be used at a later stage subsequently separated and the potential fathers withdrew consent for their gametes to be used.

CASE EXAMPLE

Evans v Amicus Healthcare Limited [2004] 3 EWCA 277

Natallie Evans was engaged to Howard Johnston and they intended to start a family together. In late 2001, she discovered she had tumours in her ovaries which required urgent treatment. Although there were different options for storing her eggs, she decided together with her fiancée to freeze fertilised embryos. Her fiancée had reassured her that there was no necessity to freeze just her eggs; they were not going to break up and he wanted to be the father of her child. Freezing her eggs alone, although more risky, would have provided her with greater options for the future. Several eggs were harvested, fertilised and then frozen. The purpose of this process was that, when she reached full health, she could have an embryo implanted with IVF. During treatment, her ovaries were removed. The following year the couple separated. Mr Johnston wanted to have the embryos destroyed and withdrew his consent to their use.

By applying Sched 3, para 6(3), the Court of Appeal found against Natallie Evans and ordered destruction of the embryos. The Sched provides that where an embryo is created *in vitro* (literally meaning 'within glass' or in a controlled environment), consent to the use of the embryo must be obtained by those who supplied the gametes. In this case, Howard Johnston withdrew his consent once the parties had separated and, thus, Natalie Evans could not implant the embryos. Her chance to become a mother had been irrevocably lost.

It was the way in which she stored her gametes which was in reality her fateful decision. She decided to store a fertilised embryo for two main reasons. Firstly, embryos store more favourable then ova and, secondly, she had been reassured by her fiancée that he wanted to have children with her. The court's decision was heart-breaking and devastating for Natallie Evans, but it was upheld by the Court of Appeal, the European Court of Human Rights and finally the Grand Chamber.

In relation to the European courts, Natallie Evans argued that her rights under Art 8 (her right to a private family life), ECHR were infringed by the provisions of the HFE Act 1990. Here was the crux of the case. There were two competing rights: the right of Natallie Evans to become a mother, and the right of Howard Johnston not to become a father. She had undergone painful IVF treatment, and endured further treatment to overcome the ovarian tumours. She had invested considerable emotional and physical effort in her only chance to mother a child genetically-related to her, but this last chance was removed when Howard Johnston withdrew his consent. There is no doubt that we feel considerable sympathy to her but we have to take into account the competing interests under Art 8. While she had the right to start a family, he had the right not to become a father if he did not wish to, and in *Evans v UK (App No. 6339/05)* (2007) the Grand Chamber refused her declaration that the HFE Act 1990 was incompatible with ECHR, stating:

JUDGMENT

'it does not consider that the applicant's right to respect for the decision to become a parent in the genetic sense should be accorded greater weight than J's right to respect for his decision not to have a genetically-related child with her.'

Thus, the court viewed the interests of the two parties as the same, but arguably they are not. This was Evans's only chance of having a genetically-related child and while Johnston argued he did not want to father a child with whom he had no daily contact, her loss was so infinitely greater that their interests seem largely disproportionate. While he could go on and father a child or any number of children in later life, she would be unable to. To father a child with someone with whom he was not living may not be ideal but, arguably, must be preferable to not permitting a child to be born. The reality of the situation is that, if she had taken the chance of freezing the eggs, it is possible she might have lost them, but it is also possible she could have had them fertilised with a sperm donor or a later partner. But, she was reassured by his desires to father her children and was pressed for time by the urgency of her medical condition.

The 1990 Act has since been amended by the 2008 Act, but one party can still oppose the use of the embryos at a later stage despite providing consent at an earlier stage. This however seems to reduce the significance of the consent in the first instance, and possibly does not fill either party with faith that their wishes at such a difficult and emotional time of their lives will be adhered to at a later stage.

The 1990 Act now provides under Sched 3 (4A) that in the event of a dispute as to the use of an embryo or embryos, no steps will be taken to use or dispose of the embryo for the period of one year. This 'cooling off' period is to allow the parties to reflect and perhaps resolve the difficulties between them, so as to avoid a similar issue to that of Natallie Evans and Howard Johnston occurring again.

A different issue arose in the case below, illustrating the application of the rules regarding consent of storage of gametes under HFE Act 1990.

CASE EXAMPLE

R v Human Fertilisation and Embryology Authority ex parte Blood [1997] 2 WLR 806

Mr Blood contracted meningitis and fell fatally ill. While he was in a coma, sperm was taken and was stored. Mr Blood had not provided written consent to the use of his sperm after his death. Mrs Blood argued that it had been discussed but provisions of the HFE Act 1990 require written consent. It was not possible for her to be inseminated with his gametes in the UK as he had not provided consent. She sought permission to take the sperm to Belgium where she hoped she could be inseminated.

At first instance, the court held that the HFEA had acted correctly. On appeal, Mrs Blood relied on her right in European Union law under Arts 59 and 60 of the EC Treaty to travel to a member state to receive treatment. Even though it was clearly a way of circumventing the strict rules under the HFE Act 1990, the court allowed her to remove the sperm out of the jurisdiction. She was successfully inseminated on two occasions, producing two sons as a direct result.

This was of course a very unusual situation, but an almost identical case occurred in 2008, just prior to HFE Act 2008. Here, in *L v Human Fertilisation and Embryology Authority* [2008] EWHC 2149 (Fam), the courts again allowed L to travel abroad for treatment. She relied, not on her rights under European Union law, but on rights under Art 8 of ECHR and thus was permitted to move the sperm to the USA in order to be inseminated.

One interesting point that arose in the case of *Blood* (1997) was that, after the successful birth of her sons, she found she was unable to register their late father's name on the birth certificate. A rushed amendment to the HFE Act 1990 was passed and Human Fertilisation and Embryology (Deceased Fathers) Act 2003 allowed children who were conceived after their father's death to have their father's name registered on their birth certificate.

Key facts on embryos and the issue of consent

Case	Judgment
Evans v Amicus Healthcare Limited (2004)	Once his consent had been withdrawn she could not use the embryos in storage. Accordingly, they were destroyed.
R v Human Fertilisation and Embryology Authority ex parte Blood (1997)	Without his consent she could not be inseminated with her deceased husband's sperm. She relied on European law and the freedom to travel to be treated in another country.
L v Human Fertilisation and Embryology Authority (2008)	L could remove sperm from her deceased husband and travel abroad for the purposes of insemination. Relied on Art 8.

ACTIVITY

Self-test questions

- How is fertility defined?
- Does a patient who wishes gametes to be stored on his or her behalf retain ownership after storage?
- Can gamete donors be identified?
- Can a person's gametes be used without their consent?

SUMMARY

▨ Perhaps this chapter more than any other demonstrates the remarkable achievements of modern medical technology.

▨ The law has acted in response to unique medical complexities as was seen in response to the cases of both *Evans v Amicus Healthcare Limited* (2004) and *R v Human Fertilisation and Embryology Authority ex parte Blood* (1997).

Further reading

Frith, L. (2001) 'Gamete Donation and Anonymity', *Human Reproduction*, Vol. 16, No. 5, pages 818–24.

7.2 Part 2: Pre-implantation Genetic Diagnosis (PGD)

7.2.1 Introduction

This procedure, PGD, can be loosely defined as embryo screening which occurs prior to implantation of the embryo into the woman by way of IVF. The questions we will be addressing in this part of the chapter are:

▨ What is PGD and when is it used?
▨ What is the legal position?
▨ Is PGD ethically acceptable?

7.2.2 What is PGD?

One way of describing PGD is to consider the process as a form of early diagnosis of an undesirable condition in an embryo. The embryo is tested or screened to identify whether it is at risk of carrying a genetic transmittable condition. Therefore, PGD screens embryos prior to implantation to avoid implanting those embryos whose genetic make-up indicates that it carries a disease or condition. Often, PGD is used to screen for a specific condition if there is a significant possibility that the couple can transmit either a hereditary disease or a chromosomal abnormality. The value of PGD in this respect is that it avoids the pain and distress of considering the option of abortion if the couple discover later that the embryo carries an inherited condition or chromosomal abnormality. A couple is then effectively choosing between an embryo which is not affected by disease or chromosomal defect and one that is affected.

7.2.3 What disease or chromosomal abnormalities can be detected?

The Human Fertilisation and Embryology Authority and Advisory Committee on Genetic Testing's *Consultation Document on Pre-implantation Genetic Diagnosis* (2000) stated in paragraph 10 that PGD can only be used in 'certain severe life-threatening disorders'.

As at March 2011, there are over 120 conditions that can be detected through the use of PGD. Some of the more commonly known conditions, each varying in severity from the other, are listed below:

- Alzheimer's disease (early onset)
- Beta thalassaemia
- BRCA 1 (the gene associated with breast cancer)
- Diamond Blackfan Anaemia
- Down's syndrome
- Gaucher's disease
- Haemophilia
- Huntington disease
- Hydrocephalus
- Muscular Dystrophy (Beckers and Duchenne)
- Sickle cell anaemia
- Tay-Sachs disease.

7.2.4 The law

A licence is required from the HFEA in order to carry out PGD. The HFE Act 2008 sets out the conditions to be applied.

Schedule 2, para 1ZA(1) states that a licence under para 1 cannot allow the testing of an embryo unless it is for one of the following reasons:

SECTION

'(a) Establishing whether the embryo has a gene, chromosome or mitochondrion abnormality that may affect its capacity to result in a live birth

(b) In a case where there is a particular risk that the embryo may have any gene, chromosome or mitochondrion abnormality, establishing whether it has that abnormality or any other gene, chromosome or mitochondrion abnormality

(c) In a case where there is a particular risk that any resulting child will have or will develop –

  i) gender-related serious physical or mental disability

  ii) a gender-related serious illness or

  iii) any other gender-related serious medical condition'

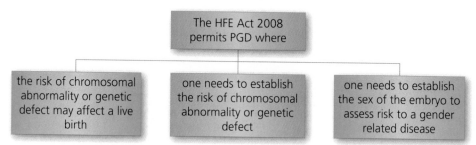

Figure 7.1 When PGD is permitted by HFE Act 2008

7.2.5 Is PGD ethically acceptable?

ACTIVITY

Applying the ethics

Edward and Margaret wish to start a family. Margaret has been told that she is a carrier of Huntington's disease. She knows that there is a 50 per cent chance that any child of hers will have the disease. In order to determine whether the baby she will carry will have this disability, they decide in conjunction with IVF to undergo genetic embryo screening. They have already decided, having learnt about the degenerative nature of the disease, that they will not implant any embryo that may be carrying this genetic disorder.

We begin from a common starting point. It is the woman's autonomous decision whether or not to proceed with the implantation of the embryo, and it is her choice to determine which embryo she wishes to be implanted with. She is now told that the first embryo tested is a carrier and the second embryo tested is not a carrier. Unsurprisingly, she wishes the embryo free from Huntington's to be implanted. While this is her autonomous choice, we must consider what message this conveys about a person who suffers a disability.

If Margaret chooses to implant the embryo free from disability, which she surely will, the embryo with the disability will be discarded. Having discarded the affected embryo, the analogy is that disabled lives are not lives worth keeping and discriminates against those who have disabilities. In reality, this is what Margaret is doing. By selecting the embryo without the disability she is discriminating, although it could be described as a form of positive discrimination as she favours the embryo that is more likely to have a happy and fulfilled life and one not full of pain and suffering. However, should Margaret and Edward be permitted to discriminate? They are not saying that it is better to have no child than a child with a disability. They are saying they would prefer to have a child free from a life of suffering by exercising their autonomy. It is important to them to avoid perpetuating disability where possible.

In our hypothetical example, the couple wished to ensure that any child they had was free from an inherited disease. There is, however, another more recent use of PGD which is considered below.

7.2.6 'Saviour siblings'

From 2001, the HFEA has permitted the use of tissue typing (also known as Human Leukocyte Antigen (HLA)) in embryos. This involves taking a cell from an embryo and testing it in a similar process to PGD. While the objective of both procedures is to establish that the embryo is disease-free, tissue typing also ensures that the embryo is an exact match to a sibling. The embryo is then implanted via IVF and when the baby child is born, the stem cells from the umbilical blood are used as potentially life-saving treatment for the sick sibling. The child born as a result of this process is often referred to as a 'saviour sibling'.

The law

The HFE Act 2008 permits embryo testing for the purpose of 'saviour siblings'. Paragraph 1Z(d) of Sched 2 states that:

SECTION

'in a case where a person (the sibling) who is the child of the persons whose gametes are used to bring about the creation of the embryo (or of either of those persons) suffers from a serious medical condition which could be treated by umbilical stem cells, bone marrow or other tissue of any resulting child, establishing whether the tissue of any resulting child would be compatible with that of the sibling, and ...'

The wording of the paragraph is very specific as it refers to blood from the umbilical cord, bone marrow or other tissue. While this may appear widely drafted, para 1ZA(4) confirms that 'other tissue' does not refer to any whole organ of the child, thereby eliminating any possible suggestion that a child born to benefit its sibling could donate a kidney.

'Saviour sibling' cases

Zain Hashmi was a three-year-old boy with beta thalassaemia. He had to undergo regular bone transplants and needed a bone marrow transplant. Beta thalassaemia is a hereditary condition, and both of his parents were carriers. The clinic which was treating the Hashmi family applied to the HFEA to carry out PGD and tissue typing. It was their intention that blood from a tissue perfect match would be used to help save Zain's life. They already had a second child who was free from the disease and was not a tissue match and this was, for them, a desperate measure to help save their child's life. A licence was granted; an embryo match was found; and when the baby was born, Zain was treated with stem cells with perfect tissue compatibility which has helped to treat him and save his life.

In contrast, the case of the Whitaker family had a different outcome. Here, Charlie Whitaker was of similar age and suffered from Diamond Blackfan Anaemia (DBA). He too required frequent blood transfusions, and a bone marrow transplant could help this incurable condition. The family asked their fertility clinic if they could test embryos using PGD. However, the difference between the Whitaker and the Hashmi case is that DBA is not hereditary. Therefore, it would be extremely unlikely that any future child born to the Whitaker family would have the same condition and, on this basis, the HFEA refused the Whitakers' application. The Whitaker family travelled to America, where tissue typing was carried out, and a baby born as a result was a tissue match for Charlie. It is, however, worth remembering that this case was decided before the HFE Act 2008 was enacted. Had it been decided post-2008, the decision is likely to have been different.

The HFEA's decision was based upon the argument that, while both parties wanted another child in any event, the Whitaker's application was based *solely* on their desire to find a tissue match to help Charlie whereas, with the Hashmi family, the purpose was also to ensure that a further child would not suffer the same condition. The HFEA were concerned about the potential effect on any future sibling of Charlie's if he or she discovered in the future that they were selected as an embryo (and the other embryos discarded) in order that Charlie's life could be saved.

More recently, in 2009, the UK's only saviour siblings were born. Connor Maguire suffered from aplastic anaemia – a condition where the immune system destroys part of the bone marrow. The only cure for the condition is a bone marrow transplant, but a match could not be found. Their other son did not suffer from the condition and was not a carrier. The Maguire famiy had the HFEA's approval to test embryos in order to identify a potential tissue match for Connor. Two such embryos were found, implanted via IVF and twins were born as a result. The stem cells from the umbilical cords were taken immediately upon the twins' birth and stored for the benefit of Connor's future health.

The legal consequences of the HFEA's decision

Following the HFEA's decision in 2001 to grant a licence to the fertility clinic treating the Hashmi family, Josephine Quintavalle, acting on behalf of Comment of Reproductive Ethics, a pro-life pressure group committed to protecting the embryo, brought an action for judicial review.

CASE EXAMPLE

Quintavalle (Comment of Reproductive Ethics) v Human Fertilisation and Embryology Authority [2005] UKHL 28

Quintavalle argued that tissue typing was not permitted by the HFE Act 1990. Section 11 of the Act stated that licences must be 'authorising such activities in the course of providing treatment services'. Treatment services are defined as 'assisting woman to carry children' and include 'practices designed to secure that embryos are in a suitable condition to be placed in a woman or to determine whether embryos are suitable for that purpose'.

At first instance, the court adopted a narrow interpretation of 'treatment services' and held that tissue typing was not a 'necessary' activity to help a woman carry a child. Applying this interpretation, tissue typing could not be licensed by the HFEA. The Court of Appeal reversed this decision which was subsequently upheld by the House of Lords.

Lord Hoffman stated that it was the intention of Parliament to define 'the licensing power of the authority ... in broad terms'. Quintavalle opposed a wider interpretation as she argued that the HFEA could then permit woman to test for a whole range of characteristics in an embryo which would invariably lead to the slippery slope of 'designer babies'.

However, the House of Lords opined that activities were permitted under the Act if they were carried out 'in the course of' providing IVF services which could be considered 'necessary or desirable'. Since it was both necessary and desirable to ensure that any embryo that Mrs Hashmi was to have implanted was free of disease, both for the benefit of the embryo itself and for the benefit of the sick sibling, the House of Lords held that tissue typing was an activity which could correctly be licensed by the Act.

KEY FACTS

Key facts on legal provisions

Case or statute	Provision or judgment
Human Fertilisation and Embryology Act 2008, Sched 2, para 1ZA(1)	Permits PGD to establish whether the embryo has or is at risk of a genetic, chromosome or mitochondrion abnormality or where there is a risk of a gender-related condition.
Human Fertilisation and Embryology Act 2008, Sched 2, para 1ZA(1)(d)	Permits PGD for the purposes of tissue typing to exclude a serious medical condition and to test for compatibility to a sibling.
Quintavalle (Comment of Reproductive Ethics) v Human Fertilisation and Embryology Authority (2005)	Claimed that tissue typing was not permitted by the HFE Act 1990. Her claim failed in the House of Lords.

The ethics of 'saviour siblings'

Is it ethically acceptable for a woman to select an embryo which is a tissue match for a sick sibling in order that, when the baby is born, the umbilical cord blood can be taken in order to treat the sibling?

One of the main criticisms of having a baby in order to benefit its sibling is that it treats the baby as a means to an end. This confirms the Kantian principle that we should 'never use people as a means but always treat them as an end'. However, this argument does not accurately interpret the Kantian principle as one should not treat a person solely as a means to an end. This suggests that it is acceptable if the baby has a purpose in being born, provided that the purpose is not the only reason why it is born. It follows that provided the baby is loved as a member of the family in their own right, then the reason how or why they were born should not be a relevant factor.

A more extreme view may suggest that the child is not born in its own right but as a source of spare parts for the existing child. Nicholson states:

QUOTATION

'we are not creating this saviour sibling to be a child in its own right. We have created it – designed it – to be a source of spare parts for the existing child.'

(Devolder, 2005)

When the saviour sibling is a minor, it is necessary for the parents to consent to any medical intervention on their behalf. Assuming that the intervention is for the benefit of the sick child, the parents have to weigh the risks of any saviour sibling's medical procedure carefully. There is clearly no benefit to *this* child, only to their other sick child. It is a difficult, maybe impossible, task to provide informed consent, free from any undue influence or pressure when this child has been born for the very purpose of helping the other.

The saviour sibling has been born for the benefit of his sibling, and being born as a saviour sibling may impose a self-made duty to serve the sick sibling's needs. When the saviour sibling reaches an age of understanding, it may resent the way it was designed to be born, and this in turn may harm the saviour sibling. Given the complexity of the sick sibling's condition, it is also possible that the saviour sibling will be needed in the future, for blood or perhaps a bone marrow transplant. The saviour sibling may feel like a commodity and, if so, the saviour sibling has invariably been harmed.

If the saviour sibling donates bone marrow at a later date and this fails to benefit the sick sibling, the saviour sibling could also be harmed as he would be aware that the very essence of his creation was to help his sibling. He may feel worthless, that he has let down his sibling and his parents, and now his life has no true value. Studies of siblings who have donated bone marrow to siblings show 'saviour donors showed more anxiety, lower self-esteem ... than did non-saviour siblings' (*The Lancet*, vol. 358, Issue 9289, page 1195). On the other hand, he may feel that he has a very special role to fulfil, that he has a unique gift that he can pass on and he may gain considerable pleasure and satisfaction if he can help his sibling live an improved quality of life.

There is little evidence to support the suggestion that a child born from PGD would be physically harmed as a result. It is suggested that 'so far embryo biopsy for PGD does not seem to produce adverse biological effects' (*The Lancet*, vol. 358, Issue 9289, page 1195). The embryo will be free from the disease it is being screened for although, of course, the embryo could be carrying another disease for which it is not tested.

Is harm caused to society if a couple can choose the genetic make-up of their embryo? It is crucial to appreciate that all the law permits is PGD or tissue typing in order to eliminate specific conditions. The law does not permit selection of embryos for any reasons such as intelligence, beauty, musical ability or sporting prowess. To permit screening for these characteristics is often referred to as the slippery slope akin to the Nazi eugenic project, where the creation of 'designer babies' is not only permitted but positively encouraged. Eugenics could occur not just where a couple desire a child with particular characteristics but where society demands certain characteristics are prevalent.

Arguments against saviour siblings

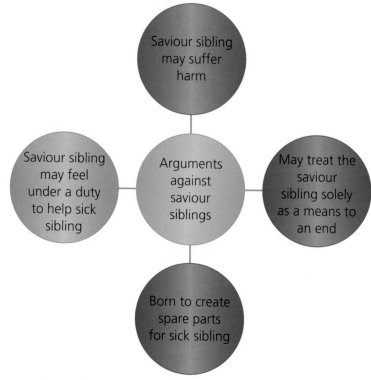

Figure 7.2 Arguments against saviour siblings

Arguments in favour of saviour siblings

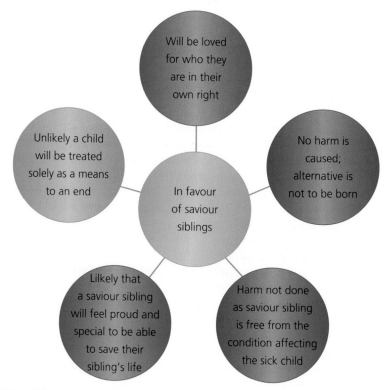

Figure 7.3 Arguments in favour of saviour siblings

7.2.7 Sex selection: the law and ethics

While the HFE Act 2008, Sched 2, para 1ZA permits sex selection of embryos for the purposes of detecting 'a gender-related serious illness', para 1ZB(1) states that a licence cannot be authorised 'to secure that any resulting child will be one sex rather than the other'. Hence it is unlawful to test an embryo for the purposes of determining its sex if the purpose would be purely social.

The United Kingdom is not alone; sex selection of embryos is unlawful in many countries to avoid the preference of boys over girls. Furthermore, Art 14 of the Convention for the protection of Human Rights and dignity of the human being with regard to the application of biology and medicine: Convention on Human Rights and Biomedicine states:

SECTION

'The use of techniques of medically assisted procreation shall not be allowed for the purpose of choosing a future child's sex, except where serious hereditary sex-related disease is to be avoided.'

We presume that if sex selection was legal in the UK it would be used responsibly. It is important however that it remains unlawful as other countries may approach sex selection less ethically. It would be much harder to argue against another country legalising sex selection, if it was permitted in the UK.

Those who embark upon parenthood may have an idea in mind of what sex their ideal family would comprise and often follow old wives' tales during conception in order to achieve that goal. Of course, few are disappointed in the sex of their child once the baby is born and almost all rejoice regardless of the sex of the child.

Given that technology exists in order to determine the sex of an embryo for the purposes of eliminating 'gender-related serious illness', to what extent is sex selection for social purposes ethically acceptable?

Some may argue that sex selection is a women's autonomous reproductive right. Arguably, it is a restriction on a woman's reproductive autonomy if she is denied the right to decide for herself what children she wishes to bear.

However, in some male-dominated societies the value of boys and men are considered infinitely more valuable than girls and women, for either religious or manual labour reasons. Here, the possibility of aborting female embryos in favour of male embryos harms the value of women by devaluing their worth and can perpetuate sexism. It is no coincidence that in countries such as India, where boys are valued more than girls for their manual labour, baby girls are often rejected at birth and the number of baby boys far outnumbers the number of baby girls. A similar problem is seen in China. However, if sex selection was permitted, it does not automatically follow that couples would select male embryos and discard female embryos. The procedure is expensive and not readily available. This would automatically exclude the population for whom sex selection is of value. Poor farm labourers in rural areas of India would not be able to afford the cost of sex selection and, where having a boy is preferable to having a girl to avoid payment of a dowry, the dowry is likely is be far less than expensive reproductive techniques.

Nevertheless, a significant ethical difficulty would arise where sex selection of embryos became state-sponsored 'for the good of the country'. This reverts to the earlier argument of the slippery slope towards abhorrent Nazi-style eugenic programmes or control of an ever-increasing population such as the one child policy in China.

Sex selection could harm a child if it was to discover that it would have been rejected if it was not the sex desired by its parents. This can devalue the child and may influence the child's behaviour to adopt a more stereotypical sexual role; for example, a girl may choose not to play football, for fear that it might portray her more 'boyish' than a girl, which was not what her parents desired.

ACTIVITY

Self-test questions

Ensure that you support your answers with case law and/or statute where appropriate.

- What is the purpose of pre-implantation genetic diagnosis?
- When can it be used?
- What is a saviour sibling?
- Does the HFE Act 2008 permit embryo testing for the purposes of saviour siblings?

SUMMARY

- PGD and tissue typing remain uncommon. Not only is it expensive but it is a stressful and time-consuming venture and, in any event, it will only be licensed in specific and limited circumstances.
- Are PGD and tissue typing ethically acceptable? Removing the possibility of great harm which can be caused by an inheritable condition or chromosomal abnormality can only benefit a child born as a result of this screening. The ethical dilemmas arise when a child is born as a result of PGD in order to benefit a sibling.
- This is more colloquially referred to as producing a 'saviour sibling' and, although there have been relatively few cases in the UK, they have sparked considerable media and legal attention.
- Provided no harm is done to the resultant child, there is positive benefit. A sick child can receive life-saving treatment and a child is born into a family and loved for who that child is. Thus far, since there is no evidence to the contrary, we can conclude that both PGD and tissue typing are ethically acceptable.
- In contrast, the use of any technology for the purpose of sex selection of embryos is unlawful and considered ethically unacceptable.

Further reading

Devolder, K. (2005) 'Pre-implantation HLA typing: having children to save our loved ones', *Journal of Medical Ethics*, 31, pages 582–6.

Jackson, E. (2001) *Regulating Reproduction: Law, Technology and Autonomy*. Oxford: Hart Publishing.

7.3 Part 3: Cloning

7.3.1 Introduction

Cloning can be defined as an individual or a creature which is genetically identical to another. Children are clones of their parents in the ordinary sense of the word, as they obtained their genetic composition from both of their parents. Hence, while they may have genetic similarities, they are not genetically identical, unlike identical twins.

Cloning has been defined by the United States' President's Council on Bioethics 2002 as being:

QUOTATION

'accomplished by introducing the nuclear material of a human somatic cell (donor) into an oocyte (egg) whose own nucleus has been removed or inactivated yielding a product that has a human genetic construction virtually identical to the donor of the somatic cell.'

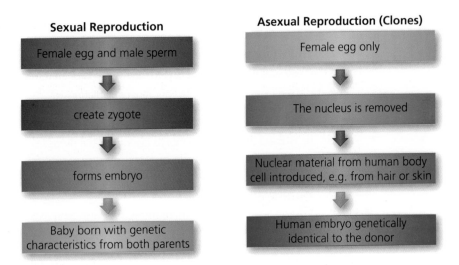

Figure 7.4 (a) Sexual reproduction (b) Cloned reproduction (asexual)

In 1996, Dolly the Sheep was the first mammal born as a result of cloning. She was cloned at the Roslin Institute in Scotland by Professor Ian Wilmut and Keith Campbell. Using the process of nuclear transfer from an adult somatic cell, Dolly lived for six years, about half the normal period of a sheep. Her premature death was not necessarily linked to the fact she was cloned, and before her death she gave birth to a number of healthy lambs.

The cloning of a mammal was not only a vastly significant scientific breakthrough but immediately generated intense worldwide speculation as to the next step forward. Could a person be cloned? Would it be possible to clone the worst of mankind, such as Adolf Hitler? As a direct result many countries took immediate steps to prohibit cloning, lest they opened the door to something society might quickly regret.

In this part of the chapter we will explore the difference between therapeutic and reproductive cloning, and in doing so will discuss the legal provisions and ethical arguments in relation to both. We will highlight how there are considerable ethical advantages to some aspects of cloning which remind us that we always need to consider arguments in detail before coming to a conclusion.

7.3.2 The immediate legal effect of Dolly the Sheep

Dolly the Sheep was achieved by cell nuclear replacement (CNR). While this process creates an embryo, the embryo has not travelled through the fertilisation process, and it would not fall into the statutory definition of an embryo in s 1(1), HFE Act 1990, which specifically refers to a process of fertilisation. The method by which Dolly was created could therefore be unregulated if embryos created by cell nuclear replacement did not fall within the s 1 definition which inferred that human reproductive cloning was not unlawful.

It was the lacuna between this statutory definition within s 1(1) and the reality of cell nuclear replacement that prompted the application for judicial review from the Pro Life Alliance Group.

CASE EXAMPLE

R (on the application of Quintavalle) v Secretary of State for Health [2003] UKHL 13

Bruno Quintavalle on behalf of the Pro Life Alliance Group claimed that the definition of embryo by ways of CNR was not covered by the Act. He was successful at first instance. Mr Justice Crane granted a declaration to the applicants stating that organisms created by CNR were not embryos within the statutory definition of s 1(1). It was held that the words were not sufficiently ambiguous to require anything other than a literal interpretation. The effect of the judgment was that the possibility of cloning was left unregulated, a truly alarming concept.

This may have been a somewhat surprising decision particularly since the Donaldson Report (*Stem Cell Research, Medical Progress with Responsibility* in June 2002), compiled by the Chief Medical Officer's Expert Group, considered that organisms that were created by CNR were in fact 'human embryonic life ... which ... could develop into a human being' and that a purposive approach should be applied when interpreting the legislation. It was not the desired intention that cloning be exposed as unregulated. Indeed, Quintavalle would have preferred a more restrictive approach. However, to some extent satisfaction was achieved when Parliament rushed through emergency legislation as a result of Mr Justice Crane's judgment – the Human Reproductive Cloning Act 2001 makes it a criminal offence under s 1(1) to 'place(s) in a woman a human embryo which has been created otherwise than by fertilization'.

The House of Lords reversed the lower court's decision, and the possibility of cloning was regulated once more. Lord Bingham adopted a purposive approach and questioned Parliament's intention, concluding that Parliament could not have 'rationally intended to leave live human embryos created by CNR outside the scope of regulation had it known of them as a scientific possibility'. The concern for the Lords was that the definition referred to both 'live' and 'human' embryos. Since those created by CNR fulfilled both criteria, they would clearly be included in the definition. The concern of the legislation was not *how* the embryo was created but whether it was both a live embryo and a human embryo. Hence as a result of the judgment, human reproductive cloning remained unlawful, a desirable response given the prevailing view that such cloning is clearly 'ethically unacceptable', according to the Science and Technology Committee in 'The Cloning of Animals from Adult Cells. Government Response to the Fifth Report 18 December 1997' (Cm 3815 1996–1997).

7.3.3 The Human Fertilisation and Embryology Act 2008

The statutory provisions replace the Human Reproductive Cloning Act 2001. Section 3, HFE Act 2008 amends the same section of the 1990 Act which prohibits activities with embryos. Section 3(2) prohibits any embryo which is not a permitted embryo to be placed in a woman. A permitted embryo is one that is fertilised by a permitted egg and sperm whose DNA has not been altered. This section therefore precludes embryos that have been altered in any way in relation to their DNA and hence prevents and prohibits reproductive cloning.

7.3.4 Reproductive and therapeutic cloning

Before we embark upon an ethical discussion of cloning, it is necessary to draw a distinction between the reproductive and therapeutic cloning. The objective of reproductive cloning is to produce a child. The cloned embryo would be implanted into the woman's womb. The objective of therapeutic cloning is to produce cells from the cloned embryo in order to use them for research purposes or to use them for the benefit of treating a medical condition of the person from whom the adult cell derived.

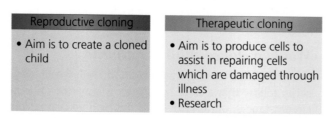

Reproductive cloning	Therapeutic cloning
• Aim is to create a cloned child	• Aim is to produce cells to assist in repairing cells which are damaged through illness • Research

Figure 7.5 The difference between reproductive and therapeutic cloning

Reproductive cloning and ethics

Human reproductive cloning is not permitted; hence no child has been born as a result of cloning and one cannot comment with any true accuracy what the effects may be. It is not disputed that cloning a child would create significant risks whether by disease or by way of severe abnormality. It should be recalled that Dolly the Sheep was only born after 277 unsuccessful attempts, so there is no reason to suggest that attempts to clone a human would not result in a similar catastrophe.

There is a concern that if cloning of individuals was permitted, it would be possible to create an exact copy of that person. This is largely erroneous as, if an individual was cloned, it would not create an identical copy of the person from whom it is cloned, just an identical copy of the **genotype** of the person. However, alarm bells have sounded at the thought of clones of distasteful characters. Indeed, there was considerable concern in the British press when the cloning of Dolly the Sheep was first reported. *The Observer* in an article entitled 'Scientists clone adult sheep' (23 February 1997) applauded the scientific breakthrough but then stated:

genotype
the genetic make up of an individual

QUOTATION

'Cloning is also likely to cause alarm. The techniques could be used on humans, drawing parallels with Huxley's "Brave New World" and the "The Boys From Brazil", in which clones of Hitler are made.'

More recently, the novelist Kazuo Ishiguro explored the potential for cloning in his novel *Never Let Me Go* (and also the film of the same name), introducing a seemingly normal, recognisable modern society in which clones have been created to provide spare parts for their body doubles.

We have already seen the immediate universal banning of reproductive cloning, but one might argue that it is not genetics that leads any tyrant to act as they did but a combination of circumstance, opportunity and prevailing social issues at that time.

We therefore cannot clone an individual and expect them to act the same way. Even if we wish to clone a person who has contributed enormous good and untold value to society, there is no guarantee that a clone would be as brilliant as the original. It is important to remember that free will and autonomous decisions have a significant role to play and it does not follow that a cloned dictator would be cloned to create a modern-day dictator. We can see this principle in action when we consider identical twins, who have the same genotype (DNA) although it is interpreted in different physical ways; they also have individual personalities and, while they may have similarities, they can also be very different. Concerns about the apocalyptic effect of reproductive cloning may simply not be of value.

Could it be argued that if we do not permit reproductive cloning then we deny women the right to procreate? Reproductive cloning is important in the sense that it can allow a woman the ability to have a child when she might otherwise be denied the opportunity. Thus, this could be particularly relevant to women who choose not to have a male partner. In denying her the right to reproductive cloning, we deny her the right to procreate and deny her the reproductive freedom to which she is entitled. However, we have already explored that one person's right has to be balanced against the rights of society as a whole and, while it is wrong to deny a woman her reproductive autonomy, if greater harm than good is caused, the restrictions can be justified.

Would a cloned child be harmed?

If reproductive cloning was permitted, we have already suggested that it does not necessarily follow that a clone would grow up to be an identical copy, as upbringing, social circumstances, opportunity and free will all play a role in determining who we are. In these circumstances, however, those who might choose to clone a child have done so with the specific intention of actually achieving an identical version of them. Hence, while we acknowledge free will and the positive effect of individual upbringing, these principles are largely shrouded in the parental expectations as to who their cloned child should be. Should the cloned child not fulfil these expectations, they could be considered by their parents to have failed, which in turn would damage the child. There are also external expectations as the cloned child will look like its clone and perceptions from others will create expectations as to how the child should act or behave. From the child's perspective, as Holm explains, 'It diminishes the clone's possibility of living a life that is in a full sense his or her life' (1998). The effect of cloning would impose upon the clone 'to be involved in an attempt to perform a complicated partial re-enactment of the life of somebody else (the original)'.

If we allow cloning of a child then we in turn deprive them of the right to be themselves; we deny them autonomy and free will to determine their own life. Hence we harm them and, if harm is done, reproductive cloning should not be ethically permitted. However, even if we conclude that harm is done, is it better to be born a clone or better not to be born at all? Burley and Harris argue that even if harm has been caused to the child, the extent of harm is relative, and:

QUOTATION

'it is none the less permissible to conceive by cloning so long as these cloning-induced welfare deficits are not such to blight the existence of the resultant child, whoever this may be'.

(1999)

The importance of genetic diversity

An argument against reproductive cloning concerns the genetic similarity of a clone and the potential psychological impact. A clone may find it difficult to regard themselves as an individual, much like identical twins can find it difficult to assert their individuality. Moreover, if cloning was permitted and became widespread, it would reduce the genetic gene pool, creating unknown havoc with genetic diversity.

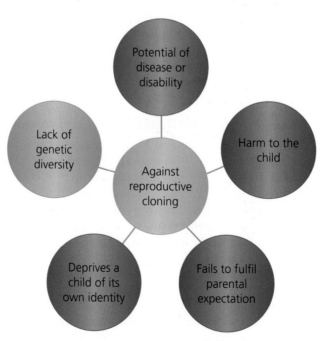

Figure 7.6 Arguments against reproductive cloning

 ### *Therapeutic cloning and stem cell research*

Cloning has an alternative function. It could be used in conjunction with stem cell research in order to help treat patients suffering from devastating and degenerative diseases. Let us imagine a person who is suffering from liver failure. If one of his cells could be cloned and allowed to differentiate to form an entire organism, this cloned cell would be almost identical to the person. If technology in the future allowed, a cloned liver could be grown which could be transplanted into the patient with positive results. The possibilities of such technology are very attractive.

Stem cells are cells which have not yet determined their specific type of tissue, although they are able to do so. Stem cells can be derived from adults, embryonic tissue, umbilical cord tissue or from foetal tissue. Opponents of using embryos for stem cell research argue that stem cells from umbilical cords at birth or adults can be just as effective and more ethical to use. However, at present, embryonic stem cells are the best source of stem cells, and are derived either at pre-implantation or from foetuses which have been aborted. These are unwanted or discarded embryonic stem cells.

Cloning also has the potential to create embryos for the purposes of research. Arguably, if an embryo is created for research purposes, it is created with the express intention of being harmed; thus it is being used as a means to an end. Surplus embryos are not created with research in mind. They are used for research as the alternative is simply to dispose of them. Perhaps it is more transparent to create embryos specifically for the purpose of research than to use embryos surplus to IVF requirements. Nevertheless, the view of the House of Lords Committee on Stem Cell Research states that:

QUOTATION

'embryos should not be created specifically for research purposes unless there is a demonstrable and exceptional need which cannot be met by the use of surplus embryos.'

(Stem Cell Research, House of Lords Select Committee 2002, para 4.28)

The therapeutic potential of stem cell therapy is both exhilarating and real, even if it is not immediate. If embryonic stem cells can be differentiated, the potential of regenerative medicine is indeterminable. The potential benefits of stem cell research are so overwhelming that they cannot be dismissed without extremely compelling arguments to the contrary. The opportunity to repair degenerative disease such as Parkinson's disease is one that cannot be ignored, as at least 120,000 people in the UK alone suffer from Parkinson's. One however has to accept that these are simply scientific aspirations and may take many years to realise but, given that their potential is so great, they cannot be readily ignored.

Ethical arguments against stem cell research

One of the main objections to stem cell research is that it involves using and sacrificing human embryos. The stage at which an embryo reaches 100 cells is referred to as a **blastocyst** and it is from within this that stem cells are taken. This is the early embryo or the pre-implantation embryo. The ethical difficulty is that if embryonic cells differentiate into **totipotent cells**, rather than **pluripotent cells**, these cells are capable of forming an embryo and therefore need to be protected.

Arguably, it may be more acceptable to conduct research on discarded embryos from IVF rather than embryos created specifically for the purposes of research. The justification here is that the discarded embryo has already fulfilled its role as it has been discarded or rejected from the IVF process. Surely it would be more beneficial to gain some use from the embryo than no use at all? However, if the embryo is to be treated as a person due to its potentiality, then it would follow that any research on embryos cannot be ethically sustained as an embryo is unable to consent and, where consent cannot be obtained, autonomy is violated. Just because something may have the potential to develop into something does not mean it should be granted full rights as if it had already fulfilled that potential. Just because you may be studying law and have the potential to become a lawyer does not necessarily mean you will, and you do not have the right to be treated as a lawyer simply because you have the potential to become one. If the embryo fails to fulfil its potential and we have failed to conduct research on it because of that potential, then we have wasted an opportunity.

Harris defines a person as a 'creature capable of valuing its own existence'; thus it follows that potential persons cannot be wronged by the killing of them because death 'does not

blastocyst

the cluster of cells after fertilisation of egg and sperm which must then move from the fallopian tube to the uterus

totipotent cells

cells which are capable of forming entire organisms

pluripotent cells

cells which cannot develop into a complete organism

deprive them of anything they can value' (1999). If embryos are not persons, they cannot be owed the same respect as persons; furthermore, since one cannot harm something that is not a creature, it follows that it is acceptable to use human embryos for research purposes. If we consider the contrary argument, while embryos may not be persons, it may still not be right to conduct research on embryos as life is valuable at all stages even a very early stage, and it is wrong if they are killed in the name of scientific research.

While embryos may have human qualities, if we accept Harris's argument, embryos are not human and cannot be owed the same moral respect as a human. Moreover, if we accept that embryos cannot feel or suffer pain, then it should be acceptable to use them for research purposes up to the point that they can feel pain.

Those who reject stem cell research argue that embryos are needlessly dying in the quest of some unknown and unspecified remedy and are therefore being treated as a means to an end, contrary to deontological values. If we accept this argument, then embryos are also being treated with a lack of human dignity which is in itself unethical and contrary to United Nations Universal Declaration of Human Rights. However, these embryos are spare and unwanted, and one might consider it preferable to utilise them beneficially rather than to waste them altogether.

It is often expressed that we should treat an embryo with moral respect, but this type of phrasing can be more placatory than hold any true value. How do we treat an embryo with respect if we have already agreed it is to be destroyed when we are done with it? It seems to be a conflict of terms to treat something with respect and then destroy it. One should therefore ensure that spare embryos, or even those created specifically for research, should be used for their specific purpose and not wasted and simply disposed of.

Legal provisions

The HFE Act 2008 permits research to be conducted on embryos, once a licence has been granted by the Research Ethics Committee. Schedule 2, para 3A(1) provides that the HFEA can only grant a licence if it believes that research is both 'desirable' and 'necessary'. It must be proved (under para 3A(2) that the 'principal purposes' for seeking a licence are:

SECTION

'a) Increasing knowledge about serious disease or other serious medical conditions
b) Developing treatments for serious disease or other serious medical conditions
c) Increasing knowledge about the causes of any congenital disease or congenital medical condition that does not fall within paragraph a)
d) Promoting advances in the treatment of fertility
e) Increasing knowledge about the causes of miscarriage
f) Developing more effective techniques of contraception
g) Developing methods for detecting the presence of gene, chromosome or mitochondrion abnormalities in embryos before implantation or
h) Increasing knowledge about the development of embryos.'

KEY FACTS

Key facts on HFE Act 2008

Human Fertilisation and Embryology Act 2008	Explanation
Schedule 2, para 3A(1)	HFEA will grant a licence if research is both desirable and necessary.
Schedule 2, para 3A(2)	Refers to the principal purposes of seeking a licence.
Part 1, s 4A(3)	Research on embryos cannot extend beyond 14 days or the appearance of the first **primitive streak**.

primitive streak
a faint white area on the end region of the embryonic disc along which the embryo will develop

Hybrid embryos

The HFE Act 2008 permits limited research on hybrid embryos. A hybrid embryo is one where the embryos are a mixture of human and animal DNA created solely for the purposes of research. The Act introduces a new s 4A which refers specifically to genetic material which is not of human origin, and states:

SECTION

'1 No person shall place into a woman –
(a) human admixed embryo
(b) Any other embryo that is not a human embryo or
(c) Any gametes other than human gametes'

Part 1, s 4A(3) provides that an embryo cannot be used for research purposes or retained after the appearance of the first primitive streak (which usually occurs about 14 days after mixing the sperm and the egg). The embryo is thus afforded the respect it is due but, until that time, the potential of research far outweighs the interest of the embryo.

admixed embryo
an early stage
embryo which
combines both
human and non-
human material

Thus, an **admixed embryo** can be created for research purposes but cannot be placed into a woman, or indeed an animal, and cannot be kept for a period longer than 14 days or the appearance of the first primitive streak.

7.3.5 Religious views on stem cell research and therapeutic cloning

All religions view a foetus with utmost respect, although their views on research differ significantly. The Roman Catholic Church states that the early embryo must be treated as if it is a person, and in line with the Roman Catholic Church's view on abortion, it condemns embryo research. The Catholic Catechism 2270 states that 'human life must be respected and protected absolutely from the moment of conception'. However there is a more liberal Catholic view which states that an embryo does not become a person and achieve that status until it reaches the primitive streak. Research up to that stage would therefore be permissible.

Within Judaism, a more gradualist view is apparent. Judaism takes a more pragmatic and progressive view towards medical advances in technology. Here, the primary question is not the ethical position of the embryo but the potential of stem cell research to save lives. This is supported by a positive requirement to save life and to take steps that life can be preserved as a person's life is of immeasurable value. In any event, a foetus until 40 days of age is not a person and so it appears to follow that destruction of embryonic cells prior to this period is permitted.

Within Islam, the position differs. The status of the embryo is important and while Islamic law considers a foetus to be a human life, this occurs at a much later stage of development than Christianity. The time of ensoulment is at the end of the fourth month of pregnancy (*Qur'an*, Chapter 23, verses 12–14) and this is the period at which an embryo can be considered human. Islamic law shares a similarity with Halachic or Jewish law since both religions consider there is a positive obligation to support scientific advances in order to help relieve human disease.

Compassion and knowledge are extremely important virtues for Buddhists, and the practice of medicine has a long history in this religious community. There would be little ethical objection to the therapeutic use of adult stem cells to help alleviate suffering and cure illness, but the use of embryonic stem cells in medical research is against their principle of causing no harm to any living creature, regardless of the researcher's benign intention to perform a good action in curing disease, and would therefore be immoral and unethical.

Interspecies or admixed embryos

Those who oppose the creation of interspecies embryos tend to share the view that it is unethical to create such entities as they offend human dignity, blur the boundaries of the species or are contrary to God's creation.

Human dignity

A body of opinion that opposes the creation of hybrid embryos does so on the grounds that it offends human dignity. The idea of human dignity is essentially deontological as it refers to a benchmark of respect or value by which all people should be treated. It therefore appears there is something special or unique about humans in relation to other species. Arguably, animals are there to serve man's purpose, whether to assist in agriculture or to be bred for food. Human dignity is notoriously difficult to define as it is such a vague concept. We will explore these conceptual ideas when considering assisted suicide later in the book, and maybe one way in which we can define human dignity is by reference to characteristics which are essentially human in nature such as language, the ability to communicate with others and to have social relationships. These are by their very essence human, but that does not assist us in deciding whether human dignity is significantly offended by the creation of interspecies embryos. Perhaps there are different levels of respect. Perhaps humans should be treated with ultimate respect and the appropriate relative respect should be granted to animals? The argument concerning human dignity presumes that embryos can be granted personhood and can therefore be identified with human dignity. But if an embryo cannot value its own existence, then how can it value or even possess human dignity?

Blurring of the species

It is argued that interspecies embryos are morally objectionable because they cross the boundaries of definition of the species. The creation of interspecies embryos is not new to science. Goat and sheep have previously been fused, creating a 'geep', and in the United States of America researchers have injected human stem cells into the foetuses of sheep, which subsequently produced human cells within their bodies. Hybrids have been created in laboratories for many years, proving invaluable to medical research. For several years, human biological cells have been put into frogs' eggs to research cell biology and, in reality, there has always been natural gene flow between species occurring naturally in nature.

It was argued that there would be no distinction between what is human and what is not, and therefore the relative standards of dignity cannot be applied. This was a view shared by the Christian Medical Fellowship who state that creating mixed human/ non-human embryos would 'undermine human dignity by blurring the boundaries of nature'. Why is human dignity so important in this respect? The answer lies in the Council of Europe Convention on Human Rights and Biomedicine, which states that the interests and welfare of the human is of paramount importance and takes precedence over the interests of science.

Mixing of the species

An Orthodox Christian view maintains that interspecies embryos would breach the biblical prohibition of mixing the species and that God created a perfect and complete world. However, Brietowitz states that 'wisdom and skill and knowledge, are in themselves gifts that come from God' (2002) and, if we accept that God created Man, then Man is endowed with the ability to improve the world that God created, and the ability should be utilised and respected.

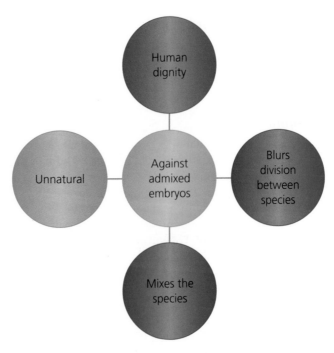

Figure 7.7 Arguments against admixed embryos

Conclusion

One might adopt a consequentialist view and conclude that research is for the greater good, and we must look to advances in medical technology for cures for diseases which could enhance the dignity of those suffering from devastating diseases. The principles of beneficence and non-maleficence are especially relevant in this regard, and it is ethically wrong to harm people if we can benefit them. Furthermore, if one concludes that it is wrong to destroy embryos for research purposes, it follows that it is also wrong to dispose of unwanted embryos in IVF treatment. However, the only way to avoid this would be if only one embryo was harvested. The consequence of this would be that IVF could be considerably less successful than it is now and would deprive many women of the hope of a child.

ACTIVITY

Self-test questions

Ensure that your answers are supported by statute where appropriate.

- What is cloning?
- Distinguish between reproductive cloning and therapeutic cloning.
- Consider whether you believe reproductive cloning is ethically acceptable. Ensure that you explore arguments for and against your view.
- Why is therapeutic cloning seen as a possible panacea?
- Is such optimism ethically justified?
- Consider whether you believe that theological views are persuasive.

SUMMARY

■ Cloning often evokes negative reactions, and it is essential to distinguish between reproductive cloning and therapeutic cloning. Reproductive cloning is not permitted and is considered ethically unacceptable despite the weakness of some ethical arguments. Nevertheless, there is an immediate reaction that it is somehow unethical to be able to create an identical copy of another.

■ Therapeutic cloning and stem cell research potentially offer research of degenerative diseases and the long-term possibility to enhance millions of patients' lives. While the therapeutic potential of stem cell research is still in its infancy, the rewards may be significant. Opponents argue that embryos are destroyed in the process.

SAMPLE ESSAY QUESTION

There is a view that therapeutic cloning can be ethically justified but reproductive cloning can never be justified. Critically evaluate this view.

- This is an essay-style question that requires you to critically evaluate the ethical arguments of therapeutic cloning and reproductive cloning.
- It is recommended that a brief knowledge of the law is demonstrated.

- In favour of **reproductive cloning**: autonomy – it enables childless couples or same sex couples to have genetic offspring. For some, this may be the only hope of a child.
- Against reproductive cloning: at this time, there are unacceptable risks. If attempted, child could suffer disease or disability. Some would argue that even if the child suffers from some disease, at least there will be life.
- Cloning will limit the genetic gene pool which in the long term will affect the population. This may be right but only if reproductive cloning was the only method of reproduction.
- Everyone is entitled to their own genetic make-up.
- A cloned person may be deprived of their own identity. We all have some of our parents' characteristics but we know we are not identical. Would a cloned person feel they have not lived up to expectations?
- Would a child rather be a cloned child or not be born at all? It depends on the harm which the child suffers.
- General feeling that it is not natural and not right.
- Religious perspective – playing God.

- Ensure that every ethical argument is critically discussed. It is not enough just to know the argument exists. For example, if one might argue that reproductive cloning is not ethical acceptable because one may be playing God, surely that means that no medical technological advances are ethically acceptable as all involve man's intervention. This would of course include vaccinations such as smallpox. By taking this approach you answer the question by providing critical analysis.

- **Therapeutic cloning:** reference should be made to the status of the embryo under the HFE Act 2008 – embryos can be used for research but cannot be implanted into a woman. Restrictions on use of embryos in research.
- This has moral implications in itself as it involves discarding unwanted embryos. Here, you should refer to some of the relevant arguments, such as the potentiality argument.

- It is necessary to then focus on the most relevant argument – the purpose of this type of cloning is to make cells, tissues or even organs that are compatible with a recipient.
- This is quite a personal view and not everyone will accept the real chance of curing devastating and debilitative disease. Of course, at present it is only a possibility, but perhaps one would appreciate that this is a possibility worth embracing.
- This is not a eugenics argument and these arguments should be avoided.
- Take care to avoid too personal an opinion developing, and always avoid letting off steam! Ensure that you have developed a cohesive and sensible discussion.

CONCLUSION

Further reading

Articles

Brietowitz, Y. (2002) 'What is so bad about human cloning?' *Kennedy Institute of Ethics Journal*, 12, pages 325–41.

Burley, J. and Harris, J. (1999) 'Human Cloning and Child Welfare', *Journal of Medical Ethics*, 25, pages 108–113.

Frith, L. (2001) 'Gamete Donation and Anonymity', *Human Reproduction*, Vol. 16, No. 5, pages 818–24.

Harris, J. (1999) 'The Concept of the Person and the Value of Life', *Kennedy Institute of Ethics Journal*, 9.4, pages 293–308.

Holm, S. (1998) 'A Life in the Shadow: One Reason Why We Should Not Clone Humans', *Cambridge Quarterly of Healthcare Ethics*, 7, pages 160–2.

Books

Deech, R. and Smajdor, A. (2007) *From IVF to Immortality: Controversy in the Era of Reproductive Technology*. Oxford: OUP.

7.4 Part 4: Surrogacy

7.4.1 What is surrogacy?

Surrogacy refers to the situation where a woman or 'surrogate' agrees to bear a child, for financial consideration, on behalf of another woman who is unable to bear a child herself. The intention is that the child born to the surrogate mother will be handed over immediately after birth to the commissioning couple. According to the Brazier Report 1998 para 6.22, it is estimated that in the UK there are between 100–180 surrogacy arrangements per year which result in approximately 50–80 births.

The issue of surrogacy 'involves an intimate and emotional area of human life' (Brazier Report) which is fraught with both legal and ethical difficulties. In early cases, the courts considered surrogacy with both distaste and disapproval, demonstrated no clearer than in the case of *A v C* [1985] FLR 445, which despite its case reference was heard in 1978. The court's view is conveyed by Cumming-Bruce J who referred to the surrogacy arrangement before the court as 'a kind of baby-farming operation of a wholly distasteful and lamentable kind'. This section of this chapter is dedicated to exploring these areas in as much detail as is permitted. It is hoped that you will be motivated to read further.

7.4.2 Distinction between forms of surrogacy

Partial or genetic surrogacy

Here, the male partner's sperm is fertilised with the surrogate mother's egg, usually through artificial insemination. Hence, the surrogate has a genetic link with the foetus she is carrying for the benefit of others. It is also referred to as partial surrogacy.

Full surrogacy

In contrast to partial surrogacy, both the egg and the sperm have been obtained from the commissioning couple and the embryo is then implanted into the surrogate mother. This form of surrogacy can also be called gestatory as the surrogate mother simply acts as a 'vessel' for the foetus to grow and develop. This type of surrogacy is referred to as full surrogacy.

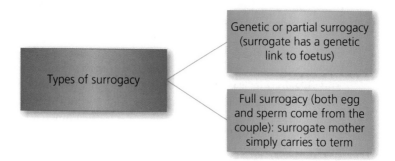

Figure 7.8 The two types of surrogacy

7.4.3 The law on surrogacy

The law on surrogacy is governed by the Surrogacy Arrangements Act 1985 and the Human Fertilisation and Embryology Act 1990 as amended by the HFE Act 2008.

Section 1, Surrogacy Arrangements Act 1985

Section 1(2) defines a 'surrogate mother' as 'a woman who carries a child in pursuance of an arrangement

SECTION

's1(2) a) made before she began to carry the child and
b) made with a view to any child carried in pursuance of it being handed over to, and parental responsibility being met (so far as practicable) by another person or other persons.'

Thus, it is not unlawful for a couple to enter into a surrogacy agreement with another.

Section 2, Surrogacy Arrangements Act 1985

There are a number of statutory provisions which can result in criminal offences if breached. It is an offence under s 2(1) for a person or an organisation on a commercial basis to:

SECTION

's2(1) a) initiate or take part in any negotiations with a view to the making of a surrogacy arrangement,
b) offer or agree to negotiate the making of a surrogacy arrangement or
c) compile any information with a view to its use in making, or negotiate the making of, surrogacy arrangements.'

However, despite the above provision, it remains lawful for a non-commercial group to arrange a surrogacy payment. Furthermore, s 2(2) states that it is not a criminal offence if the surrogate mother or the commissioning couple enter into an arrangement themselves.

Section 3, Surrogacy Arrangements Act 1985

Section 3 makes it unlawful for a person to advertise services:

SECTION

'a) that any person is or may be willing to enter into a surrogacy arrangement or to negotiate the making of a surrogacy arrangement, or
b) that any person is looking for a woman willing to become a surrogate mother or for any persons wanting a woman to carry a child as a surrogate mother.'

It is apparent that one of the primary intentions of the Surrogacy Arrangements Act 1985 is to prevent commercial bodies from involving themselves in surrogacy payments and developing a profitable business. A person or a body involved in such activity can be liable to a fine or a sentence of imprisonment not exceeding three months for each offence. It is however possible for a non-commercial body to organise a surrogacy payment. Provided that no payment other than reasonable expenses is involved, a surrogacy payment will be legal.

Human Fertilisation and Embryology Act 1990

Section 36, HFE Act 1990 amended the Surrogacy Arrangements Act 1985 by inserting a new s 1B which states:

SECTION

'no surrogacy arrangement is enforceable by or against any of the persons making it'.

Thus, while surrogacy arrangements are lawfully permitted, the provisions of the arrangement remain unenforceable.

Provisions in HFE Act 2008 amended the Surrogacy Arrangements Act 1985 still further. Section 2A makes it lawful for a non-profit-making body to be paid a reasonable fee for facilitating or making a surrogacy arrangement.

7.4.4 The legal status of the child born to a surrogate mother

In the UK, the legal status of the mother of the child born as a result of a surrogate arrangement is contained in s 33, HFE Act 2008 which states as follows:

> 'The woman who is carrying or has carried a child as a result of the placing in her of an embryo or of sperm and egg, and no other woman, is to be treated as the mother of the child.'

Thus, when the baby is born, the law is expressed with particular precision.

■ The surrogate mother is the legal mother of the child born to her as a result of a surrogacy arrangement, regardless of whether the surrogate has any genetic link to the child to whom she has given birth.

■ The surrogate's husband will be the legal father of the child if he has consented to his wife acting as a surrogate. He will remain the legal father unless parentage has been transferred to the commissioning couple. If the surrogate's husband has not consented or she has no partner, the child will have no legal father.

■ The commissioning mother will not be the legal mother of the child, even if her eggs are used.

■ The commissioning father, even if he is the genetic father, will not be the father of the child.

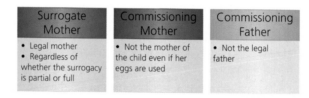

Surrogate Mother	Commissioning Mother	Commissioning Father
• Legal mother • Regardless of whether the surrogacy is partial or full	• Not the mother of the child even if her eggs are used	• Not the legal father

Figure 7.8 The legal status of parents within surrogacy

7.4.5 What are the options for the couple who engage a surrogate initially?

Since the commissioning parents are not the legal parents, they will after the baby's birth wish to ensure that one of the two options below are initiated as soon as possible:

a) Adoption parental order – this allows parenthood to be transferred from the surrogate to the commissioning couple.

b) Adoption – this will only be relevant where the commissioning parents are unable to obtain a parental order or where the surrogate mother may have changed her mind and wishes to adopt the child. It is a lengthy process and the criteria in the Adoption and Children Act 2002 must be met. Hence, the commissioning parents are more likely to seek a parental order.

7.4.6 Parental order

Section 30, HFE Act 1990 originally set out the following criteria to be applied in order to apply for a parental order:

■ The gametes must come from one or both of the commissioning couple.

■ The husband and wife must apply for the order within six months of the birth of the child.

■ At the time of making the application, the child's home must be with the husband and wife.

■ Either or both of the husband and wife must be domiciled in the UK (or the Channel Islands or the Isle of Man) and both must be aged over 18.

Section 54, HFE Act 2008 now amends the 1990 Act, s 54(2) stating that the applicants must be:

SECTION

'a) husband and wife
b) civil partners of each other or
c) two persons who are living as partners in an enduring family relationship and not within prohibited degrees of relationship in relation to each other.'

The provisions in the 2008 Act are similar save for one crucial distinction. The 2008 Act recognises the difference in modern society's demographics in the twenty-first century and the continual changing and redefinition of the family structure. Families are no longer defined simply by biology of the parties or indeed by marriage, and equality is now achieved. The change in the law has allowed such high-profile personalities as Sir Elton John and his civil partner David Furnish to have a son born via a surrogacy arrangement in December 2010. Such a case represents the acceptable face of family life in modern society.

Thus, while the wording in the 1990 Act stated that only parties who were husband and wife could engage a surrogate, the 2008 Act now permits those who are in a civil partnership and those in a committed relationship to be able to have a family.

The Act states that the following criteria must be satisfied:

- At least one of the parents is living in England and Wales and at least one must be genetically related.
- The child is living with the couple.
- The surrogate who has legal responsibility has consented to the application for a parental order and at least six weeks has elapsed since the birth of the child.
- Evidence supports that no more than reasonable expenses have been paid to the surrogate.
- The parental order must be applied for within six months of the child's birth.

A parental order cannot be made without the consent of the surrogate who has legal responsibility. If the surrogate is married and her husband consented to the surrogacy, his consent must be obtained for the parental order. A parental order cannot be made without the consent of both legal parents.

Section 54(8) states that the court must be satisfied that no money or other benefit, other than expenses which have been reasonably incurred, have passed between the parties in relation to the parental order or the original agreement.

KEY FACTS

Key facts on the law on surrogacy

Partial surrogacy	Where the surrogate has a genetic link to the foetus she carries.
Full surrogacy	Where the surrogate mother has no genetic link to the foetus.
Surrogacy Arrangements Act 1985 s 1(2) defines a surrogate mother	A woman who carries a child in pursuance of an agreement.
Surrogacy Arrangements Act 1985 s 2(1)	It is an offence for a commercial organisation, or a person on behalf of it, to be involved in a surrogacy arrangement.

Surrogacy Arrangements Act 1985 s 2(2)	It is not unlawful for a non-commercial organisation of the parties themselves to enter into such an agreement.
Surrogacy Arrangements Act 1985 s 1B	No surrogacy arrangement is enforceable in law.
HFE Act 2008, s 33	The legal mother of the child will be the surrogate mother.
HFE Act 2008, s 54	Sets out the legal requirements for a parental order and replaces s 30, Human Fertilisation and Embryology Act 1990.

Most of the cases before the courts consider s 54 parental applications from the commissioning couple who wish to become the legal parents. While most of the hearings are in private, those which do reach the public domain highlight both the complexity of the areas and the intense emotional issues which surrogacy naturally attracts.

The case below highlights the difficulties that can arise in relation to 'payment'. We have already seen that no money or payments, apart from expenses that are reasonably incurred, can be given by the couple wanting the child or in consideration of the making of the parental order. Hence, it can fall to the courts to determine whether payments are permissible.

CASE EXAMPLE

Re C (Application by Mr and Mrs X under s 30 of the Human Fertilisation and Embryology Act 1990) [2002] EWHC 157 (Fam)

Mr and Mrs X had paid the intended surrogate the sum of £12,000. It was for the court to determine whether these were expenses were reasonably incurred before a parental order could be made.

While the sum was indeed large, it was not disproportionate and the court did not feel that the couple were attempting to 'buy' a baby. The fact that the surrogate mother was on income support and also claiming 'expenses' was not a matter of which the couple were aware. Wall LJ concluded that it was in the interests of the child for the couple to be awarded parental responsibility and the payment, while large, was authorised.

A similar problem was encountered in the case below.

CASE EXAMPLE

Re X and Y (foreign surrogacy) [2008] EWHC 3030 (Fam)

A British couple had agreed with a Ukrainian woman for her to act as a surrogate. She was implanted with donor eggs which had been fertilised by the British male sperm. She gave birth to twins and handed the babies over. While in UK law the surrogate mother was the legal mother, Ukrainian law differed and the babies did not have right of entry into the UK, as the couple had no legal rights in relation to the babies. When they eventually managed to enter the UK, they applied for a parental order and the court was asked to approve the payment to the surrogate, which it was said was beyond expenses reasonably incurred.

The payment was authorised by the court despite recognising that 25,000 Euros on birth and 235 Euros in the months leading up to the birth exceeded expenses reasonably incurred. Consequently, the parental order was made as it was deemed to be in the best interest of the child.

Not only does the case illustrate the difficulties which can be encountered when engaging a surrogate in a different jurisdiction, it also highlights the need for clearer regulation of surrogacy laws and the importance of clear legal advice.

The more recent case of *Re L* (2010) below reminds us that the welfare of the child is the court's primary consideration, and the question of whether a payment is reasonable should not obscure its primary task.

CASE EXAMPLE

Re L (a child) [2010] EWHC 3146 (Fam)

The hearing, which was in private, concerned a commercial surrogacy arrangement with a surrogate in Illinois, USA. The agreement was lawful in Illinois but was unlawful in England as no payments other than reasonable expenses could be paid. The couple sought a parental order and retrospective authority to settle the payment.

While the emphasis was on the welfare of the child as the court's paramount consideration, the court was also obliged to consider the public policy issue of payments to surrogates very carefully.

Clearly, the courts are placed in some difficulty as the retrospective approval of expenses is required at the time of approving the parental order. While the welfare of the child should be the court's primary consideration, they must also consider whether any payment exceeds 'reasonable expenses'. The parental order can only be made once this is resolved.

The case below highlights the difficulties with surrogacy arrangements outside the jurisdiction. Section 54, HFE Act 2008 states that:

SECTION

'at the time of the application and the making of the order the child's home must be with the applicants, and either or both of the applicants must be domiciled in the UK, the Channel Islands or the Isle of Man'.

CASE EXAMPLE

Re G (surrogacy: foreign domicile) [2007] EWHC 2814 (Fam)

The commissioning couple could not conceive, and were Turkish nationals living in Turkey. They approached a British surrogacy agency and were introduced to a British woman who agreed to act as a surrogate mother. When the child was born, the baby was handed over to the parents who then returned to Turkey.

The difficulty concerned the fact that the parents were seeking a parental order under s 30, but were not domiciled in the UK.

After numerous court hearings in order to untangle the legal mesh, the couple obtained an adoption order and became the baby's legal parents.

However, MacFarlane J held as follows:

JUDGMENT

'Non-commercial surrogacy arrangements where neither of the commissioning couple is domiciled in the UK, while not illegal, are to be discouraged on the ground that it will not be open to the commissioning parents to apply for a parental order under HFE Act 1990, s 54 with respect to the child.'

The cases illustrated above highlight the potential pitfalls of which a couple who want a child via a surrogate can fall foul. One of the most basic problems has been where the parties have not been domiciled in the UK. The law is very clear; the applicants for a parental order must be resident in the UK. The difficulty lies where the surrogate is abroad. Assuming the surrogate agrees to honour the agreement and hand the baby over, the couple may experience considerable difficulty in returning to the UK with the baby.

More complex and distressing is where the surrogate refuses to hand over the baby once born. Surrogate contracts are not legally enforceable and therefore the commissioning couple have little legal redress. Given that the court's paramount consideration must be the welfare of the child, it would be difficult for the court to remove the baby from the surrogate's care if the surrogate has changed her mind and the mother and baby have bonded well. While this must be heartbreaking for the commissioning couple, especially where the father is the genetic father, the law offers no redress and little comfort.

The next case deals with a particularly sensitive issue, where the surrogate wished to keep the child she had given birth to. This particular issue is tricky, since the law states that the surrogate is the legal mother. In these situations, the commissioning parents are unable to apply for a parental order but will apply for a residence order instead. As a rule, the courts will not make a residence order in favour of the commissioning parents if the baby has already been living with his or her mother. The case below is an exception to the general rule.

CASE EXAMPLE

Re P (Surrogacy: Residence) [2008] 1 FLR 198

The baby was born as a result of a surrogacy arrangement where the commissioning father was the biological father. It transpired that the surrogate mother had been deceptive by telling the biological father she had miscarried. The child 'N' lived with the surrogate for the first 18 months of his life.

Coleridge J explained the issue to be determined was where the child was 'most likely to mature into a happy and balanced adult and to achieve his fullest potential as a human'. Having taken into consideration the close bond which had developed between the surrogate and the child, the welfare of the child was still best served by placing him with the commissioning couple rather than the surrogate. An appeal against the decision was dismissed.

It is worth contrasting the cases above with *Re T* (2011) below where the court determined that the best interests of the child were decided by remaining with the surrogate and biological mother. The case illustrates the unpredictable nature of a couple entering into a surrogacy arrangement.

CASE EXAMPLE

Re T (a child) (surrogacy: residence) [2011] EWHC 33 (Fam)

Mr and Mrs W were unable to bear children themselves and enlisted the help of a surrogate, having located her services over the internet. Mr W was the genetic father. The surrogate refused to hand over the baby once it was born.

In contrast to *Re P* (2008), the court held that the child's welfare was best served by remaining with the surrogate mother, with whom she had developed a close bond. It would cause the child harm to remove her from the surrogate's care and the court felt that on a balance of options, the child would be best served staying with the surrogate in any event, believing that the surrogate mother would grant the couple more visiting contact than if the roles were reversed.

Per Baker J:

JUDGMENT

'The natural process of carrying and giving birth to a baby creates an attachment which may be so strong that the surrogate mother finds herself unable to give up the child. Such cases call for careful and sensitive handling by the law.'

7.4.7 Reform: A natural way forward?

The Brazier Report was published in 1998. Having been commissioned by the government, one might conclude that reform was on the horizon, but none of its recommendations have been implemented. The report recommended that payment should cover only genuine expenses to discourage women becoming surrogates purely for financial gain, and that there should be greater clarity and transparency concerning payments before entering into any arrangement.

The report recommended a new Surrogacy Act which would repeal current piecemeal legislation and provide a much-needed comprehensive legislation on all principles of surrogacy.

A further amendment to HFE Act 2008 was made. The Human Fertilisation and Embryology (Parental Orders) Regulation 2010 took effect from April 2010 to ensure that:

- The court makes the welfare of the child the paramount consideration and introduces a welfare checklist setting out matters which the court must take into account.
- Subject to the parental order being made by the court, the child born to the surrogate will be the legitimate child of the commissioning couple.
- The parental order register will be linked to the register of live births, once a parental order has been made by the court; the register will be changed to 're-registered', to show the commissioning couple as legal parents.
- Where a parental order is made in the UK, the child will be British if one or both of the commissioning couple are British.

KEY FACTS

Key facts on surrogacy case law

Case	Judgment
Re C (Application by Mrs and Mrs X under s 30 of the Human Fertilisation and Embryology Act 1990) (2002)	The expenses incurred were large but not disproportionate. Once the payment was authorised the court could proceed to consider the interests of the child and a parental order was made.
Re X and Y (foreign surrogacy) (2008)	Significant expenses were approved and a parental order made.
Re L (a child) (2010)	A commercial surrogacy agreement was made with a surrogate in Illinois, USA. The parents in the UK were granted a parental order. Difficult questions on payments arose.
Re G (surrogacy: foreign domicile) (2007)	Highlights the difficulty which couples may have if they are not domiciled in the UK.

Re P (surrogacy: residence) (2008)	The welfare of the child was best served by moving the child to the commissioning couple despite the surrogate mother's desire to keep the child.
Re T (a child) (surrogacy: residence) (2011)	The welfare of the child was best served by remaining with the surrogate mother when she decided not to give the baby to the commissioning couple as agreed.

7.4.8 Surrogacy and ethics

Surrogacy is a highly charged and emotive area of medical ethics, often reminiscent of Aldous Huxley's novel *Brave New World* where his vision of a world in 2540 is one where natural procreation has all but been abandoned. Surrogacy is often viewed in dramatic terms of a woman hiring out her womb for money, but it is a most complex area as case law demonstrates, and ethical arguments are far from resolvable. In this section, we explore some of those ethical arguments through a hypothetical scenario.

Example

Trudy agrees to be a surrogate for Elaine and Matthew who are unable to bear children themselves. She wishes to pass on the pleasure of being able to have a family to others, and makes a clear autonomous decision to help others. Matthew has donated his gametes and is the genetic father. Trudy's husband Mike admires what Trudy has decided to do. He is the legal father of the baby as he is the surrogate's husband, and has consented. Although he has no genetic connection he remains the legal father unless parentage is transferred to Matthew. Elaine is not the legal mother and is not genetically linked to the baby.

The arrangement proceeds without difficulty. During the delivery, the baby is deprived of oxygen and is born brain damaged. Early indications suggest that the baby will be severely mentally and physically disabled. Elaine and Matthew decide they do not want to bring up a disabled child and tell Trudy that they will not honour the arrangement. Since Trudy is the legal mother of the baby she has legal responsibility. However, Trudy has not bonded with the baby during pregnancy and agreed to act as a surrogate for purely altruistic reasons.

Trudy is now the legal mother of a child she did not want for herself. The surrogacy agreement is not enforceable. She is legally responsible for all the baby's emotional and financial needs. Given its acute disability, these are likely to be extensive. If she decides not to keep the baby, the only options for the future of the child are either adoption or care.

The ethical questions that arise in this example are unlikely but illustrate the complex nature of a surrogacy agreement. Mike and Trudy are the child's legal parents and even though they have no desire to keep the child, the baby is their legal responsibility. Since the agreement is not enforceable, Elaine and Matthew can legitimately walk away from the situation.

Arguably, the child of the surrogacy suffers harm as a result as he is rejected by both the commissioning parents and the surrogacy parents and destined to a life of care or adoption. If the baby has complex mental disability it may never appreciate the true nature of its existence, but there is an argument that surrogacy harms children. Given that the alternative to being born to a surrogate is not being born at all, it is difficult to surmise that harm is actually done. In this hypothetical example however, there is no favourable result.

7.4.9 Ethical issues explored

Alternatively, let us assume that baby Sally was born to Trudy without complication and handed over to Elaine and Matthew who obtained a parental order. When Sally is old enough, Trudy explains how she was born.

Harm to the child

A child who discovers her mother is not her gestational mother could be harmed when she understands her gestational mother gave her up in return for a sum of money. Sally learns that she was given away by her gestational mother who did not want to keep her. She is a result of a commercial agreement rather than the result of a loving relationship. Is Sally harmed? She may feel rejected and resentful especially if she has no genetic physical similarity to her mother, and the fact that she was born subsequent to a commercial agreement may damage her self-esteem. She may feel like a commodity.

However, as Jackson observes, there is little information or statistical analysis on the effects of surrogacy arrangements on a child (2001). Indeed, since surrogate arrangements nearly always involve babies being handed over shortly after birth; one may conclude it is unlikely there would be any adverse impact on the child. Moreover, while it is hoped that children will always be born as a result of a loving relationship, we know that this is not always the case. Nevertheless, the Brazier Report (para 4.16) notes that surrogacy should be restricted in case harm is caused to the child:

QUOTATION

'We judge, nonetheless, that there is clear potential of risk to the welfare of such children. Research to identify and quantify that risk is needed urgently. The paramount importance of the welfare of the child is such that we believe that in making judgments about the regulation of surrogacy, the state must act on the precautionary principle. Society has a duty to minimise any such potential risk.'

Thus they conclude in para 4.29 that:

QUOTATION

'Therefore, we do not have to show certainty of major harm to potential children before we are justified, either through personal decision or legislative restriction, in avoiding conceptions on grounds of risk to the welfare of the child. It is sufficient to show that, if such lives are brought into being, they could be significantly compromised physically or emotionally. By not bringing them into being we do no harm to a child, since none exists.'

Last resort

Surrogacy is often considered as a last resort to a couple who want to have their own child naturally. If we revert to the example in the applying the law activity above, let us delve into the reason why Elaine and Matthew opted for surrogacy. Elaine was diagnosed with cancer at a young age and it was necessary to perform a complete hysterectomy which left her unable to have children. Desperate for their own family, there was little other option apart from engaging a surrogate. As Elaine cannot produce her own ova or eggs, any child born would at least have a genetic link to her husband.

Of course, Elaine and Matthew could adopt. Indeed, there are many children waiting for such an opportunity but the reality is that surrogacy provides the couple with a child genetically connected with at least one party. This cannot be condemned if having a genetically-related child is important to them. Furthermore, couples should feel under no obligation to adopt simply because there are children available for adoption. Surrogacy is simply a way to alleviate this particular couple's infertility.

Exploitation

Is Trudy being exploited? She has clear altruistic reasons for becoming a surrogate. She can provide informed consent. The money she will receive can be viewed simply in terms of financial compensation. While this may turn the agreement into a more commercial one, there is no suggestion that she is being exploited.

However, it can be argued that offering a woman money to carry a child is exploiting the would-be surrogate. The argument here is not dissimilar to that of selling kidneys. Surrogacy exploits the poor and perpetuates the economic divide between rich and poor.

Discussion point

Neha lives in India where payment for surrogacy is legal. She has two healthy children and did not find pregnancy particularly burdensome. She wishes for no more children herself but does not have enough money to feed, clothe and send her children to school. For her, schooling is a priority as it may give her children a better quality of life in the future. To carry a child on behalf of another is not problematical for her, although many would consider it unnatural and contrary to the rules of human nature. With the money she will earn from being a surrogate, she will be able to care for her children for the immediate future.

There is a concern that she will not be able to provide free and informed consent as her consent may be blurred by the attraction of the financial award, but it is difficult to appreciate why this should be an inflexible argument for condemning surrogacy. There is little ethical difference between the couple paying in order to have a child and a family, and the surrogate receiving money in order to improve the lives of her children and her family. It may be the case that she has few other options, but to deny her the options in case she cannot reach and fulfil the standards of Western informed consent is difficult to justify.

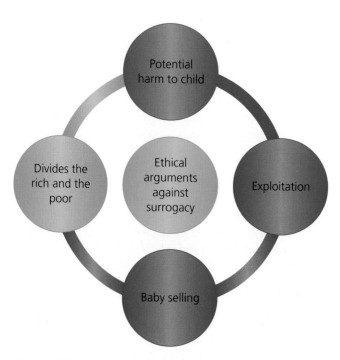

Figure 7.10 Ethical arguments against surrogacy

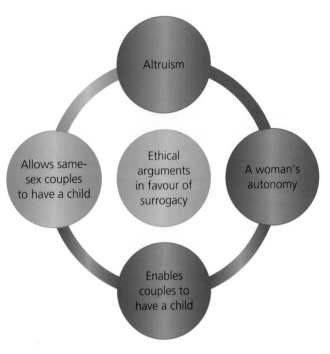

Figure 7.11 Ethical arguments in favour or surrogacy

ACTIVITY

Self-test questions

Ensure that your answers are supported by case law and/or statute where appropriate.

- What is surrogacy?
- Are surrogacy arrangements enforceable?
- Who is the legal mother – the surrogate or the commissioning mother?
- Who is the legal father – the commissioning father or the surrogate's husband (assuming he consents)?
- How can the commissioning parents achieve the legal status of the baby's mother and father?
- Can a surrogate receive payment?
- Is surrogacy ethically acceptable?

SUMMARY

- Surrogacy is a legally complex and emotionally charged area.
- Arguably the law of surrogacy is in need of reform as recommended by the Brazier Report, and recent case law demonstrates clearly the need for greater clarity and regulation. While there is some suggestion that surrogacy should be restricted, surrogacy cannot be eliminated altogether.
- Arguably, it is wrong that it should be restricted in any way. The opportunity that it can offer a childless couple is without parallel, and provided no harm is done to

the child and the surrogate is not exploited the practice should not be restricted. The practice cannot be eradicated altogether and any restriction will only move the practice underground which invariably will harm all parties.

Further reading

The Brazier Report (1997) available on the internet.
Jackson, E. (2009) *Regulating Reproduction. Law, Technology and Autonomy.* Oxford: Hart Publishing.

8

The law and ethics of abortion

AIMS AND OBJECTIVES

After reading this chapter you should be able to:

- Understand the background to the Abortion Act 1967
- Demonstrate a clear understanding of the provisions of the Abortion Act 1967
- Understand the complexity of the ethical arguments
- Be able to apply both the legal and ethical arguments to a hypothetical scenario.

8.1 Part 1: The law

8.1.1 Introduction

It is not strictly accurate to describe abortion as lawful, as in the UK abortion is still a criminal offence. The Abortion Act 1967, however, provides extensive defences and it is by virtue of this statutory provision that many thousands of abortions are carried out every year.

The most logical point to begin our consideration of the law on abortion is historically, with the provisions set out under the criminal law.

Prior to the statutory provisions set out below, abortion was governed by the common law. As early as the thirteenth century, if a woman was given a substance to help procure a miscarriage once the foetus was said to be 'quickening', this act would be tantamount to murder. Quickening is the term referred to when the foetus is first felt to move, at around 16–18 weeks' gestation (slightly later for women in their first pregnancy). By the eighteenth century, while it was no longer considered to be murder, it was regarded in a most serious manner with harsh penalties imposed by the courts.

8.1.2 Malicious Shooting or Stabbing Act 1803

The earliest legislation directly concerning abortion was more commonly known as Lord Ellenborough's Act, which in 1803 condemned those who might be involved in an abortion post-quickening to either the death penalty or transportation for a period of 14 years, such was the serious nature of the offence. The law only became slightly less restrictive with the enactment of the Offences Against the Person Act 1861, many provisions of which are still in force today.

8.1.3 Offences Against the Person Act 1861, ss 58 and 59

Section 58 states:

'Every woman, being with child, who, with intent to procure her own miscarriage, shall unlawfully administer to herself any poison or other noxious thing, or shall unlawfully use any instrument or other means whatsoever with the like intent, and whosoever, with intent to procure the miscarriage of any woman, whether she be or be not with child, shall unlawfully administer to her or cause to be taken by her any poison or other noxious thing, or shall unlawfully use any instrument or other means whatsoever with the like intent, shall be guilty of felony, and being convicted thereof.'

This section provides:

- It is an offence if a pregnant woman attempts and intends to cause herself a miscarriage.
- It is an offence if another person attempts to cause a woman to miscarry, regardless of whether or not she is in fact pregnant.
- It follows therefore that if a woman wrongly suspects herself to be pregnant and enlists the help of a friend to cause herself an abortion, only the friend can be criminally liable.

Section 59 states:

'Whosoever shall unlawfully supply or procure any poison or other noxious thing, or any instrument or thing whatsoever, knowing that the same is intended to be unlawfully used or employed with intent to procure the miscarriage of any woman, whether she be or be not with child, shall be guilty of a misdemeanour, and being convicted thereof shall be liable.'

This section provides:

- It is an offence to be concerned with the supply of drugs or instruments that could cause a miscarriage. It is worth noting that the offence applies regardless of whether or not the woman is actually pregnant.

The law was quite obviously restrictive, and abortion was unlawful even if conducted for medical reasons. With potential sentences from three years' to life imprisonment, abortion was regarded as a very serious offence.

8.1.4 Infant Life (Preservation) Act 1929

There was no change in the law until 1929 when the Infant Life (Preservation) Act was passed.

Section 1 provided as follows:

'(1) ... any person who, with intent to destroy the life of a child capable of being born alive, by any wilful act causes a child to die before it has an existence independent of its mother, shall be guilty of felony, to wit, of child destruction.

Provided that no person shall be found guilty of an offence under this section unless it is proved that the act which caused the death of the child was not done in good faith for the purpose only of preserving the life of the mother.

(2) For the purposes of this Act, evidence that a woman had at any material time been pregnant for a period of twenty-eight weeks or more shall be *prima facie* proof that she was at that time pregnant of a child capable of being born alive.'

- The offence which also carried a maximum penalty of life imprisonment referred to an intention to abort a child capable of being born alive, which at the time of drafting was deemed to be 28 weeks.
- The suggestion is that an abortion prior to the 28-week period would be lawful as it would be accepted that the foetus was not capable of being born alive. Equally, if it could be proved that a more mature foetus was *not* capable of being born alive, then presumably an abortion could also be permitted.

We can see the application of the Act in light of case law.

CASE EXAMPLE

C v S and others [1987] 1 All ER 1230

The prospective father sought an injunction on behalf of the foetus and himself to prohibit the abortion of the foetus which was between 18–21 weeks' gestation. He argued that the abortion, if it was to proceed, would breach the provisions of the Infant Life (Preservation) Act 1929, as he argued that the foetus was capable of being born alive.

The court refused the injunction, maintaining that even if the foetus had reached the normal stage of development as might be expected for its gestation, it did not follow that 'the child was capable of being born alive' within the meaning of the Act.

It is worth contrasting this case to the case below.

CASE EXAMPLE

Rance v Mid Downs Health Authority [1991] 1 All ER 801

A couple claimed damages for a negligent scan when their child was born with spina bifida. There was a suspicion when the mother had a scan at 25 and a half weeks that the baby might have spina bifida, but she was not informed. She maintained she would have sought a termination of pregnancy. The defendants maintained there was no negligence but, in any event, any abortion would be unlawful as the baby would have 'been capable of being born alive' according to s 1, Infant Life (Preservation) Act 1929.

The Abortion Act 1967 which was amended by s 37 of the Human Fertilisation and Embryology Act (HFE) 1990 states that no offence under the Infant Life (Preservation) Act 1929 can be committed if an abortion is performed by a registered medical practitioner in accordance with the provisions of HFE Act 1990.

KEY FACTS

Key facts on historical statutory provisions

Statute	Provision
Malicious Shooting or Stabbing Act 1803 (Lord Ellenborough's Act)	Abortion post-quickening unlawful. Penalty was death or 14 years' transportation.
Offences Against the Person Act 1861, s 58	Offence if the pregnant woman attempts and intends by herself or with assistance of another to procure a miscarriage.
Offences Against the Person Act 1861, s 59	Offence to supply the means to procure an abortion. Still applicable even if the woman is not pregnant.
Infant Life (Preservation) Act 1929	Offence to intend to abort a child capable of being born alive (28 weeks). Related case law: *C v S* (1987), *Rance v Mid Downs Health Authority* (1991).

8.1.5 The common law defence of necessity

R v Bourne [1939] 1 KB 687

A 14-year-old girl was raped and fell pregnant as a result. She had an abortion at St Mary's Hospital and the obstetrician who performed the procedure was charged under s 58 of the Offences Against the Person Act 1861.

The court opined that the burden is on the prosecution to prove that the operation was not performed in good faith. Thus, it would be necessary to show that the abortion was not necessary to preserve the life of the mother. The life of the mother was not limited to the physical being but also extended to whether continuing the pregnancy would render her a 'mental wreck'. Mr Justice Macnaghten directed the jury to acquit if they accepted that Dr Rees performed the operation in good faith and in order to preserve the girl's life. The jury acquitted.

The case establishes that in common law the restrictive statutory provisions against abortion could be circumvented in the case of necessity. This was, however, the exception rather than the norm. In any event, the defence is largely irrelevant in modern-day medicine as the defence of necessity is embodied in the most significant legislation – the Abortion Act 1967.

8.1.6 The Abortion Act 1967

Introduction

The 1960s witnessed a general period of social and sexual enlightenment. One significant breakthrough in this decade was the introduction of the contraceptive pill. At a similar time there came an awareness that legislation was necessary to avoid the occurrence of 'back street abortions' where, to avoid falling foul of the law or the stigma that was still associated with abortions, patients either attempted self-abortion using archaic and gruesome methods or abortions were carried out in often unsanitary and unsterile conditions, leaving the patients exposed and vulnerable to infection or even physical injury.

The Abortion Law Reform Association was formed in 1936, shortly before the case of *R v Bourne* (1939), in order to address such social injustice. Backbencher Liberal MP David Steel introduced the Medical Termination of Pregnancy Bill which later became the Abortion Act and was enacted in April 1968. The Bill was fiercely debated and was highly controversial, facing stiff opposition from religious groups. The issue of abortion remains just as controversial today as when it was first before Parliament.

The Abortion Act 1967 should probably be regarded in a similar way to the Sexual Offences Act 1967, which, in a more liberalised period, legalised homosexual relationships between two consenting males over the age of 21 in private. Of course, the provision is still restrictive according to modern-day standards but each statutory provision should be considered in relation to the social standards prevailing at the time.

The Abortion Act 1967 is drafted widely and many would argue somewhat liberally. It is only in force in England, Wales and Scotland. While abortion was now permitted, it is now argued that the circumstances in which a termination of pregnancy can be performed lacks legal clarity for medical professionals and prospective patients alike, although Keown (1988) dispels this point of view by suggesting that the judgment in *Bourne* (1939) provides any clarity that may be needed.

8.1.7 Section 1, Abortion Act 1967

Section 1, Abortion Act 1967 as amended by HFE Act 1990 states:

SECTION

'Subject to the provisions of this section, a person shall not be guilty of an offence under the law relating to abortion when a pregnancy is terminated by a registered medical practitioner if two registered medical practitioners are of the opinion, formed in good faith —'

What does s 1 tell us? See Figure 8.1.

A woman has no *prima facie* right to an abortion

A woman can only terminate a pregnancy if she fulfils one of the statutory grounds under s 1

A woman cannot terminate a pregnancy simply because she does not wish to have a child or because it is her autonomous right

Two medical practitioners must be satisfied in good faith that one of the grounds for a termination under s 1(1)(a)–(d) is made out

Section 1(1) does not mean that a termination can *only* be carried out by a registered medical practitioner

Figure 8.1 Section 1, Abortion Act 1967

CASE EXAMPLE

Royal College of Nursing of UK v DHSS [1981] AC 800

An information pamphlet from the Department of Health and Social Services permitted nurses to administer drugs for the purposes of inducing an abortion. The Royal College of Nursing sought a declaration that the wording of the direction was unlawful since the wording of s 1(1) stated that only a 'registered medical practitioner' can conduct an abortion.

By the time this case was heard, abortions were largely carried out by a drug-induced procedure rather than a surgical procedure. Thus, nurses rather than a doctor could carry out the process of inserting an intravenous line into a patient. In a controversial majority decision which relied upon use of the mischief rule to interpret the statute (see *Unlocking English Legal System*), the court held that, since the nurse was acting on the instructions of the doctor in carrying out the procedure, it was not unlawful for a nurse to 'carry out' an abortion.

The requirement of 'good faith'

Section 1 releases medical professionals of any potential criminal liability, provided that two medical professionals exercise 'good faith' in their judgment as to whether 'in their opinion' the pregnant woman fulfils one of the statutory grounds justifying an abortion. The only case to test the requirement of good faith is illustrated below.

CASE EXAMPLE

R v Smith [1974] 1 All ER 376

The patient was a young girl aged 19 years who became pregnant. She wanted an abortion and was referred to Dr Smith at a pregnancy advice centre. She saw Dr Smith for about 15 minutes. He did not examine her, and failed to ask her anything about her personal circumstances but told her that he would perform the operation for £150. The following week, when she was able to raise the money, the abortion was carried out. She alleged that at no point did she see another medical professional about the operation.

Dr Smith was convicted for breach of the provisions of the Abortion Act 1967, as he had not acted in good faith as required by s 1. He appealed against his conviction.

In upholding his appeal, Lord Scarman referring to the Abortion Act 1967 stated that:

JUDGMENT

'though it renders lawful abortions that before its enactment would have been unlawful, [the Abortion Act] does not depart from the basic principle of the common law as declared in *R v Bourne* (1939) namely, that the legality of an abortion depends upon the opinion of the doctor. It has introduced the safeguard of two opinions: but, if they are formed in good faith by the time when the operation is undertaken, the abortion is lawful. Thus a great social responsibility is firmly placed by the law upon the shoulders of the medical profession.'

While the purpose of the quote is to illustrate the importance of the element of good faith, Lord Scarman's words also show the subjectivity of whether a woman is entitled to an abortion. Remember, there is no *prima facie* right to an abortion, as two medical professionals are tasked with ensuring that the provisions of one of the grounds under the Abortion Act 1967 are met. It is not the woman who can decide on an abortion; the law is heavily weighted in favour of the medical professionals' subjective clinical judgment.
Lord Scarman continued as follows:

JUDGMENT

'The question of good faith is essentially one for the jury to determine on the totality of the evidence. A medical view put forward in evidence by one or more doctors as to the good faith of another doctor's opinion is no substitute for the verdict of the jury. An opinion may be absurd professionally and yet formed in good faith: conversely, an opinion may be one which a doctor could have entertained and yet in the particular circumstances of a case may be found either to have been formed in bad faith or not to have been formed at all. Although the Abortion Act 1967 has imposed a great responsibility upon doctors, it has not ousted the function of the jury. If a case is brought to trial which calls in question the *bona fides* of a doctor, the jury, not the medical profession, must decide the issue.'

Dr Smith's conviction was upheld on the basis that, as he had failed to obtain a second opinion, he had not balanced the risks of the abortion against the continuing pregnancy and thus had not acted in good faith. It is also interesting to note that the judgment places stress on the use of the *Bolam* test (see Chapter 1), which is to be applied despite the emphasis made by Lord Scarman on the importance of the jury in determining the criminal liability. Of course, while the jury's role in criminal trials is axiomatic, the *Bolam* test is not quite so obvious. It appears that whether a doctor has acted in good faith under s 1, Abortion Act 1967 is to be determined by the *Bolam* standards.

8.1.8 Section 1(2)

Section 1(2) states:

SECTION

'In determining whether the continuance of a pregnancy would involve such risk of injury to health as is mentioned in paragraph a) or b) or subsection (1) of this section, account may be taken of the pregnant women's actual or reasonably foreseeable condition.'

This section provides:

- When deciding whether there is a risk of injury of health to the pregnant woman, medical professionals can take into account an injury which may be reasonably foreseeable even it is not apparent at the time of examination.

8.1.9 Section 1(3)

Section 1(3) as amended states:

SECTION

'any treatment for the termination of pregnancy must be carried out in a hospital vested in the Secretary of State for the purposes of his functions under the National Health Service Act 2006 or the National Health Service (Scotland) Act 1978 or in a hospital vested in a Primary Care Trust or a National Health Service trust or an NHS foundation trust or in a place approved for the purposes of this section by the Secretary of State.'

This section provides:

■ Abortions can only be carried out in a NHS hospital, private or approved clinic as determined by the Secretary of State.

CASE EXAMPLE

British Pregnancy Advisory Service v Secretary of State of Health [2011] EWHC 235 (Admin)

An abortion in the early stages, that is, prior to 9 weeks' gestation, is carried out by prescribing the patient drugs on two occasions at intervals of between 24 and 48 hours which stimulate an abortion. The British Pregnancy Advisory Service (BPAS) argued that requiring women to attend hospital for the administration of the second drug was potentially stressful and could cause physical harm when travelling home. They sought to argue that the term 'treatment' within s 1 should refer to the overall treatment of prescribing the drugs rather than the supplying of each stage of them. If this interpretation was achieved, women could take the second set of drugs at home where they would feel more comfortable and relaxed. However, this would be contrary to s 1(3) which requires treatment to be carried out in a hospital or places approved by the Secretary of State.

The applicants sought to rely on the mischief rule, looking at the early reasoning behind the Abortion Act 1967 when the need was to avoid abortions being carried out in unhealthy and unsanitary conditions. At that time it was imperative that abortions be carried out in hospitals. However, with progress of medical technology, procedures which could only be achieved by surgical intervention could now be met by the administration of drugs. By adopting the mischief rule, the applicants argued that the term 'treatment' could be met by *prescribing* the drugs rather than the mere administration.

The words 'any treatment for the termination of pregnancy' within s 1(3) could not be interpreted in line with the applicant's argument. The true and ordinary meaning of the words included the use or administration of the drugs. Thus the court held that treatment was completed when the drugs were prescribed. It was the consequences of treatment that was relevant, which was the required abortion. Furthermore, for the purposes of s 1(3), it was Parliament's intention that the Secretary of State determined where treatment might be carried out, and this decision was a matter for Parliament and not the medical profession to determine.

8.1.10 Section 1(4): emergency abortions

Section 1(4) explains that the statutory requirement of two registered medical practitioners being satisfied that one of the grounds under s 1(1) are made out, can be dispensed with if a registered medical practitioner is of the opinion in good faith that:

SECTION

'the termination is immediately necessary to save the life or to prevent grave permanent injury to the physical or mental health of the pregnant woman'.

■ An abortion can be carried out as an emergency where it is immediately necessary to save the life of the pregnant woman.

8.1.11 Section 1(1)(a)–(d) Abortion Act 1967 as amended by s 37, HFE Act 1990

This section sets out the circumstances where an abortion is legal and represents the current law in England, Scotland and Wales.

Section 1(1)(a), Abortion Act 1967

SECTION

> 'a) that the pregnancy has not exceeded its twenty-fourth week and that the continuance of the pregnancy would involve risk, greater than if the pregnancy were terminated, of injury to the physical or mental health of the pregnant woman or any existing children of her family; or'

■ Abortion must be carried out within 24 weeks.
■ Continuing the pregnancy would involve greater risk than the termination of pregnancy, to the physical or mental health of the pregnant woman or her children.

One of the first points to note is that the termination must be carried out by the twenty-fourth week of pregnancy. Section 1(1)(a) is the only ground that specifies a time limit. There is some uncertainty as to when the twenty-fourth week may actually be, and commentators suggest slightly different options to calculate this period. In any event, given that a foetus's viability at around 22 weeks' gestation is now lower than the upper limit for an abortion at 24 weeks, many argue that the upper limit is considerably late. Hence, amendments were tabled to lower the time limit in the debate prior to the passing of the HFE Act 2008, but the proposed amendments were never enacted. Given the viability of the foetus at 22 weeks, many doctors are reluctant to perform abortions on this ground at this late stage.

Section 1(1)(a) contrasts with subs (b)–(d) as it is regarded as a social ground.

This is a common ground for abortion, as by far the majority of abortions take place very early. Department of Health statistics for England and Wales 2009 show that 91 per cent of all abortions were carried out at under 13 weeks' gestation, and 75 per cent were under 10 weeks' gestation. Thus, while this ground is regarded as a social ground, late abortions would be unusual. Section 1(2) states that doctors need to take account of the 'patient's actual or reasonably foreseeable environment', and so the interpretation of s 1(1)(a) is in fact widely drawn to encompass a wide range of social reasons.

ACTIVITY

Applying the law

Chrissie and her friends go clubbing one Friday night. She meets Dean and they have unprotected sexual intercourse. Chrissie is 16 years old and has just started college. She discovers she is pregnant and immediately regrets her actions. She is worried because she does not want to be a single mother and wants to finish college. Her parents are furious.

This example is sadly an all too familiar one. The under-18 rate of abortions in England and Wales in 2009 was 17.6 per 1,000 women, although this was slightly lower than in 2008. When Chrissie seeks an abortion she will more than likely be able to rely on s 1(1)(a), Abortion Act 1967. She would argue that if she maintained the pregnancy, there would be a risk to her mental health as, at her tender years, she is simply not ready to mother a child. Doubtless, given the situation she finds herself in, she would seek medical advice and have an abortion well within the 24-week period. However, Chrissie is relying on a risk that might or might not occur. Does the Abortion Act make allowance for speculation? If we look back at s 1(2), we can see reference to an actual or foreseeable condition. Chrissie will be able to argue and rely on the foreseeable damage to her mental health if the pregnancy was to proceed.

Section 1(1)(a) also refers to the effect that a pregnancy may have on any other children of the pregnant mother. The precise meaning is somewhat ambiguous. It could suggest that a woman finds she is pregnant again and simply does not want/cannot afford/cannot manage a further child. These are pure social reasons. It could also mean that she finds herself pregnant, has a disabled child at home who needs a high level of care and simply cannot envisage a second pregnancy. We may automatically have greater sympathy for the latter example, but they are still simply social reasons and the majority of abortions are conducted under this ground.

Section 1(1)(b), Abortion Act 1967

SECTION

'(b) that the termination is necessary to prevent grave permanent injury to the physical or mental health of the pregnant woman;'

- A medical rather than a social ground.
- Requires 'grave permanent injury' to the physical or mental health of the pregnant woman.
- The injury does not need to be physically present as s 1(2) relies upon the doctor's good faith in his belief that the injury exists or may exist.
- Unlike s 1(1)(a) there is no time limit attached; thus an abortion may be carried out late into the pregnancy.
- The wording permits the abortion only if it is *necessary* to avoid the injury. If the 'injury' to the pregnant woman can be remedied without an abortion, then an abortion will not be permitted on these grounds.

Section 1(1)(c), Abortion Act 1967

SECTION

'(c) that the continuance of the pregnancy would involve risk to the life of the pregnant woman, greater than if the pregnancy were terminated; or'

- No time limit is attached. The abortion can theoretically take place at any time before birth.
- No condition needs to be demonstrated. The section only suggests that a 'risk' to the woman's life needs to be demonstrated and that it would be greater if the pregnancy continued rather than was terminated.

Section 1(1)(d), Abortion Act 1967

SECTION

'(d) that there is a substantial risk that if the child were born it would suffer from such physical or mental abnormalities as to be seriously handicapped.'

According to Department of Health statistics, one per cent of all abortions (a total of 2,085) were carried out on the grounds of foetal abnormality in 2009. Once again, this section has no time limits, thereby allowing for late abortions. The section refers to 'substantial risk' although this is not defined in the Act; there need only be a risk. Thus, if the risk does not materialise even though it may have been regarded as substantial at some point, the abortion will still be lawful provided that the doctors have acted in good faith.

What amounts to a serious handicap? This is an undefined term both by statute and by common law, but arguably it suggests that disabled lives are not worth living and that it is better not be born than to be born with a disability. However, if the life is blighted by such an acute disability, one might agree it is more considerate to abort the foetus than permit a baby to be born into a life of pain and suffering. Moreover, if a baby is to be born with such a degree of permanent reliance upon its parents, is this too much of an ordeal to impose upon the parents?

In the House of Lords Debate on Abortion and Cleft Palate and Lip, Lord Alton referred to the Disability Rights Commission and the Disability Awareness in Action, as both groups expressed concern with the application of s 1(1)(d), as they observe:

QUOTATION

'The Section is offensive to many people; it reinforces negative stereotypes of disability and there is substantial support for the view that to permit terminations at any point during a pregnancy on the ground of risk of disability, while time limits apply to other grounds set out in the Abortion Act, is incompatible with valuing disability and no disability equally.'

A similar comment about devaluing disabled lives was made in the case of *McKay v Essex Area Health Authority* [1982] QB 1166 where a child suffered severe damage before birth as a result of her mother contracting German measles. Among other claims, the child alleged that her mother should have been advised to seek an abortion and, if this was pursued, she might never have been born at all. While this part of the claim was struck out, Stephenson LJ remarked that the effect of this allegation, should it be allowed to proceed, 'would mean regarding the life of a handicapped child as not only less valuable than the life of a normal child, but so much less valuable that it was not worth preserving ...'.

Between the years 1995–2005, there were 69 abortions due to congenital malformation of cleft palate and cleft lip, one of which was at over 24 weeks' gestation. Should such a disability justify grounds for an abortion when those born with such a condition live happy and worthwhile lives?

This very issue was tested in the case below.

CASE EXAMPLE

Jepson v Chief Constable of Mercia [2003] EWHC 3318

The Reverend Joanna Jepson applied for permission to pursue a case of judicial review. She alleged that the Chief Constable of Mercia had failed to prosecute an abortion which had been carried out on a foetus which had a cleft lip and palate. The police had investigated the abortion, concluding that it was legally justified. The applicant, who had also been born with a cleft palate, argued the facial disfigurement did not constitute a serious handicap within the meaning of s 1(1)(d) of the Abortion Act 1967 and hence the abortion was unlawful. Rose LJ and Jackson J held that the issue was one of such public importance that the court granted leave for judicial review, and West Mercia police reinvestigated the case. In 2005, the CPS concluded no prosecution would follow as the doctors had acted in good faith.

The British Medical Association (BMA) does not provide any specific guidance as to what amounts to a 'serious handicap'. However, the Royal College of Obstetricians and Gynaecologists (RCOG) has advised that each case should be considered on its merits, and has set out a number of factors to be considered:

■ the probability of effective treatment, *in utero* or after birth
■ the probable degree of self-awareness and the ability to communicate with others
■ the suffering that would be experienced.

The above factors are common to both the BMA and the RCOG's guidance. The two listed below are simply considered relevant by the RCOG:

■ the degree of assistance that would be required and performed by others
■ the probability of being able to live an independent life.

CASE EXAMPLE

Department of Health v Information Commissioner [2011] EWHC 1430 (Admin)

Soon after the case of *Jepson* (2003) above, the Department of Health in accordance with guidelines provided by the Office of National Statistics decided to no longer release precise details on late abortions on the grounds under s 1(1)(d) if the number did not exceed ten. In 2005, the Pro Life Alliance relied on the Freedom of Information Act to request statistics from 2003. The Department of Health argued that the information was personal data under s 40, Freedom of Information Act 2000 which could not be disclosed under s 44. They argued that the precise details should not be released since it concerned women who had very late abortions after the 24 weeks' legal limit. That fact, combined with the relatively small number of doctors prepared to carry out late abortions, could lead to identification of such vulnerable women.

The information tribunal found against the Department of Health, stating that the information was not personal data within s 1(b), Data Protection Act 1988 and therefore the Department of Health could not rely on s 40, Freedom of Information Act, and it followed that s 44 was not engaged. The Department of Health appealed.

The Department of Health's appeal was dismissed although the court found the tribunal wrong in finding the information to be personal data. Statistical anonymous information was not personal data and could therefore be published. Publication of the abortion statistics is now required although, at the time of writing, it is still possible the Department of Health will appeal further.

Table 8.1 Abortion Statistics for England and Wales *(Department of Health, May 2011)*

Statistics
Total number of abortions in 2010 were 189,574 (0.3% increase on 2009).
91% of abortions were carried out at under 13 weeks' gestation.
77% were under 10 weeks' gestation.
Medical abortions represented 43% of the total, an increase of 12% in 2000.

8.1.12 Section 4(1)

In this chapter we tend to focus on the woman's right to choose to have an abortion and her rights of self-determination, but let us consider the doctor's right *not* to perform an abortion. Section 4(1) provides that, where doctors have a conscientious objection, they can refuse to participate in abortions. The section states:

SECTION

'no person shall be under any duty, whether by contract or by any statutory or other legal requirement, to participate in any treatment authorised by this Act to which he has a conscientious objection.'

Although there is little definitive guidance as to what amounts to participating in 'treatment', the case below provides some assistance.

CASE EXAMPLE

Janaway v Salford AHA [1989] AC 537

A secretary objected to typing a letter relating to a patient's abortion. As a Roman Catholic who considered abortion to be murderous, she maintained she was acting as an accessory to murder and thus was participating in an act she vehemently objected to.

The House of Lords held that writing a letter did not amount to 'treatment' within the meaning of the Act; therefore she could not refuse to perform her contractual duty on the grounds of conscientious objection in the same way in which a medical professional could.

In March 2008, the GMC published *Personal Beliefs and Medical Practice* which provides some guidance as to a doctor's right to refuse to treat a patient seeking an abortion. The guidance explains that patients may consult doctors for treatment which doctors may consider unable to perform. In these circumstances, doctors must act openly and transparently, ensure that they refer the patient to another doctor, and keep in mind at all times that the patient must be treated with respect, even if their moral or religious values collide. The guidance continues by stating that where a patient is awaiting or has undergone a termination of pregnancy and requires medical care, there is no legal or ethical ground for a doctor to refuse to provide the care simply because there was a valid objection to the treatment.

KEY FACTS

Key facts on the Abortion Act 1967

Section	Provision and related cases
Section 1	A person shall not be guilty of an offence where an abortion is formed in good faith and if two medical practitioners consider the grounds in s 1(1) are met. Related case: *Royal College of Nursing v DHSS* (1981)
Section 1(1)(a)	Abortion can be carried out up to 24 weeks if the pregnancy would otherwise risk the physical or mental health of the pregnant woman or children. Social ground for abortion.
Section 1(1)(b)	Abortion is necessary to prevent grave permanent injury to the woman's physical or mental health. Medical ground. No time limit.
Section 1(1)(c)	Continuing the pregnancy would carry risk to the life of the pregnant woman. Medical ground. No time limit.
Section 1(1)(d)	Substantial risk that if the baby was born it would be seriously handicapped. Related case: *Jepson v Chief Constable of Mercia* (2003)
Section 1(2)	When assessing the grounds for an abortion, the woman's actual or reasonably foreseeable condition will be relevant.
Section 1(3)	Any termination must be carried out in a NHS hospital, private or approved clinic as determined by the Secretary of State. Related case: *British Pregnancy Advisory Service v Secretary of State for Health* (2011)

Section 1(4)	An emergency abortion does not require two medical practitioners to authorise the procedure.
Section 4(1)	Statutory provision for medical professional to conscientiously object to being involved in abortions. Related case: *Janaway v Salford* (1989)

8.1.13 The United States

In the USA, abortion is a far more controversial and political issue than in the UK. In 1973 the seminal case of *Roe v Wade* (1973) 410 US 113 held that a woman's freedom to determine for herself whether or not to have a child was a right protected under the American Constitution. Her right to privacy in this respect could not be interfered with by the State, although the Supreme Court recognised that it had legitimate interests in balancing not only the rights of the pregnant woman but also the foetus, which as the latter developed and became closer to full term its rights would grow accordingly. The court stated that in the first trimester, the decision whether to permit an abortion would be one taken by the medical professionals in conjunction with the pregnant woman. Once the foetus reached viability, the State may choose to override the woman's autonomy and impose State regulation which would promote the interests of the viable foetus over an abortion, except in circumstances where continuation of the pregnancy would adversely affect the health or life of the mother.

While the decision in *Roe v Wade* has not been overturned, subsequent decisions have sought to mitigate the initial perceived constitutional protection. In particular the case of *Planned Parenthood v Casey* (1992) 112 S Ct 2791 provided the court with an excellent opportunity to do so, as the liberal judges in *Roe v Wade* had been replaced by judges with more conservative values. The State successfully sought restrictions: henceforth it would be necessary for women seeking an abortion to be advised of the risks associated with the procedure; minors would need parental consent; and a 24-hour cooling off period would be required. The court rejected the requirement of having to advise their spouse of their planned abortion. Thus, while a woman's constitutional right to an abortion was upheld, obstacles were placed firmly in her way. The American women's constitutional right to an abortion was one which could now be tempered with 'the profound interest in potential life'.

8.1.14 Abortion in Northern Ireland

In Northern Ireland, the Abortion Act 1967 has not been adopted and the law relies mainly on the Offences Against the Person Act 1861, the Infant Life (Preservation) Act 1929 and the common law judgment of *Bourne* (1939). Thus, there are limited situations in which an abortion can be carried out, usually where continuation of the pregnancy would result in considerable risk to the mother. Consequently, many women travel to England and Wales to have abortions which would otherwise be illegal in Northern Ireland. Department of Health statistics show that over a four-year period between 2003 and 2007, there were nearly 6,400 abortions carried out on women who had travelled from Northern Ireland. This figure does not include situations where women have travelled to Scotland or other countries, or have failed to disclose their correct addresses for fear of being traced.

8.1.15 The Republic of Ireland

A strictly Catholic country, Ireland adheres to the provisions of the Offences Against the Person Act 1861, rendering all abortions illegal and subject to severe penalty. Common law precedent provides an exception, which is where the woman's life is in danger from the continuation of the pregnancy.

According to the 2009 Report of the Crisis Pregnancy Agency in the Republic of Ireland, the number of women giving Irish addresses at UK abortion clinics decreased from 6,673 to 4,422. This figure only represents those who choose to record or register their reasons for travelling to the UK. Contrary statistics suggest the figure is much higher, and that the number of Irish women seeking an abortion is rising rather than falling. One must remember that there are likely to be many women for whom travel to the UK is almost a prohibitive financial option, and others who may also wish not to disclose their Irish addresses for fear of prosecution on their return. Women may travel to other countries, not just the UK, and a reluctance to explain their reason for travelling abroad may well disguise the true nature of their journey. If a woman has grown up in a country with restrictive abortion laws, she may be extremely reluctant to publicise her pregnancy and abortion, especially where abortion still carries a significant social stigma.

Thus, abortion in Ireland is only legal where it can be proved there is a 'real and substantial' risk to the woman's life if the pregnancy was to proceed.

When the Abortion Act was passed in 1967, Irish law continued to ban abortion. The Constitution of Ireland was amended in 1983 with what is commonly referred to as a 'Pro Life Amendment'. The Eighth Amendment of the Constitution Act 1983 states:

SECTION

'The State acknowledges the right to life of the unborn and, with due regard to the equal right to life of the mother, guarantees in its laws to respect, and, as far as practicable, by its laws to defend and vindicate that right.'

However, the interpretation of this amendment was questioned in the following case.

CASE EXAMPLE

Attorney General v X and others [1992] IESC 1

X was a rape victim aged 14 and a half who became pregnant as a result of being raped. The other defendants, her parents, had decided that X should travel to the UK for an abortion. They informed the police as they wished advice on testing the aborted foetus for paternity for the purposes of the identification of the accused. The police informed the DPP, who in turn informed the Attorney-General who sought an injunction restraining X from travelling to the UK for the purposes of an abortion.

The Supreme Court held that her suicidal intentions put her life at a real risk, and they cited the Pro Life Amendment which provided the woman with a right to an abortion in certain circumstances. The wording 'as far as practicable' allowed the court to interpret the Amendment in a way that would allow the rights of the woman to usurp the rights of the foetus in limited circumstances. This was just such a situation where the real and substantial risk to life of the pregnant girl could outweigh the right of the foetus.

Subsequently, the Thirteenth and Fourteenth Amendment to the Constitution amended the law on abortion in Ireland. A woman could now receive information in Ireland relating to abortion services and could subsequently travel to the UK for the purposes of obtaining an abortion.

The Amendments became relevant in the following case.

CASE EXAMPLE

D v Ireland [2006] 43 EHRR SE16

The applicant was a 45-year-old Irish national who already had two children when she became pregnant with twins. She had an amniocentesis which identified that one foetus had died in the womb and the second had a fatal chromosome defect. She wished to have an abortion and travelled to the UK. On return she explained to her doctor and the hospital where she required further medical care that she had suffered a miscarriage. Her case concerned a complaint to the European Court of Human Rights about the lack of abortion services in Ireland. A doctor is prohibited by law from informing a woman about foetal abnormalities which may lead her to seek a termination of pregnancy abroad. She claimed that she had been discriminated against as a pregnant woman with a foetal disability.

The European Court of Human Rights rejected her complaint. They maintained that she had not exhausted the available domestic remedies. The Constitution had developed through the case of *Attorney-General v X* (1992) where it had been recognised that there was a constitutional relaxation where the mother's life was at risk through the real possibility of self-harm. Hence, the European Court of Human Rights argued that Miss D should have sought a remedy through the domestic courts, where the court could have been given an opportunity to develop the Constitution.

The most recent case to attract media attention is the case below.

CASE EXAMPLE

A and B and C v Ireland [2010] ECHR 2032

The case concerned three women referred to as A, B and C.

Woman A travelled to England for an abortion when she was nine-and-a-half weeks' pregnant. She had believed her husband was infertile. She had four children, one of whom was disabled and all of whom were in care. She was poor, suffered from depression and was a recovering alcoholic trying to regain custody of her children. She believed that a further pregnancy would exacerbate her depression and jeopardise her recovery from alcoholism and the return of her children from care. She borrowed money, travelled in secret abroad for an abortion and was careful not to miss a contact visit with her children. She returned to Ireland the day after the abortion but needed further hospital care.

Woman B was seven weeks' pregnant, having unexpectedly fallen pregnant after taking the morning-after pill. There was initially concern about an ectopic pregnancy but by the time she travelled to England for the abortion she knew she was no longer at risk. On return from Ireland, she needed further care in hospital.

Woman C had a history of cancer and was advised by her doctor that a foetus could be injured by the effects of chemotherapy. While in remission, she fell unexpectedly pregnant and was concerned about any potential side-effects on the foetus from her condition. She was unable to secure any clear advice due to a lack of information. Having been forced to investigate the risks herself, she felt she had little alternative but to seek an abortion in the UK. Much like the other women, she was forced to seek medical advice on her return to Ireland.

All three women argued that the restriction in the Irish Constitution was incompatible with their human rights. They argued that Art 3, ECHR (right against inhumane and degrading treatment) was violated, together with Art 8 (the right to a private and family life) and Art 14. Woman C also argued that the restrictions against abortion violated Art 2, her right to life.

In a decision given by the European Court of Human Rights in Strasbourg, the Court held that Art 8, ECHR 'cannot be interpreted as conferring a right to abortion'. However, with regard to Woman C, it confirmed that the woman's rights had been violated and she was awarded 15,000 Euros. The specific difficulty in Woman C's case was that there was nowhere she could go to for advice as to what her rights were in the situation. In this regard Irish legislation was considered to have a 'significant chilling factor'. The claimants' other arguments and claims of Article violations were dismissed on the grounds of being manifestly ill-founded.

From this judgment it is clear that Member States have a significant margin of appreciation when determining whether abortion is prohibited. The lack of interference from the European Court of Human Rights indicates not only the court's reluctance to intervene but maybe to some observers, an endorsement of Ireland's restrictive abortion laws. One aspect is clear. Given the success of Woman C with reference to Art 8, it is apparent that Irish law in this respect lacks accessibility. It is unlikely to be too long before further clarification is needed as to when an abortion is required to protect a pregnant woman's life.

8.1.16 Selective reduction of multiple foetuses

If a woman is carrying more than one foetus, can she legally elect to abort one of them? Selective reduction can be used in one of two ways:

■ Firstly, if one foetus is suffering from an abnormality, selective reduction may be an important decision as a continuing pregnancy may have an adverse effect both on the mother and on the development of the other foetus.

■ Secondly, the pregnant woman may choose to reduce the number of foetuses she is carrying. Strong opinions may be held about women who may choose to abort a foetus in a multiple pregnancy, but it should be remembered that multiple foetuses are often the direct result of fertility treatment. While one may think that any child born from fertility treatment is a blessing, one should not ignore the significant stresses – physical, psychological and financial – that also inevitably flow from multiple births. But how easy is it for a woman to select a foetus to abort? Which foetus would she choose? How can a person choose between two potential offspring?

The procedure for selective reduction was not developed until the 1980s and there is a view that this cannot be considered to be abortion, as the aborted foetus is not expelled from the uterus in the normal way but simply absorbed.

The HFE Act 1990 remedied the lack of clarity in the law. Section 37(5), HFE Act amended the Abortion Act 1967 in order that s 5(2) now reads as follows:

SECTION

'For the purposes of the law relating to abortion, anything done with intent to procure a woman's miscarriage (or, in the case of a woman carrying more than one foetus, her miscarriage of any foetus) is unlawfully done unless authorised by s 1 of this Act and, in the case of a woman carrying more than one foetus, anything done with intent to procure her miscarriage of any foetus is authorised by that section if –
(a) the ground for termination of the pregnancy specified in subsection (1)(d) of that section applies in relation to any foetus and the thing is done for the purpose of procuring the miscarriage of that foetus, or
(b) any of the other grounds for termination of the pregnancy specified in that section applies.'

■ An abortion of one foetus, if more than one is being carried, is lawful if it complies with s 1, Abortion Act 1967 and grounds within s 1(1)(a)–(d) are satisfied.

8.1.17 Abortion and the incompetent patient

We have previously explored the circumstances in which a medical professional will act in the patient's best interests if he or she considers the patient lacks capacity as defined in the Mental Capacity Act 2005. Although an application to the court in these circumstances is not required, it may fall to the doctor to determine whether the pregnant woman's best interests are served by a continuation of the pregnancy. As far as possible her wishes must be taken into account, alongside other matters such as the likely impact of the pregnancy and subsequent birth.

The case below indicates the court's approach, although it is important to note that the case was decided prior to the Mental Capacity Act 2005, hence its value in terms of precedent may be limited.

CASE EXAMPLE

Re SS (An Adult: Medical Treatment) [2002] 1 FLR 445

S was suffering from schizophrenia and was being detained under the Mental Health Act 1983. She was a mother of four children, was 24 weeks' pregnant and wished to have an abortion. Given the fact that the pregnancy was far advanced, it would not be in her best interests to undergo an abortion given the trauma that would be associated with such a late termination. Despite S's desire to have a termination, on a finely balanced decision, the court decided that giving birth and the baby being removed would be less traumatic for the patient than a termination of pregnancy.

8.1.18 Abortion and the minor child

In cases where the child is not *'Gillick* competent', due to their tender years, it is commonplace for medical decisions to be taken by their parents. In these circumstances it is also possible for the courts to overrule a parental decision, as occurred in the case below.

CASE EXAMPLE

Re B (wardship: abortion) [1991] 2 FLR 426

B was 12 years old and became pregnant by her 16-year-old boyfriend. She wanted to have an abortion and her grandparents with whom she lived supported her decision. Her mother did not accept her decision. She was made a ward of court by the local authority who then applied to the court for an order to allow her to have the abortion she wanted.

The court took into account the mother's views but explained that if her mother's wishes were respected, B would have to go through a pregnancy which she did not want to endure. The court explained it would be necessary for her to leave school, albeit temporarily. Given her age, she might not bond with the baby once born and, even if she did, it would not be practical for her to raise a child herself. She would have to place the baby up for adoption or have it cared for by other family members. Despite her mother's wishes to the contrary, the court concluded that it was in her best interests for her wishes to be followed and an abortion was carried out.

8.1.19 Does a foetus have a legal status?

A foetus only obtains full legal personality and status once it has been born and exists independently from its mother. Until that time, common law demonstrates a foetus has little, if any, rights.

CASE EXAMPLE

Paton v British Pregnancy Advisory Service [1978] 2 All ER 987

Mrs Paton became pregnant and unbeknown to her husband sought medical advice for an abortion. Two doctors in good faith certified that continuation of her pregnancy would adversely affect her physical or medical health and certified an abortion under s 1(1)(a), Abortion Act 1967. Mr Paton had not been consulted and once he became aware that his wife was eight weeks' pregnant, he applied for an injunction to stop the termination from proceeding on the basis that he had a right to express his views with regards to his child's future, and she could not have a termination without his express consent.

The court refused to grant an injunction and Sir George Baker observed that he had 'no legal right enforceable in law or in equity to stop his wife from having this or to stop the doctors from carrying out the abortion'.

As far as the rights of a foetus are concerned, Sir George Baker famously said:

JUDGMENT

'The foetus cannot, in English law, in my view, have any right of its own at least until it is born and has a separate existence from the mother.'

Hence, a foetus has no independent rights and no legal personality until such time as it can survive independently from its mother.

The case further demonstrates that a husband has no rights in relation to his wife's termination of pregnancy. Provided that the provisions of the Abortion Act 1967 are adhered to and two medical practitioners have approved 'in good faith' the grounds for the woman's termination of pregnancy, neither the courts, the spouse nor a partner can interfere with this decision. Sir George Baker expressed this principle as follows:

JUDGMENT

'not only would it be a bold and brave judge ... who would seek to interfere with the discretion of doctors acting under the Abortion Act 1967, but I think he would really be a foolish judge who would try to do any such thing, unless, possibly, where there is clear bad faith and an obvious attempt to perpetrate a criminal offence. Even then, of course, the question is whether that is a matter which should be left to the Director of Public Prosecutions and the Attorney-General.'

Hence, in law, a woman's right to terminate a pregnancy will be respected and permitted so long as it can, in good faith, be supported by one of the grounds in s 1(1), Abortion Act 1967.

Mr Paton then took his case to the European Commission on Human Rights.

CASE EXAMPLE

Paton v UK (1981) 3 EHRR 408

Mr Paton argued that he had standing as the father and could seek to protect the right to life of his unborn child under Art 2, ECHR. Furthermore he argued that his right to respect for family life was violated under Art 8.

Although the issue of whether a foetus had a right to life had been left open in *Brüggemann and Scheuten v Germany* (1981) 3 EHRR 244, the court rejected Mr Paton's complaint as being 'manifestly ill-founded'. Article 2 was rejected on the basis of the existence of legislation which justified the termination of a pregnancy in order to protect the life and health of the pregnant woman. His right to a family life was rejected under Art 8 as the derogation under Art 8(2) was essential in order to protect the right of the mother. Moreover, the court rejected an interpretation that was so widely construed as to enable a father to have any right to be consulted about an abortion.

The decision is not difficult to justify. Firstly, it is the woman who is affected by pregnancy and, since it is her body, she should have the right to say how it is treated. Secondly, if the European Commission had decided that Mr Paton did have a right to be consulted about his wife's wishes to have an abortion, it would open the gates for continual oppression of women in violent or abusive relationships where they would not be able to decide for themselves whether to abort a foetus. Self-determination would effectively be eroded.

A woman's right to determine the fate of her foetus was confirmed in the case below which we have already considered in Chapter 2 on Consent (page 48).

CASE EXAMPLE

St George's Healthcare Trust v S [1998] 3 All ER 673

A woman was 36 weeks' pregnant and was diagnosed with pre-eclampsia, a severe condition with potentially fatal consequences for both herself and her baby. She was advised to have a Caesarian section in order to deliver the baby with haste but she refused. She was sufficiently competent to make a decision and simply wished nature to take its course. However, she was detained under the Mental Health Act 1983 due to a previous episode of moderate depression, and it was considered in her best interests to have her baby delivered by Caesarian section. After the baby's birth she appealed and the court in an overwhelming endorsement of her personal autonomy held that detaining her under the Mental Health Act 1983 was unlawful and that a battery had been committed.

As far as the status of the foetus was concerned, the Court of Appeal said as follows:

JUDGMENT

'while pregnancy increases the personal responsibility of a woman, it does not diminish her entitlement to decide whether or not to undergo medical treatment. Although human, and protected by law … an unborn child is not a separate person from its mother. Its need for medical assistance does not prevail over her rights. She is entitled not to be forced to submit to an invasion of her body against her will, whether her own life or that of her unborn child depends on it.'

Thus, even if the foetus is viable, every woman has a right to refuse medical treatment and the rights of a pregnant woman are not outweighed by a viable foetus. Autonomy rules!

The case below further confirms that the foetus has no independent legal personality.

CASE EXAMPLE

Attorney-General's Reference (No. 3 of 1994) [1997] 3 All ER 936

A woman was 24 weeks' pregnant when she was stabbed by the father of the foetus. He had not intended to harm the foetus. Although both the mother and the child survived the attack, the mother went into labour and delivered the child at 26 weeks' gestation. It transpired that one of the wounds had caused the foetus injury and, once delivered, she underwent surgery. The baby subsequently died.

The defendant could not be guilty of murder because Coke's accepted definition of murder requires the death of a person '*in rerum natura'*, translated as 'a person in being' or a baby existing independently from its mother. When the baby was born, the defendant could not be convicted of murder as he lacked the necessary intention to kill or cause grievous bodily harm (*R v Vickers* [1957] 2 QB 664) as required by the criminal law. He was convicted of manslaughter but even if the foetus had died *in utero* from the stab wounds, the defendant would still not have been guilty of either murder or manslaughter.

Lord Mustill, while referring to the 'emotional bond' between mother and child as 'very special', confirmed that the relationship was based upon this bond and not on 'identity'. He further said:

JUDGMENT

'The mother and the foetus were two distinct organisms living symbiotically, not a single organism with two aspects … the foetus does not have the attributes which make it a 'person'; it must be an adjunct of the mother.'

It is hopefully now clear that domestic law does not grant a foetus any rights, but the case below explored whether a foetus has any rights under ECHR.

CASE EXAMPLE

Vo v France [2004] 2 FCR 577

Due to a negligent mix-up in patient names, a doctor accidentally and unintentionally ruptured the pregnant applicant's amniotic sac, leading to a loss of amniotic fluid. Due to further errors, the amniotic fluid was not replaced and the pregnancy was terminated on medical grounds shortly afterwards. Ms Vo brought a case before the European Court of Human Rights, arguing that there was insufficient protection of the foetus's life under Art 2 which protected an individual's right to life.

In a majority decision, the court held that there was no violation of the foetus's right to life in French law. They refused to commit themselves as to whether there could ever be such a violation, stating that another Member State could conclude that, in a similar situation, a foetus could be endowed with a right to life under Art 2, ECHR. Although the dissenting judgment argued that it would still be possible to recognise a woman's right to an abortion even if a foetus was protected under Art 2, it must be suggested that this would invariably lead to a Goliath-scale conflict between two crucially significant principles. Thus, whether or not a foetus's right can be violated under Art 2 remains largely unresolved.

KEY FACTS

Key facts on the legal status of a foetus

Case	Judgment
Paton v British Pregnancy Advisory Service (1978)	A foetus does not have any rights independent of its mother until it is born.
Paton v UK (1981)	A father has no rights in relation to whether or not the mother of his child can terminate a pregnancy.
St George's Healthcare Trust v S (1998)	An unborn child is not a separate entity from its mother. A competent adult has the right to bodily integrity even if it risks the life of the foetus.
Attorney-General's Reference (No. 3 of 1994) (1997)	Confirmed the foetus was not a separate legal entity.
Vo v France (2004)	A foetus was not protected under Art 2, ECHR in French law.

ACTIVITY

Self-test questions

Ensure that your answers are supported by case law and/or statute where appropriate.

* What is the statutory provision governing abortion?
* Explain the grounds which permit abortion.
* What is provided by s 1(4), Abortion Act 1967?
* What is provided by s 4(1), Abortion Act 1967?
* Does a foetus have a legal status? Ensure that your answer is supported by case law.
* How does the law of England and Wales differ from the law in Northern Ireland and the law in the Republic of Ireland?

8.2 Part 2: The ethics of abortion

8.2.1 Introduction

It is an understatement to say that abortion is one of the most controversial ethical areas of medical law and ethics. Readers tend to have pre-conceived opinions which they regard as unyielding. When you read this section, challenge yourself. Try to keep an open mind and formulate logical arguments. There is no problem in considering abortion either acceptable or unacceptable provided you can support and clearly explain your reasoning.

People's views tend to attract commonplace labels. Some consider themselves to be pro-life, where they maintain above all else the right of the unborn child. To them, abortion is simply murder. Others who regard themselves as pro-choice maintain that a woman has a right to determine what happens to her body. Deeply engrained with self-determination and bodily integrity, they believe that it is a woman's right to determine what happens to her body.

When considering the ethics of abortion there are therefore two distinct areas: the status of the foetus, what it is and when it becomes a person, balanced against the rights of the pregnant woman.

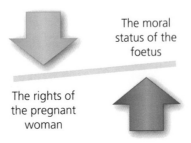

Figure 8.2 Balancing rights between the foetus and the woman

In this section we consider the moral status of the foetus. We look at the foetus alone and in a direct relationship with the woman who carries it, upon whom it is entirely dependent. We consider some of the ethical views of the status of the foetus and we follow the foetus from conception through to birth, at each stage considering its moral status.

8.2.2 The foetus at conception

Conception occurs when the sperm enters the ova or egg. Fertilisation of the egg does not take place until approximately 24 hours after fertilisation. Some believe that the foetus is a person from conception. While this is regarded as a largely religious view, the view also gains secular support as well.

J Finnis (1973) argues that:

QUOTATION

'two sex cells, each with twenty-three chromosomes, unite and more or less immediately fuse to become a new cell with forty-six chromosomes, providing a unique genetic constitution ... which thenceforth throughout its life, however long, will substantially determine the new individual's makeup.'

The above quote conveys clearly that once conception takes place (even though fertilisation is slightly later), a new individual is created. Because of the fusion of the chromosomes, the foetus has its own unique identity. But why does he accept that conception is the morally acceptable point at which to identify the foetus? After all, one might argue, a foetus has no physical identification apart from genetic make-up and, furthermore, many eggs fail and simply do not continue to develop. He continues:

QUOTATION

'To say that *this* is when a person's life began is to not work backwards from maturity, sophistically asking at each point, "How can one draw the line *here*?". Rather it is to point to a perfectly clear-cut beginning to which each of us can look back.'

Hence, it appears to be an entirely logical approach. There is a fixed point in time at which we can determine that life begins, and after that point abortion is not permissible. However, if you accept abortion to be permissible, ask yourself at what stage in a foetus's development you consider it to be so.

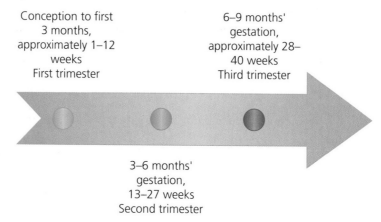

Conception to first 3 months, approximately 1–12 weeks
First trimester

6–9 months' gestation, approximately 28–40 weeks
Third trimester

3–6 months' gestation, 13–27 weeks
Second trimester

Figure 8.3 The three trimesters of pregnancy

Is abortion permissible at nine months? You might quickly agree that it would not be ethically acceptable as the foetus is a baby. Certainly, it is viable and can exist independently. This is the argument that is illustrated by C. E. Koop (1978), who asks us to work backwards. Would abortion be ethically acceptable at eight months? You are likely to consider it is not. A foetus is fully-formed and identifiable; it is almost a person. Ask yourself, would abortion be ethically acceptable at seven months? Six months? This is the difficulty that Koop illustrates. It is almost impossible to pinpoint the stage at which the foetus is ethically acceptable to abort, as at each stage the foetus is special and develops uniquely. Thus, what Finnis explains is that one cannot draw the line at which abortion is ethically permissible. There is no ethical difference in aborting a foetus at any stage of development after conception and birth. Life begins at conception.

The above view which is supported by philosophers is also a religious view. If one accepts that life begins at conception, this represents the staunch Catholic view which regards abortion as morally reprehensible and tantamount to murder.

If we adopt the ethical argument that life begins at conception and abortion after that point is not morally permitted, it must surely follow that other medical techniques where the embryo is involved such as IVF, PGD and embryo research cannot be permitted as they too will at some point involve the destruction of the embryo.

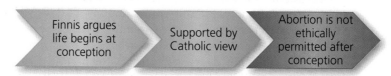

Finnis argues life begins at conception

Supported by Catholic view

Abortion is not ethically permitted after conception

Figure 8.4 Finnis's argument

8.2.3 Is the foetus a person?

We have seen that Finnis argues that personhood begins at conception because that is the stage at which a new individual is formed. M. A. Warren argues that the foetus is not a human person and cannot be treated as one. Just because it may have the potential to become one, does not mean that it should be considered a more dominant force than the pregnant woman. She argues that while the foetus is biologically human and can develop into a human being, it does not follow that a foetus is a human in the moral sense. So how do we identify what amounts to something that is entitled to be considered a person? She addresses this question, listing the following features as essential to be considered a person:

1. consciousness and the capacity to feel pain
2. reasoning (the *developed* capacity to solve new and relatively complex problems)
3. self-motivated activity
4. the ability to communicate
5. the presence of self-concepts, and self-awareness.

This is not a definitive list, and not all of the elements need to be present in order to conclude that the status of a person has been achieved. She continues by explaining that if a foetus cannot display any of the above then it cannot be a person and thus cannot have any rights.

In summary, she maintains that a foetus:

QUOTATION

'is a human being which is not yet a person, and which therefore cannot coherently be said to have full moral right ... But even if a potential person does have some *prima facie* right to life, such a right could not possibly outweigh the right of a woman to obtain an abortion, since the rights of any actual person invariably outweigh those of a potential person, whenever the two conflict.'

Thus she reaches a conclusion that the rights of a person who is living cannot be outweighed by the right of a potential person who may exist at some point in the future. Hence, abortion is permissible.

Mary Ann Warren → A potential to become something should not be treated as if that something has already been achieved → The rights of an actual person outweigh the rights of a potential person. Abortion is permissible

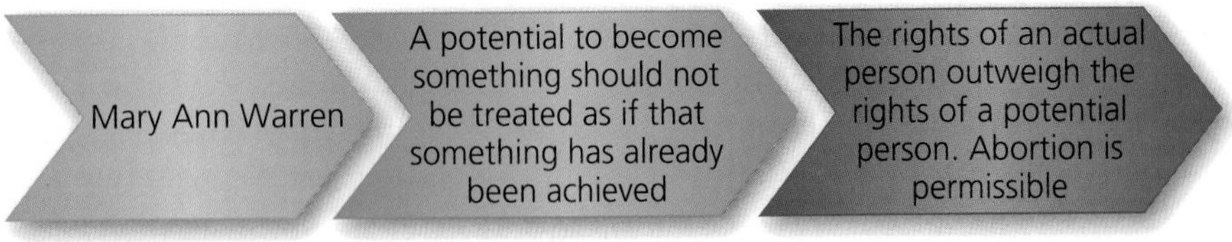

Figure 8.5 Warren's view

Let us jump forward slightly from conception to the appearance of the primitive streak which occurs at approximately 14 days. It is at this period that an embryo can divide in order to create twins. Can we conclude that the embryo becomes a person at 14 days? One advantage of adopting this approach is that we have previously seen that embryo research is permitted until a 14-day period. Thus, accepting that a foetus becomes a person at approximately 14 days would permit IVF, PGD and embryo research, all of which are arguably essential procedures. The difficulty with this approach is that since the appearance of the primitive streak is not clear, one cannot state with any degree of accuracy the precise moment at which life definitely begins.

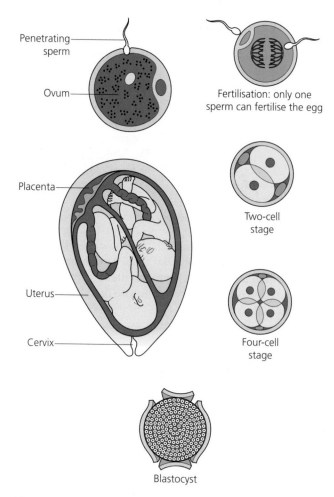

Penetrating sperm

Ovum

Fertilisation: only one sperm can fertilise the egg

Placenta

Uterus

Cervix

Two-cell stage

Four-cell stage

Blastocyst

Figure 8.6 The early days of life

 ### 8.2.4 Academic debate

Marquis's argument is essentially a secular one and takes a different perspective altogether (1989). Without any reference to personhood, he takes a pro-life approach. He states unequivocally:

QUOTATION

'abortion is, except possibly in rare cases, seriously immoral ... it is in the same moral category as killing an innocent adult human being.'

He accepts there are some limited circumstances where abortion is acceptable, such as abortion subsequent to rape, but to kill a foetus deprives it of a valuable future and the 'experiences, activities, projects, and enjoyments' it would have had. His argument rests on the principle that it is morally wrong to abort a foetus because of the potential it has. He does not accept that there is a distinction between the killing of a person who is already living his life and the killing of a foetus which is yet to live their life. Their current experiences, he argues, should not be distinguished from a foetus's future experiences.

He expresses the argument as follows:

QUOTATION

'When I am killed, I am deprived both of what I now value which would have been part of my future personal life, but also what I would come to value. Therefore, when I die, I am deprived of all of the value of my future'.

Hence, we can conclude, if we adopt Marquis's argument, that abortion is immoral.

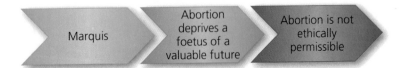

Figure 8.7 Marquis's argument

In response, Savulescu (2002) acknowledges Marquis's argument but maintains that although a foetus's potential may be one reason not to have an abortion, it does not follow that abortion is fundamentally wrong. He acknowledges that 'abortion and embryo destruction prevent a future of value, but that does not make them wrong' and argues that:

QUOTATION

'Abortion before 20 weeks is like contraception. It is no different from discarding a sperm and an egg, or an embryo, or a skin cell. Preventing a person from coming into existence does prevent a future of value, but it is not the same as killing.'

He draws a distinction between stopping something from coming into existence and deliberately ending life, maintaining that they cannot be regarded as the same.
Furthermore, he states:

QUOTATION

'In sum, Marquis establishes an argument that there are reasons against having an abortion (and by extension to contraception and embryo research). But that argument is defeasible. It is an argument that identifies one important property associated with killing foetuses or embryos. But it does not establish that either abortion or embryo destruction is wrong, all things considered. There are other important considerations that outweigh our obligation not to destroy embryos or foetuses. In the case of embryonic stem cell research, the enormous potential to save people's lives and to improve their quality of life outweighs the wrong of the destruction of some embryos.'

Savulescu points out that Marquis's argument is limited to one particular avenue, but there are other issues that may be more significant than an obligation not to destroy a foetus. Without the moral authority to destroy a foetus, embryo research would simply not be possible.

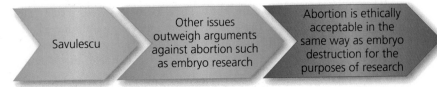

Figure 8.8 Savulescu's view

Another prominent critical analysis of Marquis is found in Brown (2000) who argues that a foetus only has the potential that Marquis describes because it is dependent upon the 'reproductive system of a woman'. In order to realise its potential, it has to occupy and to be reliant upon the pregnant woman's womb, but Brown argues that that does not mean that it has a right to do so at the 'expense of the autonomy, bodily integrity, and wellbeing of another person'. Brown does not accept that the right of the foetus automatically trumps the rights of the pregnant woman to her self-determination. He draws a useful analogy and states:

QUOTATION

'If I need a bone marrow transplant in order to realise my potential future of value, I do not thereby gain a right to your bone marrow, even if you are my mother.'

Just because there is a potential future does not mean that one automatically has a right to that future; hence abortion is permissible.

Peter Singer's approach (in Kuhse and Singer, 2001) to the ethical question of abortion differs from other philosophers. Unlike other thinkers, his focus is not dominated by when life begins. He observes that the question of the moral status of the foetus is often overlooked by those who simply define themselves as being pro-choice or pro-life. Thus, by that distinction, the emphasis is on the personal autonomy of the woman. Singer explains that this approach is not correct as we cannot assume that a woman has a right to an abortion until we determine the moral status of the foetus.

He continues by explaining what is often regarded as the focus of the debate, as shown in Figure 8.9. He maintains that the focus of discussion tends to revolve around when we deem the life of the foetus to begin, and from that point determine whether abortion is ethically permitted. Indeed, we have already discussed several philosophical arguments that adopt just this approach.

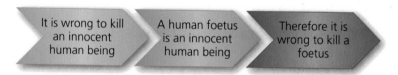

Figure 8.9 Singer's argument

There are some ethicists who regard a foetus as a human being at conception as this is one of the few points in development that can be pinpointed with a degree of accuracy. The problem with defining an embryo as a human being at the point of fertilisation, or even before, is that it is simply hard to comprehend. A fertilised egg does not share any characteristics with a human being. Nevertheless, whatever you may conclude a foetus is, all philosophers agree it is worthy of utmost respect.

A stage at which Singer observes it is common to define a foetus as a human being is the stage of viability, where the foetus may survive independently of the mother, albeit with the help of medical technology. This is at around 22 weeks. However, as he points out, a foetus which may be viable with the benefit of Western medicine may not be viable in another less developed country whose facilities for neonatal care are not as advanced. Therefore, if the stage at which a foetus is viable is consequent upon the quality of healthcare, which in turn depends on which country the pregnant woman lives in, and the ethical acceptability of abortion is dependent upon determining viability of the foetus, it must follow that the rule is inconsistent, which questions its very ethical acceptability. In any event, he argues, there is no specific time to determine when life begins as it is a developing and ongoing process.

We believe we can easily accept that it is wrong to kill a human being, but Singer queries what precisely is wrong about killing a human being. Is it just because the foetus is human that causes abortion to be wrong? Just because the foetus is both human and alive, it does not automatically follow that it is wrong to kill a foetus. He argues that the relevant issues are whether a human being has certain characteristics, more specifically a capacity for thinking which separates a person who is alive from a foetus yet to be born. As living individuals, we have capacity for thought and of simple awareness that we are indeed living. This can be distinguished from the foetus which, as Singer indicates, does not have consciousness at the time at which the majority of abortions are performed, and even later abortions still involve foetuses that have not developed the capacity to think or the ability to determine that they wish to continue living.

While this may be logical, one only need look at a newborn baby to realise that it does not have this capacity either, and thus Singer states that killing a newborn baby cannot be the same as killing a person who has the ability to understand the value of the life he lives. Even if one accepts this argument, one could also maintain that it does not take long before a newborn baby is able to express its own autonomy even in a limited way parallel to its experiences and, thus, even when a baby is very young, it does not follow that it would be preferable to kill a young baby than to kill an adult.

Singer takes a utilitarian approach to abortion and attempts to balance the views or preferences of the foetus with the views or preferences of the mother. However, preferences are those that can be expressed; for example, I prefer strawberries to bananas. A foetus cannot express any preferences. It cannot express itself until at least 17 weeks when it can feel or suffer pain. At this point it is clear that it would prefer not to suffer pain and therefore it follows that it has a preference or a view. Now we balance this preference against that of the woman. She can feel pain and she has opinions and views. She has made a decision that she wants to terminate the pregnancy. It follows that if one adopts a utilitarian approach of where the best possible outcome is achieved, it follows that the woman's wish to have an abortion is that which should be respected and thus it follows, according to Peter Singer, that abortion is ethically permissible.

8.2.5 The gradualist view

It is possible you have found it difficult to determine the stage at which you consider abortion to be morally acceptable (if at all). You might agree that such a task involves some imaginary timeline at which you must place an 'X' at the point you consider ethical permissibility for abortion is determined. Try and decide using the timeline in Figure 8.3 and considering the graphic figures below the point at which you consider abortion ethically acceptable.

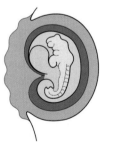

Figure 8.10 Embryo 4–5 weeks

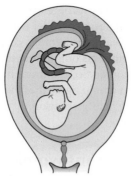

Figure 8.11 Foetus 15–22 weeks

There is however another perspective called the **gradualist** view, which instead allows us to focus on the development of the foetus during pregnancy. The gradualist view is also sometimes called the developmental view and, as Mary Warnock explains, the more the foetus has developed, the more protection we feel towards it to prevent it from being destroyed; the closer it becomes to its birth, the more urgent the reason needs to be for its destruction. Of course, you might argue that if the mother's life was in immediate peril and the foetus was threatening the mother's very existence, an abortion at a late stage is entirely acceptable.

There is logic in the gradualist approach. While we might easily accept that there is value to every potential life, one might consider it more morally acceptable to abort a foetus in its early stages of development than in the last trimester. That is not to say we should not respect a foetus when it is first formed, but the respect develops almost in relation to the foetus. C. MacKenzie (1992) explains that 'the foetus is not a free floating entity' but one 'whose existence and welfare are biologically and morally inseparable from the woman in whose body it develops'. As gradualists argue, the more respect can be attributed to the foetus; the more ethically challenging it becomes to abort it.

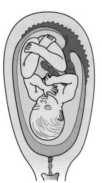

Figure 8.12 Foetus 31–40 weeks

MacKenzie continues with reference to the mother:

QUOTATION

'She is no longer just herself but herself and another, but this other is not yet separate from herself.'

The more a pregnancy progresses, the more respect the foetus is owed. Increased respect for the foetus runs parallel with development. As the foetus begins to grow and pregnancy is physically discernible, contemplating abortion becomes more emotionally difficult as the mother becomes more emotional connected and the foetus imposes itself more upon the mother. So, the more the foetus develops, the greater respect it should attract. Maybe you would agree that the longer the pregnancy progresses, the more difficult it is to morally justify abortion.

8.2.6 The pregnant woman

What rights does a pregnant woman have? Does she have the right to determine whether she carries the foetus to full term and delivery? Figure 8.13 shows how her rights may be expressed.

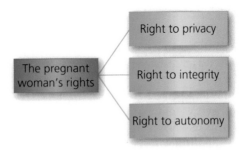

Figure 8.13 The rights of the pregnant woman

8.2.6.1 Privacy

It is for the pregnant woman and her alone to determine whether she allows the pregnancy to continue. This is an intensely personal decision which will affect the rest of her life. One can therefore argue that since it is her life that will be affected, no one but she can or should make the decision as to whether a foetus is aborted. How true is this? We have already learnt that a woman has no automatic right to an abortion, and can only have an abortion if two medical professionals certify one of the grounds in s 1(1)(a)–(d), Abortion Act 1967 in good faith. Perhaps one might agree that she has neither privacy nor personal autonomy.

Closely entwined with the right of privacy is the right to bodily integrity, the right to define for ourselves what we do with our bodies. Hence, if we are denied the right to abortion, one may argue that such action may violate Art 8 (the right to a private and family life), ECHR.

This point was specifically raised in the case heard in the European Court of Human Rights below.

CASE EXAMPLE

Tysiac v Poland [2007] 22 BHRC 155

A Polish woman who had severe visual impairment was denied an abortion which she sought on medical grounds. She argued with the support of her doctors that pregnancy would damage her eyesight further. Initially she was refused a certificate for an abortion and, when finally granted one, went to a hospital in Warsaw, only to be told that she would not be given an abortion. She had no alternative but to give birth. Her medical condition worsened and her eyesight deteriorated. She argued that the Polish Government failed to ensure that her rights under Art 8, ECHR were adequately respected as they failed to grant the abortion which doctors had authorised.

The European Court of Human Rights accepted her argument finding that the Polish Government, in failing to ensure that there was an adequate system in place for appeals and reviews from medical decisions, had violated her right to a private and family life under Art 8. She was awarded Euros 25,000 in damages for pain and suffering.

Although she was denied an abortion which had significant and serious consequences on her health, the court concluded there was no inhumane or degrading treatment and hence no violation of Art 3.

The decision is a controversial decision and, while it cannot be interpreted by saying that the court confirmed the existence of a right to abortion, the decision does make interesting steps in that direction.

8.2.6.2 *Equality*

How is abortion relevant to equality of women in contrast to the role of man in society? It has to be considered in terms of how a pregnant woman may be treated in some societies. We can only really appreciate the true nature of this idea by removing ourselves from our comfortable perceptions of what a 'normal pregnancy' should be and imagine ourselves instead in a society where there is little concern for the role of women generally in society, where sexual intercourse may not necessarily be a matter of free will or choice, where the pregnant woman is regarded with disdain, where there may be little recourse to facilities for abortion and limited healthcare during pregnancy and birth. Women who endure such experiences are truly oppressed and, in so being, are not treated equally to men. Furthermore, there is substantial evidence to support the claim that there is a nexus between domestic violence and abortion. In one study it was reported that nearly 40 per cent of patients seeking an abortion admitted being abused (Glander, 1998). These victims were unlikely either to consult or involve their partners in an abortion decision. In these circumstances, women are not equal to men because they are oppressed. There is an inextricable, unavoidable and distasteful link between the two concepts of oppression and inequality.

8.2.6.3 *Autonomy*

As we saw earlier, Warren argues that a woman's right to autonomy must prevail over any rights which may be claimed by a foetus. The reasoning is that as people we have full moral standing, and foetuses cannot be described in that same way. Indeed, she graphically describes a foetus at eight months' gestation as a 'fish' and in these terms a foetus cannot outweigh the rights of a person. To her an abortion has no more moral significance than the cutting of one's hair.

8.2.7 The Violinist Analogy

One of the most significant and well-known arguments relating to self-determination of the pregnant woman is found in an article by Judith Jarvis Thomson, a moral philosopher. *A Defense of Abortion* was published in 1971 and presents one of the most discussed theoretical arguments on abortion.

For the purposes of the debate, Thomson starts from the assumption that the foetus is indeed a person. If the foetus has rights, she explores whether they are more or less important than the rights of the pregnant woman. Her debate adopts the vision of a famous violinist. An extract appears below:

'You wake up in the morning and find yourself back-to-back in bed with an unconscious violinist. A famous, unconscious violinist. He has been found to have a fatal kidney ailment, and the Society of Music Lovers has canvassed all the available medical records and found that you alone have the right blood type to help. They have therefore kidnapped you, and last night the violinist's circulatory system was plugged into yours, so that your kidneys can be used to extract poisons from his blood as well as your own. The director of the hospital now tells you, "Look, we're sorry the Society of Music Lovers did this to you – we would never have permitted it if we had known. But still, they did it, and the violinist is now plugged into you. To unplug you would be to kill him. But never mind, it's only for nine months. By then he will have recovered from his ailment, and can safely be unplugged from you"'.

She asks, 'Is it morally incumbent on you to accede to this situation?' Do you unplug yourself from the violinist? There are probably few readers among you who would happily remain connected to an unknown but dependent violinist for the next nine months of your life. Only if you were extremely altruistic would you even consider it. You might quite easily come to the conclusion that you should not be obliged to remain physically committed to the life-form that is reliant upon you if you do not wish to do so. As Thomson says, 'If you do allow him to go on using your kidneys, this is a kindness on your part, and not something he can claim from you as his due'. If you agree with this idea then you are entitled to unplug yourself from the violinist. By unplugging yourself, you confirm that you have a right to self-determination and to bodily integrity. This is Thomson's argument: the foetus is not entitled to life as of right, and all you are doing is simply denying the foetus the right to use your body by denying the foetus its parasitic existence.

Commentators find difficulties with parts of this analogy with abortion. If you unplug yourself from the violinist, he will die. If you abort a foetus, this does not have the same effect as the foetus is intentionally killed. While the outcome may be the same, the intention is very different.

The argument presupposes you had no wish or desire to become attached to the violinist. This is emphasised by the fact that you have been 'kidnapped'. If however, you had attended concerts by the violinist and began to know him personally, for example by admiring his work, your answer may be different. How does one draw an analogy between kidnapping and abortion? Commentators remark that this is analogous to rape. The sexual intercourse in which a woman engaged is not voluntary and desired; hence the pregnancy is unwanted – the woman is pregnant through no fault of her own. In these circumstances, abortion is justified. Many consider that the violinist example can only be relevant in this respect. In all other respects, it is considered unsatisfactory. Thomson addresses this anticipated response by continuing thus:

QUOTATION

'people-seeds drift about in the air like pollen, and if you open your windows, one may drift in and take root in your carpets and your upholstery. You don't want children, so you fix up your windows with fine mesh screens, the very best you can buy. As can happen, however, and on very very rare occasions does happen, one of the screens is defective; and a seed drifts in and take root ... Someone may argue that you are responsible for its rooting, that it does have a right to your house because after all you could have lived out your life with bare floors and furniture, or with sealed windows and doors. But this won't do – for by the same token, anyone can avoid a pregnancy due to rape by having a hysterectomy.'

What does this mean? It metaphorically represents a vision of sexual intercourse. The mesh screens symbolise contraception and the defective mesh screen represents failed contraception. It seems to suggest the arguments presented in the Figure below.

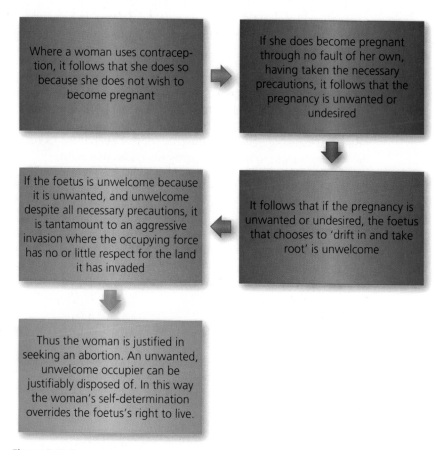

Figure 8.14 Thomson's argument

The reference to a hysterectomy to avoid pregnancy due to rape suggests an extreme and unacceptable method of preventing pregnancy.

However, many also argue that contraception is known to have its failing, and if one engages in sexual intercourse then one runs a risk, however small, of falling pregnant. In this situation, where contraception may fail, it does not necessarily follow that one is entitled to abort a foetus. Nevertheless, if a woman ensures that she is protected against the risk of pregnancy, she demonstrates a desire not to become pregnant. If pregnancy then follows, that is clearly an undesired event and abortion should be ethically justified.

Thomson further demonstrates the arguments of abortion by referring to a child growing inside a tiny house, rather like an *Alice in Wonderland* vision of a child growing who cannot stop. The room does not get bigger.

QUOTATION

'Suppose you find yourself trapped in a tiny house with a growing child. I mean a very tiny house, and a rapidly growing child – you are already up against the wall of the house and in a few minutes you'll be crushed to death. The child on the other hand won't be crushed to death; if nothing is done to stop him from growing he'll be hurt, but in the end he'll simply burst open the house and walk out a free man. Now I could well understand it if a bystander were to say, 'There's nothing we can do for you. We cannot choose between your life and his, we cannot be the ones to decide who is to live, we cannot intervene.'

This seems to suggest the following:

1. The third party, that is, the medical professional, states that he cannot help the pregnant woman.
2. This suggests that the woman does not have a right to an abortion as such but that an abortion is entirely dependent upon the doctors' agreement.
3. It follows that the above statement is accurate; the woman lacks both autonomy and self-determination.

Thomson then explains how the pregnant woman 'owns the house'; the foetus simply rents it. She states that even though a third party cannot intervene, the person who is threatened, the mother, can do so and it is therefore ethically justifiable if she aborts the foetus.

Thomson does not attach any moral responsibility to the woman's act of becoming pregnant, focusing instead on the concept that even if the foetus does have a right to life, the woman's right to bodily integrity overrides that right.

ACTIVITY

Self-test questions

Ensure that you can clearly explain the following people's ethical arguments concerning abortion:

- Finnis
- Warren
- Marquis
- Savulescu
- Brown
- Singer
- Thomson.

SUMMARY

- The law relating to abortion was historically restrictive, and abortion was punished by severe penalties. In more recent years, while abortion is still not permitted by right, numerous abortions are carried out every year by relying on one of the four grounds in s 1(1), Abortion Act 1967.
- The foetus has no legal right in law until it exists independently from its mother. The biological father of the foetus does not have any legal rights in relation to whether the mother can terminate a pregnancy.
- The ethics of abortion require a balancing act between the moral status of the foetus and the rights of the pregnant woman.
- There is a plethora of philosophical debate as to whether a foetus is a person at conception or at any point during a woman's pregnancy until its birth. Any commitment to an ethical position will conflict with the right of a pregnant woman to determine what happens to her body and the use of the foetus.
- Accordingly, in debates about the status of the foetus, we may neglect the pregnant woman's rights to privacy, integrity and autonomy.

SAMPLE ESSAY QUESTION

Sarah and Bob already have two children when Sarah discovers she is pregnant. The couple are happy as they have always wished to have a larger family. The pregnancy proceeds without difficulty until she has a routine blood test for Down's syndrome. While this usually takes place 11–20 weeks, she has been extremely busy and does not have the test done until 19 weeks. There is a family history of genetic abnormality in Bob's family; indeed Bob's sister suffers from Down's syndrome. She has had routine tests in previous pregnancies and both were negative. This time, however, the test is positive and further tests are required. At 22 weeks' she has an amniocentesis test which is positive. The medical professionals are as sure as they can be that their baby will suffer from Down's syndrome. Sarah and Bob are extremely distressed. Sarah wishes to have an abortion but Bob does not want her to. Advise Sarah and Bob on their legal rights and what ethical issues arise from this situation.

- As always, the first advice is to plan your answer. One of the difficulties that students encounter with problem-style questions is that multiple issues arise. If this is the case then ensure that you can separate the issues and plan your answer for each part of the answer.
- So what are the issues in this question? See Figure 8.15:

Does the law allow Sarah to have an abortion?	What are Bob's rights?	What is the moral status of the foetus?
• You will need to consider s 1, Abortion Act 1967 • You will need to consider whether any grounds under s1(1)(a)–(d) • Does the foetus have any legal rights? This will link in conveniently to Bob's rights.	• Does Bob have any rights? • This is important to discuss as Bob does not want Sarah to have an abortion.	• Here, you will need to consider the ethical acceptability of an abortion. • You will need to consider the competing and conflicting interests of the moral status of the foetus and Sarah's right to an autonomous decision to have an abortion. • You will need to explore the ethical arguments relating to the status of a foetus and then the rights of Sarah as the pregnant woman.

Figure 8.15 The issues of this question

- A model answer appears below. You may consider it to be too lengthy or too concise. It is simply designed to illustrate how this question may be answered. Of course, greater focus could be paid either to the law or ethics, although a balanced answer should address both areas equally.

- Sarah does not have a *prima facie* right to on abortion. Section 1, Abortion Act 1967 as amended by the HFE Act 1990 states that a person will not be guilty of an offence if two medical professionals are of the opinion formed in good faith that Sarah satisfies one of the grounds in s 1(1)(a)–(d). The requirement of good faith is generally not an issue although the case of *Smith* (1974) illustrates the importance of ensuring that two medical professional opinions are sought.
- Although s 1(2) allows for 'reasonable foreseeable conditions' to be taken into account by the medical professionals, we are here concerned with an actual condition as Sarah's test results confirm the baby will be born with Down's syndrome.
- Sarah is unlikely to fulfil the grounds under s 1(1)(a) as the time limit for abortions under this ground is 24 weeks; she did not have the amniocentesis test until 22 weeks so it is possible that she will exceed this period. While the majority of abortions take place under this ground (Department of Health statistics in 2009 show that 91 per cent of all abortions fell into this category), it is more commonly considered to be a social ground for termination of pregnancy and involves a physical or mental risk to Sarah or to her children if the pregnancy was continued.
- She might argue that continuing the pregnancy would affect her mental health and indeed could have an adverse effect on her children.

- It would however be more appropriate if she relied on s1(1)(d), Abortion Act 1967 which refers to a substantial risk that if the child were born it would suffer from such physical or mental abnormalities as to be seriously handicapped. We do not know at this stage the extent of the potential disability, but we do know that Down's syndrome manifests itself both mentally and physically, and any baby would require considerable care. Serious handicap is not defined in the Act and the only clear guidance is from the BMA and the RCOG. The factors set out by the professional bodies apply to Down's syndrome in several ways.
- Any baby born with the condition may lack an ability to communicate with others to some extent, and it is a possibility that there could be associated suffering if there was physical disability as well. Sarah and Bob would inevitably be required to provide significant assistance to a Down's syndrome child and it is possible the child would not in the future be able to live an independent life. Hence, it would appear that the grounds under s 1(1)(d) seem to be satisfied and importantly, since there is no time limit referred to in this ground, time is not of the essence.
- One however should advise Sarah and Bob that it is a late abortion and it is possible that a doctor may refuse to perform an abortion. While this may not be likely, one should advise them that a doctor can, by virtue of s 1(4), conscientiously object to participate in any treatment connected to an abortion.
- If this is the case, the GMC guidelines state that the doctor must refer them to another medical professional who can assist. A doctor however cannot refuse aftercare.

- We are told that Bob objects to the abortion, probably as his sister has Down's syndrome. He has no rights in relation to the foetus. Sir George Baker observed in *Paton v British Pregnancy Advisory Service* (1978) that a father has no enforceable legal or equitable rights to stop his wife from having a termination of pregnancy. Moreover, the slightly later case of *Paton v UK* (1981) also shows that a foetus has no right of life under Arts 2 and 8, ECHR and these could not be relied upon to stop Sarah from having an abortion.
- The decision of *Vo v France* (2004) confirmed the view that a foetus does not have a right of life under Art 2. A similar decision was reached in *St George's Healthcare Trust v S* (1998) which illustrates that an unborn child is not a separate entity from its mother and hence does not have prevailing rights. This judgment is seen as a significant authority to support the premise that the mother has the right of self-determination and the right to make the autonomous decision to have an abortion, which takes precedence over any rights of life of a foetus.

- In advising Sarah and Bob of the ethical arguments in relation to a potential abortion, the essential issue is a balancing act between the moral status of the foetus and Sarah's rights as a pregnant woman. Sarah should be advised that she has a right of privacy. It is her decision on whether or not to have an abortion.
- The case of *Tysiac v Poland* (2007) demonstrated the seriousness with which a violation of Art 8 was regarded, although it cannot properly be interpreted as saying that there is a formal recognition of a right to life. She also has a right to

self-determination, and Thomson's violinist analogy explores her rights of self-determination. Thomson asks us to imagine that we wake up in the morning to find ourselves in bed with an unconscious violinist, whose circulatory system has been plugged into ours. We are entitled to unplug ourselves from him but he will die if we do. As this is an analogy to a foetus's dependence upon ourselves, we are asked to question whether it is morally permissible to unplug ourselves. Thomson suggests that it is, although critics often draw a parallel between being kidnapped and pregnancy as a consequence of rape. Anticipating this argument, she continued by her 'pollen seeds' analogy explaining that if a woman protects herself against pregnancy then she is fully entitled to abort an unwanted foetus. While this may not be an unwanted foetus for Sarah and Bob, it does emphasise the self-determination and how, while a woman is engaged in a balancing act, her autonomy should prevail. This last point is supported further by Warren who regards a foetus as a form of a fish which cannot override a woman's autonomy.

- She continues by explaining that just because the foetus has the potential to become a human does not mean that it should be treated as a human in the moral sense. She sets out criteria to be applied to determine whether the foetus should be entitled to be treated as an equal to us. Although it is likely at over 22 weeks' gestation Sarah's foetus can feel pain, it has no ability to reason, cannot communicate and has no self-awareness. Accordingly, it cannot be treated as a person and have moral rights. She concludes that even if it did have rights, it could not outweigh Sarah's rights to have an abortion since an actual person outweighs a potential person.

- We should advise Sarah and Bob of the view held by Finnis that a foetus is a person from conception due to the unique genetic identity being established. Hence, abortion is not ethically acceptable at any time after conception. This may be a view Sarah and Bob may accept, particularly if they believed in a theological approach that abortion is tantamount to murder.
- Koop questions the point at which we can effectively draw the line and say that abortion is or is not ethically acceptable. If Sarah and Bob find it difficult to accept abortion at nine months when a foetus is born, then they should adopt Finnis's argument, work backwards and ask themselves at what point they can pinpoint moral acceptability. Can they consider it morally accept able to abort their foetus at over 22 weeks' gestation?

- Savulescu argues that although he recognises that a foetus has potential, this is not reason in itself not to abort a foetus, and there are more compelling reasons to justify abortions other than simply the potential value of a foetus. Diametrically opposed to this is Marquis who argues that only in very limited circumstances can a foetus be aborted as this deprives the foetus of a valuable future. He specifically refers to 'experiences, activities, projects and enjoyment'. Here, we know that Sarah and Bob's foetus has several abnormalities and therefore we have to question the extent to which it could fulfil the experiences referred to above. However, that is to suggest that a disabled person's life is not worth living and is valueless, a principle opposed by Harris. Given that Bob has a sister with Down's syndrome, he is unlikely to agree that a disabled life is not worth living.

- Determining the point of the moral permissibility of an abortion is fraught with difficulties. Sarah and Bob may prefer the gradualist approach which argues that the more the pregnancy progresses, the more respect should be owed to the foetus.
- However, Sarah is already nearing the end of the second trimester and this may be an emotionally challenging approach for her as her pregnancy is significantly advanced. She may prefer Singer's approach which, rather than attempting to determine the moral status of the foetus, attempts to balance views or preferences of the mother.
- Adopting a utilitarian approach, Sarah may conclude that an abortion is ethically acceptable. She has made a decision that she wishes to terminate the foetus, while the foetus cannot express a view.

Thus we can conclude that the Abortion Act 1967 will permit Sarah to have a lawful abortion, Bob has neither a legal nor an equitable right to determine whether his wife has an abortion, and case law shows that the foetus has no rights in law. The moral status of the foetus is particularly difficult to determine, although since Sarah wants an abortion, there is considerable support for her rights of self-determination and autonomy.

Further reading

Brown, M. (2000) 'The Morality of Abortion and the Deprivation of Futures', *Journal of Medical Ethics*, 26, pages 103–7.

Finnis, J. (1973) 'The rights and wrongs of abortion', *Philosophy and Public Affairs*, 2, pages 117–45.

Glander, S. (1998) 'The prevalence of domestic violence among women seeking abortion', *Obstetrics and Gynecology*, vol. 91, issue 6.

Keown, J. (1988) *Abortion, Doctors and the* Law. Cambridge: Cambridge University Press.

Koop, C. E. (1978) *The right to live, the right to die*. Wheaton, IL: Tyndale House Publishers; Cape Town; New York: Oxford University Press.

MacKenzie, C. (1992) 'Abortion and Embodiment', *Australasian Journal of Philosophy*, vol. 70:2, pages 136–55.

Marquis, D. (April 1989) 'Why abortion is immoral', *Journal of Philosophy*, Vol. 86, No. 4, pages 183–202.

Savulescu, J. (2002) 'Abortion, Embryo, Destruction and the Future of Value Argument', *Journal of Medical Ethics*, 28, pages 133–5.

Singer, P. (2001) 'Killing and Letting Die' in Kuhse, H. and Singer, P. (2001) *Bioethics. Oxford Readings in Philosophy*, edited by John Harris. Oxford: Oxford University Press.

Thomson, J. (1971) 'A defense of abortion', *Philosophy and Public Affairs*, autumn, pages 47–66.

Warren, M. A. (1973) 'On the Moral and Legal Status of Abortion', *The Monist*, 1, pages 43–61.

9

Organ transplantation

AIMS AND OBJECTIVES

After reading this chapter you should be able to:

- Appreciate the necessity for the Human Tissue Act 2004 and understand its provisions
- Understand the reasons for the acute shortage of organs available for transplantation
- Be able to understand the 'opt in' system of organ donation in the UK and appreciate the alternative systems that could be introduced
- Appreciate the law in relation to live organ donors
- Be able to demonstrate a clear understanding of the issues in relation to the buying and selling of organs.

Organ transplantation can transform the quality of a person's life, and often save it. Organs are transplanted into patients who are on an organ donor waiting list but there is an acute shortage of available organs in the UK – a situation which we will examine in this chapter. This chapter examines the Human Tissue Act 2004 (HT) with its emphasis on consent in Part 1, and then considers the legal and ethical issues that arise in organ transplantation in Part 2.

9.1 Part 1: The Human Tissue Act 2004

9.1.1 Background: the Alder Hey scandal

One of the most fundamental issues addressed in the provisions of the HT Act 2004 is the issue of consent. Before we take a closer look at the provisions of the Act, it is worth considering why consent had become such a focal point in the legislation.

The Kennedy and Redfern Inquiries were set up to investigate the care of children who had been treated for cardiac conditions between 1994 and 1998 at the Bristol Royal Infirmary and Alder Hey Children's Hospital, Liverpool. The findings are largely beyond the scope of this chapter, but during the inquiries' investigations, one particular area of concern attracted considerable alarm.

During a hearing in 1999 it became apparent that, without the parents' consent, hospital pathologists routinely removed human organs from children who had died during heart surgery. Vast number of hearts from children that had died were stored at the hospitals. The fact that parents were not asked for their consent does not necessarily mean that the practice was deliberately deceptive, simply that the law was unclear and there was no statutory provision to indicate that consent was required.

Understandably, the parents of the affected children were extremely distressed that material from their children had been retained by the hospital without their consent or without them even being aware that body parts were being retained. Unsurprisingly, this discovery was so scandalous that the media quickly picked up on it.

Headlines were dramatic and conveyed the nation's distress and revulsion. 'He stripped the organs from every dead child he touched' (*The Guardian*, 31 January 2001) referred to the pathologist Van Velzens, who was alleged to have removed almost every organ from every child that a post mortem was carried out on between the years 1988–95. *The Sun* newspaper ran the headline, 'We buried our daughter like a jigsaw at three funerals'.

Regardless of the other issues surrounding the inquiries, one of the most important concerns was that hospitals were not acting in accordance with medical practice of the 1990s. The hospitals never even considered the importance of seeking the parents' consent, believing it would be too distressing to the parents to ask them. This paternalistic style of medicine which is now largely rejected was still prevalent in the hospitals during the relevant period. The doctors did not consider they were doing anything unlawful or improper. From the hospital's perspective, not only does the removal of an organ assist in establishing the cause of death, but there are other projects where such organs are invaluable, such as education and research.

However, even while the media was reeling from the scandals in Bristol Royal Infirmary and Alder Hey Hospitals, the *Chief Medical Officer for England Report* in 2000 and the *Isaacs Report* in 2003 (which concerned the issue of the retention of adult human brains) reported that the practice of organ retention which was thought to be isolated to these two hospitals was in fact widespread, and thousands of organs had been retained without appropriate consent.

In reality, law and medical practice were taking diverging, not complementary paths, and it was this issue that needed to be addressed by urgent legislation.

As a result of the scandals at the two children's hospitals, many families began litigation for the wrongful retention of hundreds of hearts, brains and other organs. Where it was possible, organs were returned and parents were forced to undergo separate burials for their children's organs. Through mediation, the hospitals compensated every family, publicly apologised and gave a sizeable charitable donation. For the purposes of this chapter, however, it is beyond doubt that clarity in the law was required and that the scandal galvanised the government into action.

The scandal highlighted that the two areas of primary concern were a) the retention of body parts and b) the issue of consent. The Department of Health's consultation report entitled *Human Bodies, Human Choices* followed in 2002. It set out guiding principles underpinning future organ retention. Paragraph 1.28, section 2–5 set out the principles as shown in Figure 9.1.

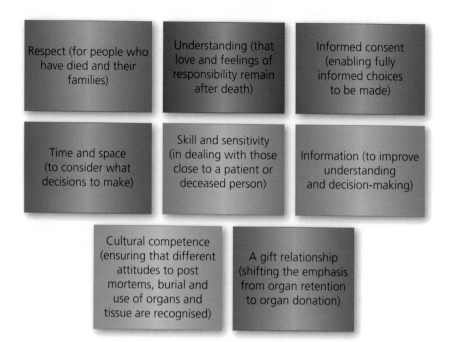

Figure 9.1 The principles underpinning future organ retention

The consultation report observed that the Human Organ Transplants Act 1989 (which regulated the live organ transplants) and the Coroners Act 1988 and Coroners Rules 1984 (which regulated post mortems) did not complement the other two statutory provisions – the HT Act 1961 and the Anatomy Act 1984.

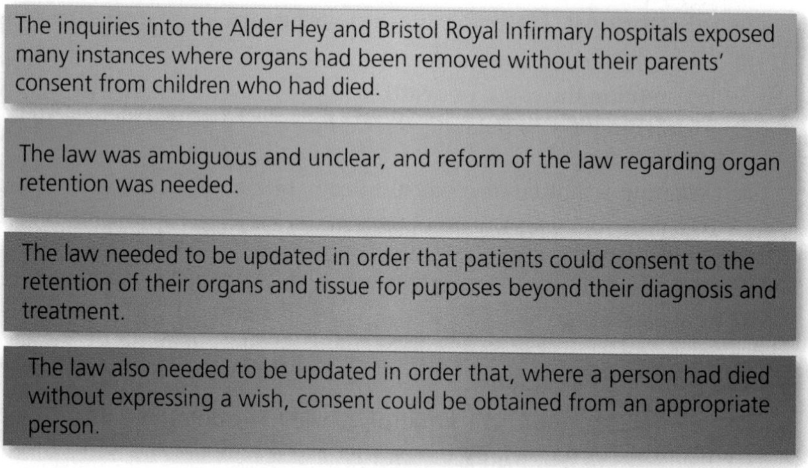

The inquiries into the Alder Hey and Bristol Royal Infirmary hospitals exposed many instances where organs had been removed without their parents' consent from children who had died.

The law was ambiguous and unclear, and reform of the law regarding organ retention was needed.

The law needed to be updated in order that patients could consent to the retention of their organs and tissue for purposes beyond their diagnosis and treatment.

The law also needed to be updated in order that, where a person had died without expressing a wish, consent could be obtained from an appropriate person.

Figure 9.2 The inquiries' findings

9.1.2 The Human Tissue Act 2004

The HT Act 2004 received Royal Assent on 15 November 2004 and took effect from 2006. According to the Department of Health, the purpose of the HT Act was:

> 'To provide a consistent legislative framework relating to whole body donation and the taking, storage and use of human organs and tissue'.

The Act introduced new requirements and provided a framework for the regulation of the removal, storage and use of human organs and tissues which applies in England, Wales and Northern Ireland. Similar provisions apply in the Human Tissue (Scotland) Act 2006.

The Act replaces the Human Tissue Act 1961, the Anatomy Act 1984, The Corneal Tissue Act 1986 and the Human Organ Transplants Act 1989. It is specific in its wording and only deals with the use and storage of human material.

The Act regulates:

- the removal, storage and use of human organs from living persons
- the removal, storage and use of human organs and tissues from the deceased.

The Act also introduced a new offence of 'DNA' theft.

What is 'relevant material?'

The Act only applies to 'relevant material'. This is defined in s 53 and states in subs 1 that 'relevant material' means material, other than **gametes**, which consists of or includes human cells. Subsection 2 explains that relevant material from a human body does not include embryos outside the body, or hair and nails from a living person. It follows therefore that blood would be regulated by the Act as it contains cells.

What does the Act permit?

Providing there is 'appropriate consent', under Part 1, s 2 for children and Part 1, s 3 for adults, the Act permits the storage of the body of a deceased person and the removal of any 'relevant material'. However, this can only be carried out if it relates to any of the following:

- anatomical examination
- determining the cause of death
- establishing after a person's death the efficacy of any drug or other treatment administered to him
- obtaining scientific or medical information about a living or deceased person which may be relevant to any other person (including a future person)
- public display
- research in connection with disorders, or the functioning, of the human body
- transplantation.

The issue of consent

As previously stated, the issue of consent is one of the most important aspects that needed to be addressed by the HT Act 2004.

The phrase 'appropriate consent' is all important and is needed for all removal and use of tissue. We now consider what amounts to appropriate consent by considering the different categories, as there are different requirements for each.

1. Where the adult is living

Unsurprisingly, 'appropriate consent' means the person's consent according to Part 1, s 3. This means that a person can consent to activity which involves his body or the removal of material from his body.

2. Where the adult is deceased

Where the adult has died, consent is required if his body or removal of material from his body concerns public display or anatomical examination. If he did not expressly consent, a personal representative may consent on his behalf. If there is no personal representative, a person with a 'qualifying relationship' under s 27(4) may consent.

gametes
reproductive cells, either eggs (or ova) or sperm

3. Where the adult is incapacitated

In these situations, the law is governed by the Human Tissue Act 2004 (Persons who Lack Capacity to Consent and Transplants) Regulations 2006. There will be deemed consent to some use and storage of 'relevant material' if it is compatible with the provisions of the Regulations. Where a person lacks the capacity to consent, the Mental Capacity Act 2005 must be applied.

4. Where the child is living

As with an adult, Part 1, s 2 states that 'appropriate consent' refers to the child's consent. However, by virtue of s 3, if the child is not competent to make a decision or has not made a decision, then a person with parental responsibility can do so on their behalf.

5. Where the child has died

If the child did not consent, a person with parental responsibility can do so after their death. If there is no one with parental responsibility then a person with a qualifying relationship can provide the required consent.

What amounts to a 'qualifying relationship?'

Section 27(4) sets out the relationships which will amount to a 'qualifying relationship'. They are to be considered as ranked in order, and therefore if the first preferred relative is not available, one may move to the next available relative to seek consent. The Act also provides that a person's relationship can be left out altogether if that person does not wish to deal with the question of consent, is unable to or it is not reasonably practicable to discuss it with him given the available time.

The 'qualifying relationships' are:

- spouse or partner
- parent or child
- brother or sister
- grandparent or grandchild
- child of the brother or sister
- step-father or step-mother
- half-brother or half-sister
- friend of long standing.

Situations where consent is not required

We have already seen that a person's consent to the use of their 'relevant material' is the bedrock of the Act. There are a number of specific but limited areas where the Act states that consent is not specifically required. As they are relatively uncommon, only two will be outlined in any detail. They are:

- Section 7(1), HT Act 2004 provides that there are some circumstances where consent is not required for the storage and use of 'relevant materials'. If the Human Tissue Authority (see below, page 282) is satisfied that it is not possible to trace the donor of material and it is in the interest of another person, either now or in the future, that the material be used for either scientific or information-gathering purposes, then the material can be used without the donor's consent. It would also be necessary to establish that the donor has not died, had expressly not consented or lacks the capacity to consent.
- Section 7(2) provides that if the Human Tissue Authority is satisfied that relevant material has come from a living person and where reasonable efforts have been made to get the donor to decide whether to consent to the use of the material, the material can be used for the purpose of obtaining scientific or medical information about that person. Thus, where a person can no longer be traced in order to obtain his consent, the material donated can still be used.

In reality, neither of these two provisions is expected to be widely used. The other situations where consent is not specifically required are:

- where storage of material from a living but unidentified person is desired for research purposes which has been approved by the Secretary of State
- where there is a High Court order for appropriate consent for research on material obtained from a deceased person
- where the storage of material concerns clinical audit, education and training
- where there is surplus material from treatment or diagnosis or research. In these circumstances, consent is not required for disposal of the material
- if the body has been imported from abroad or the 'relevant material' has been imported, there is no need for consent to be given
- if 'relevant material' was held by the hospital before the Act came into force, consent is not required for the continued use or storage provided that they are not anatomical specimens. The Code of Practice has been issued by the Human Tissue Authority to deal with existing holdings
- the HT Act 2004 does not govern coroners' activities and therefore use of any material in connection with coroners' acts does not require consent.

Criminal offences created by the Human Tissue Act 2004

Breach of the HT Act 2004 can result in criminal liability. The range of criminal offences mirrors the serious nature with which the issue of consent is now treated.

Earlier we considered obtaining 'appropriate consent'. Section 5 provides that if the appropriate consent is not obtained or a person carries out an activity to which s 1(1), (2) or (3) applies, a criminal offence is committed.

Since s 1 refers to storage or use or the 'material' of a deceased person, it therefore follows that should an organ be retained without the person's consent or the consent of an appropriate person in the alternative, a criminal offence is committed. If we reflect on the Alder Hey scandal, where organs were retained without the person's consent, the government has responded appropriately to the scandal by the imposition of criminal sanctions. There is a defence of reasonable belief which a medical professional can rely upon, and it is entirely correct that an offence of such seriousness allows a defendant a statutory defence especially given that the issue of consent, where it is derived from and how it is granted can sometimes be far from clear. The maximum sentence is three years' imprisonment and/or a fine. The sentence is far from modest and the fact that the case can be tried in either the Magistrate's Court or the Crown Court shows the potential seriousness of the offence.

However, this is not the only criminal offence that can be created under the Act. The following activities are also illegal:

- to store or use a body for anatomical examination without a death certificate
- to use or store 'relevant material' for a purpose other than that stated in the Act
- to analyse the donor's DNA without 'appropriate consent' being given unless one of the exceptions apply
- to falsely represent the existence of appropriate consent
- to conduct licensable acts without a licence granted from the Human Tissue Authority
- to sell or be involved in the selling of human organs (an area we will consider in more detail shortly).

9.1.3 The Human Tissue Authority (HTA)

The HTA was set up by Sched 2 of the HT Act 2004 and became effective in 2005. Its purpose was to regulate certain activities set out in the Act through a system of licensing. The purpose of the licensing was to restore damaged public confidence as a result of the Alder Hey scandal and to ensure that human organs and tissue were managed with appropriate and effective consent.

In brief, the Authority 'regulates and licenses the removal, storage, use, import and export and disposal or human bodies, organs and tissue'. It also has authority to issue and revoke licences and has statutory powers of inspection with the ability to search and seize.

The activities within its remit are set out in Part 2, s 14. Some refer to:

- removal, use and storage of 'relevant material' from the body of a deceased
- storage of an anatomical specimen, the import or export of bodies or relevant material which has come from a human body for use for a scheduled purpose
- the disposal of the body of the deceased which has been imported, stored or used for a scheduled purpose
- the disposal of relevant material which has been removed from a person for the purposes of his treatment.

Having explained the importance of the HT Act 2004, it is therefore a little difficult to fathom the motivation behind the current government's proposal to dismantle this Act. We have seen the important role played by the HTA but yet it is the current government's intention to dismantle the authority. A letter to *The Guardian* (4 March 2011) by a group of surgeons expressed the sentiment clearly:

QUOTATION

'As consultant surgeons we are concerned about the dismantling of the Human Tissue Authority, as proposed in the public bodies bill. The HTA regulates all living donor transplants and is of huge importance in reassuring surgeons and patients that proper checks and balances exist.

The HTA has had an important role in enabling us to progress with new technologies. The removal and/or division of such an entity, which has helped increase the number of successful transplants year on year, would be a huge loss to the public confidence it has helped to create.

Abolishing this independent body would undermine professional and public confidence in the area of medical consent – the issue it was set up to address. Within the government's arms-length bodies review there are no proposals for where transplants approvals sit. We urge the government to think again and stop trying to operate on things that aren't broken.'

Conversely, there is a body of opinion that considers that the HTA is overly bureaucratic. The Royal College of Pathologists in July 2010 stated that abolishing the HTA was a 'sensible economy'. The HTA budget is over £6 million a year and since the funds come from the allocation from patient care, the potential saving should be directed back into NHS services. Apart from the obvious saving, the college observes that, while there is a need for a regulatory framework, 'the current system is disproportionate and extends its demands beyond the areas envisaged when the Human Tissue Authority was planned'.

Equally, in a letter to the *Sunday Times* on 20 February 2011, leading academics Margaret Brazier, David Price and Jean McHale suggested that the proposals to abolish the HTA risk 'confusion and error in the implementation of the HTA' which will result in a loss of public confidence. Remarking that the HTA has brought 'flexibility and sensitivity to the regulation process', one hopes that the abolition is not a misguided move to save costs which could not only damage public confidence but also have a detrimental effect on organ donation for the future.

It is true that the provisions of 'appropriate consent' are somewhat laborious but as the authors of the letters observe, 'how will "appropriate consent" be interpreted consistently' without the HTA?

In an era of austerity and cuts in public spending, the HTA will soon be disbanded. One must wait to see whether any possible financial saving outweighs risk in public confidence and whether there is, indeed, a detrimental effect on organ donation.

Key facts on provisions of the Human Tissue Act 2004

Statutory provision	Definition
Ss 2 and 3	Defines appropriate consent.
S 27(4)	Defines what amount to a qualifying relationship.
S 7(1) and (2)	Consent to use of relevant material is not specifically required.
S 5	A criminal offence is committed if appropriate consent is not obtained.
Sched 2	Established the Human Tissue Authority.
S 53	The Act refers to 'relevant material'. Defined in s 53(1), refers to material other than gametes which consists of or includes human hair. Does not include embryos outside the body or hair or nails.
Part 1, s 2 for children and s 3 for adults	There must be 'appropriate consent'.
Part 2, s 27	A 'qualifying relationship' may be necessary in the case of a deceased.
Part 1, s 7	There are some situations where consent is not required.
Part 1, s 5	Criminal offences: this section underlines the seriousness of lack of consent
Sched 2	Human Tissue Authority established. Effective in 2005.
Part 2, s 14	HT Authority's activities: regulates and licenses the removal, storage, use, import and export and disposal of human bodies, organs and tissues.

Reason for introducing the Human Tissue Act 2004: Alder Hey scandal, organ retention and lack of consent.

The Human Tissue Act repeals Human Tissue Act 1961, Anatomy Act 1984, Corneal Tissue Act 1986, Human Organs Transplants Act 1989.

9.2 Part 2: The law and ethics of organ donation

9.2.1 The shortage of organs in the UK

It is indisputable that the number of patients awaiting transplants far outweighs the number of organs that are available for transplantation. It is simply a matter of demand outstripping supply. Statistics supplied by the NHS show that, in March 2007, 7,234 patients were waiting for organ transplantation, the highest number ever recorded – although, during that same period, 3,074 transplantations were carried out, also the highest number recorded. However, many patients do not receive organs and, sadly, die. Data supplied by the UK Transplant Support Services Authority show that, between April 2010 and February 2011, although 2,363 patients had received transplantations, a further 7,736 were still on the waiting list. By far the most common organs sought after for organ transplantation are kidneys, liver, lungs and heart.

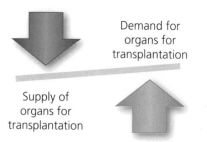

Figure 9.3 Demand outstrips supply

However, the NHS Blood and Transplant statistics show a record number of 3,706 transplants in 2009–2010, an increase of seven per cent in the number of deceased organ donors to 959 and a ten per cent increase of living donors to 1,061.

The subject of organ transplantation is of crucial importance as many patients wait for organs to become available in order to improve their quality of life, or often to save their life. The available organs which derive largely from cadavers (literally meaning a dead body) must be of a 'quality' that can be transplanted; hence those who die from conditions such as cancer do not have organs suitable for transplantation. The 'quality' however, is often dictated by the fact that the organs are still 'alive': in order words, the organs are still receiving an adequate supply of blood.

The quality of organs from brain-stem dead patients is of preferable quality to those in patients where the heart has stopped beating. In brain-stem dead patients, the heart can be artificially maintained so as to ensure the all-important blood flow. In this way the following organs can be preserved and used for transplantation: heart, lung, liver, kidneys, small bowel and the pancreas. However, in patients where the heart has stopped beating, only tissue can be donated. This includes the eyes, corneas, joints, tendons, ligaments, heart valves, skin and bone. While this is still valuable, the demand is largely directed towards heart, lung and liver transplants. Hence, for the purposes of organ transplantation, it is infinitely preferable if a patient is brain-stem dead.

In recent years, since there is a significant shortage of kidneys and the demand far outstrips the supply, there has been an increase in the use of non-heartbeating donors.

9.2.2 What are non-heartbeating donors?

Traditionally, the definition of death was cardio-respiratory failure, where the heart stopped beating and the lungs ceased to breathe. Since brain stem death has been accepted, far fewer organs have been sought from non-heartbeating donors. These are patients who either die of cardiac arrest while in hospital or who are brought into hospital and declared dead. Thus, there is no chance to maintain such a patient on a ventilator in order to preserve his organs prior to retrieval for transplantation. As organs from brain-stem death patients were preferable, the demand for organs from non-heartbeating patients fell. The difficulty was however that the pace of demand far exceeds the pace of supply. Hence in recent years, there has been an increase in the number of non-heartbeating donors.

While it is widely accepted that kidneys from brain-stem death patients are preferred, a study reported in *The Lancet* (October 2010) suggests that kidneys transplanted from non-heartbeating donors may be equally successful. The study records the outcome of 9,000 recipients of kidney transplants from 2000–2007. From this figure, approximately one-third of the kidneys had come from non-heartbeating donors, with the remainder coming from brain-stem death donors. It was noted that over the two- to three-year period preceding the report, there had been an increased use of organs from cardiac-deceased donors.

There were, however, concerns about the long-term success of kidneys from non-heartbeating donors compared to those kidneys from brain-stem death donors. The study concluded that the results of kidneys from non-heartbeating donors were very positive, and there was little difference in the set of results from the different types of donors.

9.2.3 The definition of death

For the purpose of this chapter we focus on the relevance of the definition of death to the period in which an organ may become available for transplantation. If organs are to be used for transplantation then it becomes imperative to be able to pinpoint the precise moment of death in order that the organs due to be transferred maintain their viability. The difficulty is that, while death may be instantaneous from a lay perspective, in reality it is not. The organs do not all die or cease to function at precisely the same moment. They cease to function consecutively rather than concurrently.

There is no 'formal' definition of what amounts to being dead, and on first glance this may seem obvious as it amounts to the final cessation of life, but a further reflection will illustrate that it is not that straightforward. In the UK there is no statutory definition of death but the definition which is now accepted by both lawyers and doctors alike is referred to as 'brain-stem death'.

Historically death was usually diagnosed using a **cardio-respiratory/cardiopulmonary** criteria which meant, once there was no evidence of breathing and heartbeat which was irreversible, the patient was dead. There seemed no difficulty with this definition; the entire person was dead once the heart and lungs ceased to function, as shortly afterwards the organs would die as well.

However, as medical technology advanced, patients could be kept alive artificially by use of a ventilator which assisted breathing and by heart bypass machines which artificially maintained a beating heart. The latter development was particular significant as it meant that, if the heart could be stopped entirely or bypassed, the patient would still remain alive. The first heart transplant was carried out in 1967. However, even earlier in 1954 in Boston, the first organ transplant of a kidney was successfully performed.

It follows that, if the heart could be kept artificially alive, then the lack of a heartbeat could not amount to death and, if a patient's heart and lungs could be made to work artificially, the definition of death was not reflecting medical reality. So what other function of the human body could provide an appropriate explanation of death? The answer was the brain. When we refer to brain-stem death, the loss of function must include the entire brain – both the upper and the lower brain.

The definition of brain-stem death began to evolve in the 1960s, when in 1968 the Ad Hoc Committee of the Harvard Medical School Report made specific reference to it. In the UK in 1976 the Conference of Medical Royal Colleges published *The Diagnosis of Brain Death*. This definition appeared to be the discrete justification for the removal of a patient from a ventilator. By 1995 an article appearing in the *Journal of the Royal College of Physicians* suggested that the definition of death should be considered to be the:

QUOTATION

'irreversible loss of the capacity for consciousness, combined with irreversible loss of the capacity to breathe'.

The Code of Practice for the Diagnosis of Brain Stem Death by the Department of Health 1998 now states that death involves 'the irreversible loss of those essential characteristics which are necessary to the existence of a living human person'. The above definition was adopted.

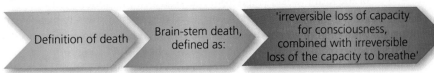

Figure 9.4 The definition of death

cardio-respiratory/cardiopulmonary relating to the heart and lungs

9.2.4 Criteria for brain-stem death

The Code of Practice sets out the criteria to be met in order for brain-stem death to be satisfied:

■ The patient must be 'deeply unconscious' or comatose, and doctors must ensure that this state has not been drug-induced.
■ The patient must be unable to breathe spontaneously.
■ It is beyond doubt that the patient's condition is due to permanent brain damage.

9.2.5 Diagnosis of brain-stem death

The diagnosis of brain-stem death must be carried out as follows:

■ by two medical practitioners who must be five years' post-registration
■ one must be a consultant
■ neither must be members of the organ transplant team
■ two sets of tests must be carried out by the doctors
■ these tests can be carried out together; it is not necessary for them to be carried out separately
■ the tests are done twice to avoid any element of subjectivity in diagnosis
■ death is not pronounced until both sets of tests are completed, but the legal time of death is given according to the first set of tests.

A cynic may suggest that it is no coincidence that the Code of Practice for the diagnosis of brain-stem death is contained within the same document as issues concerning organ donation and, indeed, the two are inextricably linked since the vast majority of organs may only be donated if a person is declared brain-stem dead, meaning that all brain function has stopped. The heart can continue to beat but artificial assistance must be used in order to keep the blood flowing to the organs. The organs must effectively be 'alive' even if the patient is actually dead. With this is mind, the major organs can be donated – the heart, lungs, liver, kidneys, pancreas and the small bowel. However, if one applies the cardio-pulmonary definition of death, then a patient can only donate tissue such as the corneas, eyes, joints, skin, bone and heart valves.

It perhaps then comes as no surprise that brain-stem death has been readily accepted as the legal definition of death for both the medical and the legal profession, allowing a significant number of organs to be donated to help others to live. Doubtless, if cardio-pulmonary failure was still applied as the accepted definition of death there would be a catastrophic lack of organs.

9.2.6 Is the definition of brain-stem death an acceptable one?

While the definition of brain-stem death is widely accepted, it is not universally accepted. It is worth briefly considering the stances of a few countries which do not accept brain-stem death as the definition of death.

Iran

In contrast with many other Islamic countries, in 1995 the Iranian Parliament voted to reject the brain-stem death criteria as a definition of death. It was acknowledged that organ retrieval and the acceptance of brain-stem death as the appropriate criteria are inextricably linked, but a refusal to accept the modern definition undoubtedly results in death for many of those who urgently require transplantations. In Islam, death is deemed to be the separation of the soul from every part of the body, but the question remains:

at what point does this occur? There is an argument to support the more orthodox Islamic view that cessation of brain-stem function cannot amount to death as the heart still beats and therefore the soul is not separate from the body. The Council of Islamic Jurisprudence (appointed by the government) in Iran states that a person is dead when the pulse and the heart have stopped and, according to Sharia law, brain-stem death is incompatible with separation of the soul from the body.

Japan

The Japanese Organ Transplantation law of 1997 only applies if a decision needs to be made in relation to organ transplantation. The approach in Japan is somewhat unique as the individual patient has the autonomy to determine whether they wish to choose loss of brain function or the cessation of cardio-respiratory function as the definition of death.

However, the importance and significance of Japanese culture is apparent as, while it would appear that a patient can decide which form of death to opt for with a view to organ transplantation, the family's wishes are taken into account and they can accept or reject the patient's wishes. Should a patient elect brain-stem death with a view to organ donation, this wish should be in writing made during his lifetime. A patient can therefore determine during his lifetime that he wishes to donate his organs on death by signing an 'Organ Donation Decision Card' upon which he then indicates which definition of death he accepts.

While Japan demonstrates a truly unique approach by providing the patient with the autonomy to determine at what point life ends for him, the family can still overrule the deceased's wishes. Nevertheless, the true value of Japan's approach lies in the flexibility of its approach which allows an individual to genuinely choose the manner of his death, taking into account his lifetime choices, cultural and religious views.

ACTIVITY

Self-test questions

Ensure that you refer to statute where appropriate.

- Explain why the Human Tissue Act 2004 was introduced.
- Broadly describe what the law permits.
- Why can criminal sanctions be imposed?
- Explain why there is a shortage of available organs for transplantation.
- Briefly describe the accepted definition of death.

9.2.7 The ethics of organ transplantation

It is already apparent at this early stage that the definition of brain-stem death is intimately linked with organ transplantation. Indeed, Singer (1994) comments that the definition of brain-stem death appears to some to be a mythical creation for the purposes of transplantation, and refers to it as 'a convenient fiction' as the truth probably lies somewhere there.

Truog (2007) observes that if we could obtain organs from somewhere else, such as animals, then there would be no need to have cadaver donors as their purpose would become redundant. The definition of death could then revert to the cardio-respiratory/cardiopulmonary definition – a far less contentious and more widely accepted definition.

Clearly, the current definition of death is a more utilitarian approach as it suggests that harvesting organs from brain-stem death patients causes the greatest happiness to the greatest number of people, as there are more organs available, although still insufficient to satisfy demand. Arguably no harm has been caused to the brain-stem dead patients (although there is a view that disagrees with this), and the number of people that benefit are significant: the donee himself, his family, the hospital and so on. Perhaps also this is a benefit to the deceased's family as well (who would have consented to donating his organs, if he had not consented himself), knowing that some good has come of their loved one's death.

From a health economic perspective, the allocation of resources is largely satisfied. Kidney transplantation, while expensive, is infinitely cheaper than maintaining a patient on long-term kidney **dialysis**, and by returning a patient to full health, the NHS, the patient's family and society as a whole are benefitting.

By adopting brain-stem death, a patient is not kept alive for long periods of time on a ventilator and life support machine which is costly, with no hope of recovery. In turn it frees a valuable bed for other patients who may have a more pressing and urgent need. The definition of brain-stem death may also be beneficial to the family of the deceased as it can be difficult to appreciate that their loved one is really 'dead' when they are being kept alive by artificial means.

dialysis
a way of cleaning the blood by passing it through a machine to replace the normal function of a kidney

9.2.8 Incentives to increase organ donors

Would more people be willing to donate their organs if incentives or rewards were given to them? At present, those who donate their organs after their death do so for largely altruistic reasons, feeling that something good may come out of their death.

Here, we explore whether a person would be more likely to donate an organ if in return they or a close family member of theirs would be placed in higher priority if they needed an organ themselves.

This suggestion appears to be attractive and has a pleasant tone of reciprocal altruism, in that there is a mutual understanding of donation to one another. A positive aspect of this approach is that those who indicate they are prepared to donate will be placed in a higher priority to receive than those who have not, reducing the feeling of resentment against those who would receive an organ but not donate an organ. Of course, this would not be the only criteria, and clinical indications would still remain the most important reason for placing a person higher than another one on a waiting list.

Israel, a country that has one of the lowest organ donation rates in the Western world, is embarking on a scheme similar to the one described above. This is in order to challenge the chronic shortage of available organs, as according to the Israeli National Center for Transplantation only four per cent of the population carries an organ donor card.

The scheme introduced by the Israeli Organ Transplant Law and outlined by Lavee, Ashenazi, Gurman and Steinberg (2009) is due to come into force in 2012 and will offer privileges to those who donate over those who do not. Once a person has agreed to become a donor, both they and their first-degree relatives are given priority over those who have not agreed to become organ donors.

However, this is not as fool-proof a scheme as it may first appear. Any potential donation is not legally binding and still largely depends on the family's consent. There is also the suggestion that the scheme will encourage 'gaming': that is, donor cards will be signed to gain priority without any real intention to donate. Another difficulty relates to one of the attractions: if signing up to become a donor is attractive because it provides both the donor and his first-degree relatives with a potentially higher priority, this becomes a disadvantage if a potential donor comes from a smaller family who would then find the incentive scheme less attractive. Nevertheless this is a brave and innovative scheme that has every potential of increasing the amount of available organs and being successful.

In reality, any non-financial incentive scheme is likely to be based upon some form of prioritisation on the organ donation transplant list. It would however be unethical if this was the only criteria and, while prioritisation is a worthy incentive, any transplant waiting list can only be equitable if its primary consideration is a patient's clinical needs.

In the UK, the Nuffield Council on Bioethics considered very similar issues. The consultation had been exploring the ethical issues in trying to increase the number of organ donors, in order to combat the numbers of patients waiting for organ donations combined with an increasing ageing population. While they explored whether more significant financial incentives will increase the number of potential donors, they also considered whether it is ethical to pay donors cash, pay their funeral expenses on death or provide them with priority in the event that they require an organ at some future point. Bearing in mind that women can already get free IVF treatment from some private clinics to encourage them to donate eggs, these ideas are potentially ethical. Having undertaken a consultation paper in April 2010, the council reported with recommendations for policy in late 2011, that eliminating the costs of funeral expenses for families may encourage organ donation.

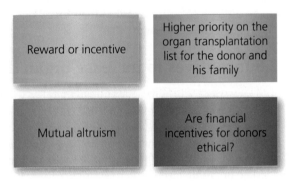

Figure 9.5 How can we increase the potential number of organ donors?

9.2.9 Live organ donors

There can be few legal or moral objections if a person wishes to donate regenerative tissue, such as bone marrow or blood. The latter is considered both commonplace and a caring and altruistic act. It is hardly intrusive, does not harm us and (should) cause us no ill health. The donation of bone marrow is a slightly more intrusive procedure, involving the removal of some of the donor's bone marrow either by general or local anesthetic (general anesthetic is more normal). Donating compatible bone marrow can potentially save a patient's life although there is a small risk of complication either from the anesthetic or from the associated procedure.

In situations where a person wishes to donate a non-regenerative organ, such as a kidney, both the law and the ethical position become more complicated. For the donor, it is largely a low-risk procedure and a person can live comfortably with one remaining kidney. For the recipient, a kidney from a live donor is preferable to a kidney from a cadaver as the transplant team can coordinate both the donor and the recipient so that the transplant operation is done at the optimum period for both of them.

In recent years, the numbers of living donor kidney transplants have increased significantly. Statistics from the NHS Blood and Transplant show that there were 1,038 live kidney donations in 2009–2010 which represented approximately one-third of all kidney transplants. While the demand for kidneys continues to outpace the supply, there really is no alternative but to accept donations with enormous gratitude and recognise the significant sacrifice that live organ donors make.

Ethical issues

The donation of a kidney is an altruistic act and is entirely self-sacrificing. The donor puts himself at some degree of risk, albeit minor, to donate an organ to help save another. While the element of risk may be small, the donor still has to undergo a general anesthetic with associated risks. The donor will also appreciate that there may be some effect on his general health. While the donor's intentions are laudable and exceptional, perhaps it would not be too unkind to suggest that it is also a little uncomfortable, both from a legal and an ethical view.

Largely for policy reasons, the criminal law in England and Wales limits the boundaries of the degree of harm that we may consent to. We may not consent to grievous bodily harm being inflicted upon us. Although surgery is an exception to this rule, this is not surgery to benefit our own health but indirectly to harm us in order to help others. Nevertheless, organ transplantation is academically recognised as falling within this exception.

From an ethical point of view, the doctor who undertakes to 'above all do no harm' clearly harms the donor by removing his organ from him. There can be no positive implications on the donor's health, only potentially negative ones. This is not to suggest that the donor's health will be definitely harmed as one can happily live with one kidney. However, if that kidney was to fail, the donor would require dialysis – a costly and time-consuming procedure. He may even require a kidney donor himself! On the other hand, the principle of beneficence imposes a positive obligation to act in the person's best interests. The question that follows is: in whose best interests is the doctor acting? It is in the recipient's best interests to obtain a healthy kidney but it is not in the donor's best interests to lose one. It could also be the case that doctors would experience difficulty in intentionally inflicting harm on a healthy patient and, while this may respect the donor's autonomous and altruistic wishes to assist another, the paternalistic instinct may sit uncomfortably with this.

Example

Dr Rognons has two patients: Patient A, who is desperately ill and awaiting a kidney transplant, and Patient B who is willing to donate his kidney and is compatible. Dr Rognons is concerned about how ethical it may be to remove B's kidney. He knows that it will benefit A and it is likely that it will save his life, but he is aware of his Hippocratic Oath and the principle of non-malfeasance that he should do no harm. By removing B's kidney, he is harming B.

Two essential principles are in conflict – that of non-malfeasance and beneficence which imposes a positive obligation to act in a person's best interests. Patient A has made an autonomous decision to donate his kidney, and to overrule his wish, other than for medical reasons, would be acting paternalistically. In reality, the kidney which A wishes to donate is such a valuable commodity that it is unlikely to be refused. The benefits of the procedure to A outweigh the risks to B; hence it can be ethically justified.

9.2.10 Consent

It is essential that a live organ donor consents to the procedure. As the procedure is not for their benefit and is non-therapeutic, it is imperative that consent is fully informed. There is an inherent difficulty with this as the basis of informed consent is that consent must be free of any coercion, pressure or influence. While a donor may be making an autonomous decision to help another, when the recipient may be a close relative or a loved one the donor's motivations are more clouded. They may feel they wish to help their relative regardless of the risk to themselves, or they may feel pressurised to donate a kidney and could not contemplate letting their family down. The fundamental principle of informed consent therefore becomes less transparent when there are other motivating factors.

Thus far, we have assumed that the donor is a competent adult, but what if the potential donor is incompetent or a child? Can that individual still be a kidney donor?

Children

In the UK, it is unlikely it would be considered in a child donor's best interest to donate a live kidney to another family member. If the child was 'Gillick competent' and could demonstrate the necessary level of maturity, intelligence and understanding then, in theory, he or she could give a valid consent to organ donation. However, it is worth bearing in mind Lord Donaldson's *obiter* views in *Re W (a minor)* [1992] 3 WLR 758 where he indicated that the Family Law (Reform) Act 1969 which provides the minor with the ability to consent to treatment and diagnosis would be unlikely to extend to organ donation. While the morality of this is entirely acceptable, it may be difficult to act contrary to a 16- or 17-year-old child with mature understanding who wishes to donate a kidney to save a family member's life. We have seen, however, that the courts will act paternalistically towards a young adult, intent on protecting them until they are 18, when the courts no longer have jurisdiction.

ACTIVITY

Applying the law

How should the courts respond in this hypothetical example? Boy A is on the kidney transplant waiting list. His condition is deteriorating. Boy B is 16 and a half years of age, and an older brother to Boy A. He is a positive match and is happy to donate his kidney to save his brother's life. The boy's parents would be extremely grateful if Boy B was to help save his brother's life but would be concerned about any impact it would have on Boy B. Boy B admits he feels pressurised to consent as the loss of his brother would devastate both his parents and himself. His parents know that the risk to Boy B would be minimal, but a risk nonetheless. The kidney would save Boy A's life.

How would you decide the case if you were the judge?

Your first natural inclination might be to allow Boy B to consent to donate his kidney. Indeed, medically the benefits to Boy A outweigh the risks to Boy B. However, if Boy B was to donate his kidney then he would be treated as a commodity and a deontologist would consider this unethical. On the other hand, the utilitarian argument seems to gather strength as the greatest happiness would be caused to the greatest number of people. Boy A (we assume) will recover, the family unit would in intact and the status quo would remain. This latter alternative seems very attractive.

The courts would have to consider how the potential organ donation would affect the older brother. While there is no doubt that he would be happy that his brother would live, what adverse psychological effect would it have upon him? This would have to be taken into account – would he grow up to resent his parents for encouraging him to donate his kidney (especially if his own health is compromised), or would he feel as if his bodily integrity has been violated? We know that the approach of the courts is to err on the side of protecting the minor from any harm and will not allow a minor to refuse any life-saving treatment. It is also relevant to bear in mind Lord Donaldson's *obiter* comments in *Re W* (1992). Nevertheless, the court, if satisfied that Boy B consented and the benefits outweighed the risks, may approve the organ donation as in the US case of *Hart v Brown* (1972) 289 A 2d 386 (Conn Sup Ct).

Section 2(3), HT Act 2004 states as follows:

SECTION

'Section 2(3) Where —
(a) the child concerned is alive,
(b) neither a decision of his to consent to the activity, nor a decision of his not to consent to it, is in force, and
(c) either he is not competent to deal with the issue of consent in relation to the activity or, though he is competent to deal with that issue, he fails to do so,'

If a child lacks the capacity to consent and where a person with parental responsibility seeks to consent on his behalf, the approval of the courts will be required. We have already explored the ethical issues in the previous section on page 290, where it was indicated that it was only in the most extraordinary of circumstances that this may be considered.

The Codes of Practice confirm this, stating in para 46 that 'children can be considered as living organ donors only in extremely rare circumstances'. Approval of the HTA Panel would be required in the case of children under the age of 18 in England and Wales, and 16 in Scotland by virtue of the Human Tissue (Scotland) Act 2006. The Codes further state that any decision regarding a child donor will be made by applying common law rules and the Children Act 1989, confirming that the child's best interests are the paramount consideration.

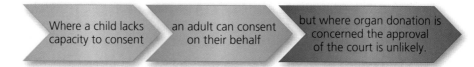

Figure 9.6 Children and consent

The incompetent patient

As the incompetent patient lacks capacity, under the Mental Capacity Act 2005 it would be necessary to seek authorisation from the courts.

Earlier in this book we considered the unusual case of *Re Y (Mental Patient: Bone Marrow Donation)* (1997) where the court authorised a patient who lacked mental capacity to donate bone marrow for the benefit of her sister. It was held to be in the patient's best interests as the wider picture had to be taken, which included her social and emotional interests.

However, would the court have allowed a kidney donation in the same circumstances? The indication from *Re Y* is that they would not allow a non-regenerative organ to be transplanted, although in the well-known US case of *Strunk v Strunk (1969) 445 SW 2d 145,* the court did allow an organ to be transplanted from an incompetent patient into his brother. While this type of issue has not been dealt with by the UK courts, the reasoning in *Strunk* is similar to that in *Re Y*: although it would not be in the donor's best interests to donate a kidney, the risk of any medical complications would be outweighed by the emotional and social interests that would be irreversibly damaged if his brother was to die. Best interests therefore are not necessarily determined on a purely medical criteria but having taken all the circumstances of the case into account. It may be the case that if the courts in the UK were to hear a similar case, they might authorise a non-regenerative organ to be transplanted.

Children as kidney donors

- *Re W* indicated it was unlikely that a child's consent when '*Gillick* competent' would extend to organ donation but the US case of *Hart v Brown* has permitted it. It is possible a court in England and Wales would overrule a child's consent, acting paternalistically until the child became an adult.

The incompetent patient as an organ donor

- Donation of bone marrow was permitted in *Re Y* as the entire circumstances needed to be considered, not just the clinical factors. Organ donation was permitted in the US case of *Strunk v Strunk* S.W.2d 145 1969 but has not been permitted here.

Figure 9.7 Consent from children and the incompetent adult

The competent adult and consent

We have already seen as a basic principle that a competent adult must consent to donation of a live organ.

Subsections 1(1)(c) and (f), HT Act 2004 provide that the storage and use of material from a live body is lawful if it is conducted with the donor's consent. Although we have already seen that s 3(2) refers to 'appropriate consent' and means 'his consent', a more detailed explanation of what amounts to consent is provided in the HTA's Codes of Practice 2 (Donation of Solid Organs for Transplantation) which confirms under para 32 that an offence will be committed if an organ is removed or used from a living person for transplantation unless the requirements of the HT Act 2004 and the Regulations are met.

Consent is to be found in para 71 which confirms that the HT Act 2004 requires consent before an organ can be donated from a living person for the purposes of transplantation.

Paragraph 72 explains that a competent adult's consent must be:

- given voluntarily
- by an appropriately informed person
- who must have appropriate capacity.

Paragraph 78 states that in order to determine whether the person is competent, the provisions of the Mental Capacity Act 2005 must be applied. There is, however, a presumption of capacity but the likely donor must be able to:

- understand the information given to them that is relevant to the decision
- retain that information long enough to be able to make the decision
- use or weigh up the information as part of the decision-making process
- communicate their decision by any means.

The donor cannot be fully informed unless the procedures together with associated risks are fully explained to him, and he is given an opportunity to withdraw his consent at any time.

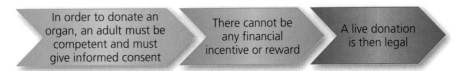

Figure 9.8 Consent from a competent adult

9.2.11 The trade in live organs

The law

In the UK, as in most other countries, it is unlawful to pay a person for a human organ. As we will see shortly, there is undoubtedly a trade in live organs, together with large sums of money to be made. UK legislation is tightly drafted to ensure that, where necessary, the courts can take appropriate actions with criminal sanctions to ensure that any potential market is quickly eliminated.

Section 32, HT Act 2004

This provides that a person commits a criminal offence if he:

SECTION

'a) gives or receives a reward for the supply of, or for an offer to supply, any controlled material;

b) seeks to find a person willing to supply any controlled material for reward;

c) offers to supply any controlled material for reward;

d) initiates or negotiates any arrangements involving the giving of a reward for the supply of, or for an offer to supply, any controlled material;

e) takes part in the management or control of a body of persons corporate or unincorporated whose activities consist of or include the initiation or negotiation of such arrangements.'

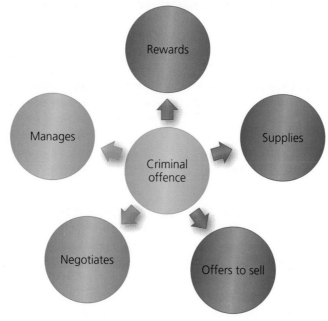

Figure 9.9 Ways in which an offence can be committed under s 32, HT Act 2004

Section 32(2) continues by stating:

SECTION

'(2) Without prejudice to subsection (1)(b) and (c), a person commits an offence if he causes to be published or distributed, or knowingly publishes or distributes, an advertisement —

(a) inviting persons to supply, or offering to supply, any controlled material for reward, or

(b) indicating that the advertiser is willing to initiate or negotiate any such arrangement as is mentioned in subsection (1)(d).'

The prohibition against the trading in organs covers whether the donor is a live donor or is a cadaver (subs 32(8) and (10)), and the maximum penalty on indictment under s 32(1) is three years' imprisonment. The section is drafted in such a way as to punish and ultimately deter both the person who may sell organs and ultimately the recipient.

Lawful trade

Section 32(3) allows an authority such as the National Blood Service to lawfully engage in acts which might otherwise be unlawful.

Nevertheless, as far as the restriction on payment is concerned, subsection 32(6) confirms that payment in money or money's worth should not be treated as a reward where that payment is connected to the 'transporting, removing, preparing, preserving or storing' costs involved in controlled material.

Subsection (7)(c) allows a donor to be compensated but not paid for expenses incurred and losses suffered when he donates.

Section 33, HT Act 2004 states that taking a human organ from a person who is alive is a criminal offence *unless* the conditions in subsections 33(3) and (5) are satisfied. These conditions include that the HTA is satisfied that the regulations and requirements are met and no reward has been given to the parties concerned, although costs can be reimbursed.

KEY FACTS

Key facts on s 32, HT Act 2004

Statutory provision	Definition
S 32(1)(a)	Makes the trade in organs for financial reward a criminal offence.
S 32(1)(b)	Seeks to find a buyer.
S 32(1)(c)	Offers to supply.
S 32(1)(d)	Negotiates an arrangement.
S 32(1)(e)	Takes part in the management of.
S 32(2)	Is involved in the advertisement for sale or purchase.
S 32(8)	Prohibition on sale from a live donor.
S 32(10)	Prohibition on sale from a cadaver.
S 32(3)	Allows lawful trade for an approved body subject to compliance with regulations and conditions.

KEY FACTS

Key facts on the law of organ donation

The law of organ donation	
Demand for organs far outstrips demand	In 2009–10: • 3,706 transplants • 959 deceased organ donors registered • 1,061 living donors registered.
Definition of death	Traditionally cardio-respiratory, now brain-stem death.
Criteria for brain-stem death	A non-drug-induced deeply unconscious or comatose state. Unable to breathe spontaneously and unquestionable brain damage.
The definition is widely but not universally accepted	See countries such as Iran and Japan.
Non-financial incentives to increase organ donation	Idea of reciprocal altruism: higher priority if required on the organ transplantation waiting list.
Consent: children	If '*Gillick* competent' but see *Re W* (1992). Allowed in *Hart v Brown* (1972) (US case). S 2(3), HT Act 2004
Consent: the incompetent patient	Mental Capacity Act 2005 would apply. *Re Y (Mental Patient: Bone Marrow Donation)* (1997) *Strunk v Stunk* (1969) (US case)
Consent: adult	S 3(2), HT Act 2004 Codes of Practice confirm that consent is required before an organ can be donated from a living person for the purposes of transplantation.
It is a criminal offence to take an organ from a person who is alive	S 33 unless subs (3) and (5) are satisfied.
It is a criminal offence to trade in live organs	S 32(1), HT Act 2004
Exceptions to the above	S 32(3), HT Act (2004)

ACTIVITY

Self-test questions

Ensure that you refer to case law and/or statute where appropriate.

• How can we increase the number of available donors?
• For what does the criminal law impose sanctions?
• Can an incompetent patient donate an organ?
• Can a child donate an organ?

9.2.12 The ethics

Thus far, we have seen it is unlawful to conduct or be involved in the purchase or sale of a live organ. We now consider the trade in organs and consider the ethical issue. It is likely that we have a gut reaction that selling organs is instinctively wrong. It is a concept that fills us with revulsion. These instinctive reactions are however inadequate for us to determine whether it is in fact unethical. We now explore the arguments.

The black market in organ trade

Although we began this discussion by explaining that the market in buying and selling organs is unlawful, it is apparent that there is a black market in the supply of organs. Making an activity unlawful does not prevent people engaging in the activity altogether; rather it moves the activity out of the reach of the law. The difficulty is that, if the market is being conducted 'underground' away from the watchful eye of authorities, poor people who donate their organs are less likely to receive appropriate levels of care for fear of being detected.

We must accept that the trade of organs is a flourishing trade. Indeed, numerous incidents have been exposed over recent years. In 2007, *The Observer* newspaper exposed a cash-for-organs trade in India and, in the same year, a man in the UK was convicted under HT Act 2004 for attempting to sell his kidney in order to pay off his gambling debts. In 2008, an Indonesian man in Singapore was convicted for organ trafficking, and several people from different countries were similarly charged in 2010.

We have thus far only considered whether a poor person should or should not donate an organ but, if we conclude that a poor person can donate his organ for money, it is only right and equitable that such a person should be paid a fair sum. The cases above show that, where a donor has been paid sums of $8,000–10,000, the recipient or donee pays a considerably larger sum and the middle man who arranges it takes an extremely healthy profit. If a poor person is to donate an organ, he or she must be afforded the same level of healthcare as the rich recipient, including continuing aftercare.

It is not possible to remove a black market altogether; thus Harris and Erin (2002) argue that an ethically sustainable market in human body parts could be established. They propose creating a market in the buying and selling of organs where the vulnerable are protected against wrongful exploitation and would be ensured protection. In order to avoid unnecessary competitive practices, which would drive prices up, they propose establishing a monopsony (a market where there is only one buyer but a number of sellers of goods or services). They argue that the NHS could represent the appropriate market, setting a fair price to protect the poor, compensating them appropriately, and perhaps being afforded greater priority on the transplant waiting list should they ever require an organ themselves.

In turn, since the price for organs would be fixed, the rich would not be competing for available organs. In other words, the richer man does not necessarily get the available organ. If the authority responsible for this market, even set up with this trade in mind, was a respectable ethical body that genuinely cared for both the donor and the recipient, Harris and Erin argue that such a market could be ethical.

Of course, to some the idea of an ethical market in the trade of organs can never be ethical because it can never be even remotely acceptable for a poor person to sell a body part in order to survive, and it clearly is not an ideal scenario. However, where there is significant and desperate need, either medically or financially, no amount of legislation will ever effectively control a black market trade; hence it may be more beneficial to legislate in favour of organ sales under controlled and ethical conditions.

We have thus far focused on the very poor, and have tried to argue that a trade which may originally cause revulsion may become a little more acceptable when we consider the circumstances of those who feel compelled to sell. But should the donor's circumstances be relevant? The only conviction in the UK under HT Act 2004 was in 2007 when Daniel Tuck, aged 26, was convicted when he agreed to sell his organ for £24,000 in order to pay off his gambling debts. More recently, *The Sunday Times* exposed a lady from Ireland who wished to sell her kidney in order to buy a new home. If we are to argue that it is *prima facie* acceptable to sell one's organ, it should follow that we cannot stand in judgment of what the money earned is used for. Thus, it is arguable that it may cease to be solely a poor man's donor market and could easily equally be a rich man's donor market. Wealth is only relative, and we have already seen by the situations in the UK that neither of those who were exposed was truly destitute; they just wanted better lives. Hence the rich person may choose to sell his organ in order to enhance his own wealthy life even further.

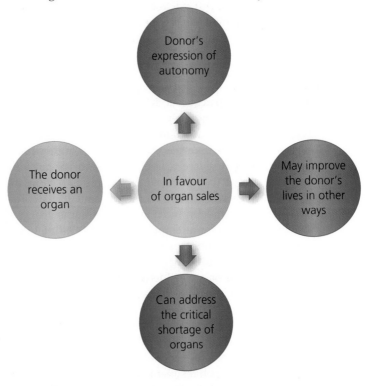

Figure 9.10a Arguments in favour of organ sales

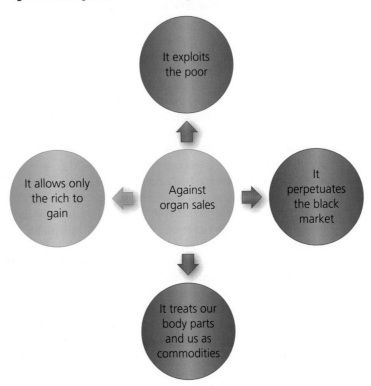

Figure 9.10b Arguments against organ sales

9.2.13 Presumed consent

In the UK, organ donation is managed by an 'opt in' system. This means that if a person does not consent to donate their organs after death (or indeed, has never even considered it), they need not take any steps at all. Conversely, if a person does want to donate their organs to another person after their death then they merely apply for and carry with them an Organ Donor Card or, since 1994, sign up on the computerised Organ Donor Register run by the NHS.

By implication, only those who have truly considered organ donation will make the effort to opt in. There are likely to be many people who are not organ donors, not because they have any particular objection but because they are either apathetic or have simply never considered becoming an organ donor.

Presumed consent or 'opting out' is a way of attempting to increase the number of potential donors. Whereas with opting in a person only consents to donating one's organs if positive steps are taken to become an organ donor, with opting out a person's consent is presumed *unless* they choose to opt out.

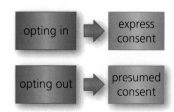

Figure 9.11 The difference between opting in and opting out

The relatives' wishes

It is perhaps worth pointing out at this stage that, on death, if a person has not expressed any wishes during his lifetime, then HT Act 2004 allows a relative to indicate that a person may have wanted to donate organs even if he had not expressly 'opted in'. Conversely, even if the person has indicated their wish to donate their organs, the relatives are asked on death whether they object. If they do not wish the deceased's organs to be taken for transplantation, the relatives can overrule the express wishes of the deceased during his lifetime. In fact, refusal by the deceased's relatives is one of the primary reasons of transplant teams missing out on potentially viable organs from those who had died. Bird and Harris (2010) explore these statistics, explaining that the relative refusal rate has recently increased to 40 per cent. Therefore, despite the donor consenting to donating his organs on his death, 40 per cent of all families when asked after the person dies refused consent for those organs to be harvested.

One advantage of opting out is that relatives would no longer have to be asked whether they are content for their loved ones' organs to be taken, further to their specific request. There is an advantage for both the doctors and the family. The doctors are relieved of the responsibility of asking intensely difficult questions at a very personal time, and the relatives who are just having to come to terms with their loved ones dying do not have to face any further stressful and emotional issues. However, if presumed consent was introduced in the UK it would be likely to incorporate a system whereby families would not be asked if they consented to organs being removed, but will be told that the donor had consented and the transplant will proceed unless there is a particularly significant reason why it should not do so.

Another more ethical advantage of this process is that while the family maintains some level of control over what may happen to the deceased's organs, they are less likely to object, enabling the deceased's autonomous wishes to be respected.

Why choose 'opting out'?

The reasoning behind a scheme of opting out is that there could be a significant increase in the amount of available organs. Surveys indicate that far more people are actually willing to donate organs than are registered, and logic thus dictates that an opt out system would be preferable.

One of the difficulties with this system is that it presupposes that everyone has the appropriate level of education to appreciate the clear implications about organ donation and transplantation. This is a fundamental error. There would have to be a significant and ongoing programme of education with a high level of public awareness in order for the subject matter to be fully understood. There is also an understandable reluctance of people to consider what may happen to them once they have died, as it suggests a certain vulnerability which most people do not care to think about. Even if there is sufficient high-profile education about an opt out system, there may still be the endemic problem of people not opting out either through apathy or because they cannot understand what is likely to be a complicated system. People who would fall into this category – the vulnerable and the poorly educated – would have failed to 'opt out' and their consent would be presumed, which would not reflect their actual consent.

Statistics supplied by the Council of Europe, National Transplant Organisation suggest that countries which exercise presumed consent (an 'opt out' system) also have the highest number of donors; for example, Spain has an opt out system and, in 2003, 33.8 organ donors per million population. These statistics have remained consistently high, even rising to 34.4 per million inhabitants before dropping to 32 per million in 2010. However, the reason why Spain's donor statistics remain so high is largely connected not only to their opt out system but also to their organ transplantation infrastructure. According to the Parliamentary Office for Science and Technology (October 2004, no. 231), Spain's success is largely reflected by the way that organ transplantation is coordinated. Spain has a large number of transplant centres, highly trained physicians in charge of the entire process of organ transplantation, and in general a population which has been educated to a greater understanding and appreciation of the needs of organ transplantation.

However, recent reports in the *BMJ* (vol. 242, page 194) confirm the recent reduction of both organ donors and corresponding transplantations in 2010. Ironically, one of the main reasons for this (itself a cause for celebration) is the recent noticeable decrease of fatalities from road traffic accidents in Spain. Combined with this, there are also fewer brain deaths in intensive care units. Nevertheless, Spain represents a success story of presumed consent. Other countries which have adopted presumed consent, such as Austria, Belgium, Finland and at least five other European countries, have noticeably high organ donor rates.

Ethical critics of presumed consent

While the doctrine of presumed consent appears to fulfil its intention of increasing the number of organ donors, Kluge criticises the concept, suggesting that it renders our bodies public property unless we demand otherwise (2000). She explains that if we applied presumed consent to our everyday lives,

QUOTATION

'it would mean that someone who did not want to be interfered with physically, whether that be sexually or in any other fashion would have to inform potential trespassers to the individual's person of that fact'.

Is it time for presumed consent in the UK?

There are no current proposals to introduce presumed consent in the UK. However, the Welsh Government has expressed their interest in moving towards presumed consent, and will be publishing a white paper setting out their intention to introduce presumed consent by 2015.

While statistics suggest that presumed consent increases the number of potential donors significantly, the Organ Donation Taskforce appears not to be as convinced. Their report, *The potential impact of an opt out system for organ donation in the UK – an independent report from the Organ Donation Taskforce* (2008) stated that they were

QUOTATION

'… not confident that the introduction of opt out legislation would increase organ donor numbers and there is evidence that donor numbers may go down'.

There is indeed, some evidence that an opt out system would actually decrease potential donors. The taskforce provides particular examples:

- Sweden which adopted presumed consent in 1996 has one of the lowest rates of organ donation in Europe.
- Brazil adopted presumed consent in 1997 where opt out was indicated on an individual's driving licence or an identification card. However, in a climate of mistrust of the government and concerns about body-snatching, the scheme was abandoned the following year.
- France too has had negative experiences. In 1992, a young man died in a road traffic accident, at which point his corneas were removed. However, his parents had only consented to limited organ donation and the subsequent negative press publicity damaged the image and trust of presumed consent.

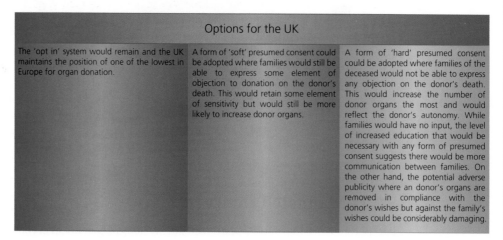

Options for the UK		
The 'opt in' system would remain and the UK maintains the position of one of the lowest in Europe for organ donation.	A form of 'soft' presumed consent could be adopted where families would still be able to express some element of objection to donation on the donor's death. This would retain some element of sensitivity but would still be more likely to increase donor organs.	A form of 'hard' presumed consent could be adopted where families of the deceased would not be able to express any objection on the donor's death. This would increase the number of donor organs the most and would reflect the donor's autonomy. While families would have no input, the level of increased education that would be necessary with any form of presumed consent suggests there would be more communication between families. On the other hand, the potential adverse publicity where an donor's organs are removed in compliance with the donor's wishes but against the family's wishes could be considerably damaging.

Figure 9.12 Options for the UK

The BMA, however, is supportive of introducing a system of presumed consent. In 1999, the BMA set out their reasoning as follows:

QUOTATION

'It is reasonable and appropriate to assume that most people would wish to act in an altruistic manner and to help others by donating their organs after death.

Studies show that the majority of people would be willing to donate but only a small number of these are on the NHS Organ Donor Register or carry a donor card. While this level of apathy exists, people will continue to die while waiting for donor organs.

Given that the majority of people would be willing to donate, there are good reasons for presuming consent and requiring those who object to donation to register their views.

A shift to presumed consent would prompt more discussion within families about organ donation.

It is more efficient and cost-effective to maintain a register of the small number who wish to opt out of donation than of the majority who are willing to be donors.

With such a shift, organ donation becomes the default position. This represents a more positive view of organ donation which is to be encouraged.

Despite the acknowledged difficulties of obtaining meaningful data about the success of presumed consent in other countries, the BMA believes that, as one part of a broader strategy, a shift to presumed consent is likely to have a positive effect on donation rates.'

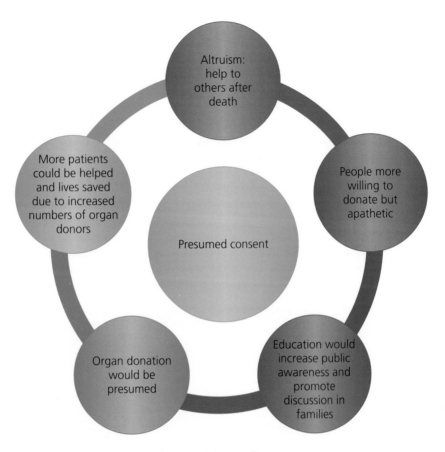

Figure 9.13 Presumed consent

9.2.14 Mandated choice

Part of the criticisms of the 'opt in', 'opt out' systems is that not everyone makes a decision to either donate or not to donate. The opt out system has an entrenched problem in that, even if considerable sums were spent on education, some may find it just too complicated or troublesome to opt out. Mandated choice involves trying to make it possible for everyone to make a decision either to donate their organs after death or not. Everyone would have to make a decision. How practical is this? On the face of it, it may seem an almost impossible task. However, there are certain aspects of our life that we are compelled to do such as paying taxes and, while a system would have to be established in order to maintain a complex database, it is possible to ensure that everyone makes some decision. There would, of course, have to be extensive education in order to ensure that the subject of organ transplantation ceases to be a subject that is not discussed and becomes an issue which has a higher profile.

However, the Organ Donation Taskforce did not find mandated choice an acceptable alternative, stating:

QUOTATION

'In general in the UK, we do not require people to make choices ... A system of mandated choice on organ donation would be a significant departure from established UK norms.'

Furthermore, the taskforce was uncomfortable with considering the possible penalties for non-compliance, and was concerned about a possible backlash with potential donor numbers falling if mandated choice was introduced.

9.2.15 Should we need the consent of a deceased person in order to utilise his organs?

We have seen that the main reason why organs are required is that they are desperately needed either to help others live or, at the very least, to improve their lives. We also know that, until a potential donor expressly consents in the UK, his organs will be wasted. As there is no presumed consent in the UK, we cannot presume that a person will consent unless he has opted out. If presumed consent was introduced in the UK, it would be likely to increase the number of available organs and, if 'soft' presumed consent was introduced, it is also less likely that families would object.

There is one question remaining to be explored – should we need the consent of a person who has died in order to harvest their organs? We know that morality holds that the bodily integrity of the deceased should be revered, and this is evidenced by the way in which we respect the bodies of our loved ones once they have died. Admittedly, there is a certain natural revulsion in contemplating organ retrieval in the deceased, and we have already explored the scandal at Alder Hey hospital when organs of children were removed without parental consent.

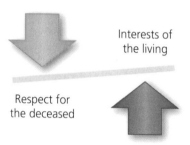

Figure 9.14 A balancing act

The real issue for consideration is, what is more critical: the interests of those who are living, or respect for those who have died?

ACTIVITY

Applying ethics

Stephanie's father has suffered a stroke and is unlikely to live. He has never considered organ donation. Her sister Serena has been waiting for a kidney transplant for two years and spends a considerable amount of her time on dialysis. She is therefore unable to work and needs help looking after her two young children. If we assume that they have a perfect tissue match, consider whether you accept it is ethically permissible to harvest the father's organ once he has died to help Serena. A transplant means she is likely to be able to care for her children and also return to work. She will be able to live a normal life.

It is likely that you would conclude that it is morally acceptable even though you may be concerned that the father may not have consented. If there was presumed consent in the UK, it would be legally acceptable to harvest his organs for her benefit. You are therefore concluding that the interests of the living outweigh the interests of the dead.

Would it matter if he had not spoken to Serena for the past ten years? If he had disowned her? It should not, because we are not taking personal emotions into account, simply exploring where the greatest utility is required.

Sheddon (2009) places the principles of fairness and utility over consent and autonomy, arguing that any system that places the importance of the integrity of the dead over the living has to be inherently unfair. This is fundamentally true, and maybe one could even argue that we shouldn't even need consent from a person once they are dead. However, the impacts of such arguments are quite significant.

Firstly, we may feel uniquely displaced if we do not know what will happen to our bodies when we die, although a pragmatist might readily conclude that it would not matter as the person is dead. Secondly, the feelings of the family need to be taken into account and, if there was objection from the family, it would be very difficult to morally harvest these organs in the face of such opposition. Thirdly, there is a real risk that there could be growing distrust of the medical profession.

If we revert to the activity above, Stephanie's father has had a stroke and is unlikely to live. How would the family feel if the medical professional did not do all in their power to preserve his life, and instead even hastened his death in order that his organs could be harvested? Simply from an ethical perspective, one could have a growing distrust of the medical profession as it could place their own subjective interpretation on the value of a person's life.

9.2.16 Xenotransplantation

We have established that there are insufficient available organs for those who are waiting for an organ transplant. One method of addressing this shortage could be by the use of xenotransplantation. This form of transplantation involves using the cells, tissues or organs from one species and transplanting them into another. The use of pig organs has the potential to resolve the severe shortage.

One of the best known cases of whole organ transplant from animal to human took place in California in 1984 and involved a transplant of a baboon's heart into a 14-day-old baby girl. 'Baby Fae' as she was known was born with a fatal heart deformity, and it was felt that a baby who had an immune system which was not fully developed was less likely to reject foreign tissue. She survived a period of 20 days. More recently, also in the US, Parkinson's and Huntington's patients received pig tissue to aid therapy.

During the 1990s there was a real growth in interest in the possibility of xenotransplantation. Although organ transplantation is still in its very early stages, pig valves have been used in heart valve operations for the past few decades. It appears that pigs are the best source of organs for a variety of reasons with greater potential to be accepted by humans than our closer relatives – the primates. While xenotransplantation of whole organs is still just a scientific possibility, the development of better immune-suppressant drugs and procedures to help avoid rejection has brought the possibility a stage closer.

Hammerman (2011) observed that the need for immune-suppression which has traditionally complicated transplant proceedings could be a step closer to being alleviated. Having explored the use of embryonic pig kidneys and pancreas with some success, it is possible in the future that they could be used effectively and supply an unlimited number of donor organs.

Thus the potential complications of xenotransplantation are both significant and complex. The risk of rejection poses real and immediate difficulties and can be fatal for the recipient. It is possible that diseases which may have originated in animals could be transmitted to the recipient, which may have acute consequences not only for the recipient but the whole of society if the disease was then transmitted from person to person.

Hence, if a disease could be transmitted from animal to human and then transmitted from person to person, is it ethical to proceed with xenotransplantation in light of potentially devastating consequences?

9.2.17 Ethical arguments

Using animals for organs is not natural

Some argue that, while it may be acceptable to eat the meat of animals, using their organs for transplantation is not acceptable because it is not natural. Downie (1997) argues that eating animals is 'natural' in the sense that many other species, including ourselves, eat meat.

He continues by explaining that the transplantation of animal organs into humans is 'unnatural' in itself but it does not follow that it is inherently wrong, suggesting that 'every medical intervention is in that sense unnatural'. It can be wrong if the potential risks outweigh any possible benefits, but it does not automatically follow that it is wrong simply because it is unnatural. While the process of 'a) inserting the genes of one species into those of another and b) transplanting organs so treated into the human species' may seem unnatural, so do many other examples of medical intervention, and it may seem unnatural because they are simply new scientific developments.

Playing God

A common argument against any new technology is that we are playing God, and we were not intended to have the hearts of pigs transplanted into us. While this may so, it is an argument that has little basis. This could be applied to any new medical intervention or vaccination that has been introduced. Without the introduction of mass vaccinations against smallpox, we may have witnessed many more millions dying, but we are still 'playing God' by removing this disease. Some may argue, however, that since man was created in God's image, the work of medicine is in fact directly the work of God. Moreover, and with reference to the argument above that xenotransplantation is unnatural, it is because of man's unnatural interference that some diseases have been eradicated, many are being contained and limited, and lives are consequently being saved as a direct result.

Animal rights

Animals do not have the same rights as humans and, while we must ensure that we care for them and cause them as little suffering as we can, they are not equal. The point made above is relevant to animal rights; if one accepts that we are made in God's image then we must be considered to be superior to animals. Throughout history, man has used the animal for his benefit; before modern transport people used donkeys and camels (and still do). Animals work for us; they feed us and clothe us; and they are subservient to us. It is possible they may allow many more of us to survive. This is not morally wrong. We however must ensure that, if xenotransplantation is ever a reality, animals are cared for humanely. This is no simple task as they would have to be treated as research animals, living in sterile laboratory conditions used solely for the purposes of science.

9.2.18 Legal issues

The issue of informed consent poses a particular dilemma. How can we consent to xenotransplantation when we do not know all the risks that it may entail? If we consent to the risk of infection, the risks to the patient may justify the benefits, but what about the risks to the wider society? Do the patient's family and friends consent to the risk of disease from his colleagues or the stranger whom he sits next to on the train to work? If we do not know what the potential risks are, then how can we provide informed consent? Who should consent to this risk? This suggests an apocalypse scenario although it is not intended to be alarmist. However, the Nuffield Council on Bioethics explained as follows:

QUOTATION

'Most of the concern about the risks of infection from xenotransplantation focuses on viruses. This is because ... viral infections may have a long latent period during which the person has no symptoms of the disease ... If a new disease were to emerge as a result of xenotransplantation, it might be several years before the problem was identified. During this time the infection might be spreading throughout the population.'

Thus, given the risks are unknown, it is extremely difficult to establish how informed consent can be given.

KEY FACTS

Key facts on the ethics of organ donation

The ethics of organ donation	
Is it ethical for a person to sell their organs?	Deontologists would not consider it ethically acceptable because it would be treating a person as a commodity. Utilitarians may consider it acceptable as it creates happiness for the most number of people.
It is not acceptable because:	• it harms the poor • it exploits the poor • only the rich benefit • it encourages and sustains the black market.
It is acceptable because:	• it is the donor's wishes and self-determination, but can they truly consent? • it makes more organs available for transplantation.
Organ donation in the UK operates an opt in system	A person must register to be an organ donor.
An alternative is presumed consent:	It will be presumed that a person consents unless they opt out. Presumed consent will increase the number of organs available.
Families can veto the deceased's wishes to donate organs	A opt out system will make this less likely.
Mandated choice	Will impose upon everyone to decide whether they opt in or opt out.
Xenotransplantation	The use of animal organs in human transplantation. Unproved but would increase number of available organs.

ACTIVITY

Self-test questions

- Is it ethically acceptable for a person to sell their kidney? Consider the arguments for and against.
- In order to increase available donors in the UK, should we introduce presumed consent?
- If you do not believe that the UK should introduce presumed consent, what alternatives could be considered?
- Consider the acceptability of xenotransplantation.

SAMPLE ESSAY QUESTION

Nikita is destitute living in the slums of Mumbai; her husband has recently died and she does not have enough money to feed her children. She also has to care for her elderly ailing parents. She has heard that if she sells her kidney, she will be handsomely rewarded. This will enable her to feed her children, buy the essentials and care for her parents for a considerable period. After careful consideration, she wishes to proceed. She knows that it is unlawful but is aware that the practice carries on regardless. Moreover, she is aware that a rich buyer is waiting.

Is it ethical for Nikita to sell her kidney?

- Is Nikita being exploited? While on the surface it is her autonomous decision, there has to be something fundamentally wrong with our society if it is necessary for a person to sell an organ in order to buy food, the most basic commodity of all.

- Does she need to be protected against the rich buyer? Some may argue that she does. Although she considers this to be the only option available to her to feed her family, how can we be sure that her choice is a truly autonomous one? She sees donating her kidney as a last resort, in which case we may argue that her decision is not free from outside pressures or influences. Since her decision is motivated by her desire to feed and protect her family, her consent may not be real and genuine. Furthermore, if she does not understand the risks that she may be undertaking then she cannot provide informed consent, in which case once again her consent is not real. But, is it reasonable to impose such standards on Nikita? If she does not sell her kidney, she will be poorer and unable to feed her children and care for her parents. By imposing Western standards of informed consent and denying her wishes to her, we are denying her a chance to improve her life.

- How realistic is it that adequate information could be provided to her in order to satisfy informed consent? In reality, it is unlikely that those who live in mass poverty and are illiterate and uneducated could be educated sufficiently to satisfy our Western standards of informed consent. However, it does not necessarily follow that if people are not educated they should be denied their autonomous wishes. For some, it is a far simpler equation and, even if she was educated and understood the consequences of her actions, the reason for donating her organ is more compelling than anything else, and no amount of education would influence her.

- The risk to her is far outweighed by the potential benefit and she is aware that, the more money she has, the better all her family's health with be. For her, it is not a difficult decision. In reality, the poorer she is, the more she needs to sell her kidney and the less she would care about the possible risks.

- If one adopts a utilitarian approach, the sale of organs can probably be supported ethically, because the greatest happiness is caused to the greatest number of people. The recipient is happy because he has a chance to recover and lead a normal life, and the donor is happy because her standard of living is being improved. To a deontologist, however, the sale of organs is unethical because it treats people's organs as valuable assets and therefore people as commodities.

- We may feel morally superior if we act to protect the poor from exploitation but this serves only two purposes: firstly, it satisfies our own sense of morality to allow ourselves to feel vindicated; but secondly, and more importantly, it will only do harm to the poor person who sees organ donation as a last resort. This does not mean that we applaud the circumstances of the poor in participating in a market for much needed organs; rather there is nothing to be achieved in denying a person a better life even if the path to the better life is potentially hazardous. If we deny her autonomy we may feel virtuous, but in reality we have harmed her.

SUMMARY

- The Human Tissue Act 2004 was introduced to remedy defects in the common law and to ensure that there was appropriate consent for those who donated their organs after death.
- The acute shortage of organs in the UK needs to be addressed. Patients die while waiting for organs to become available. Arguably, a reformed system is essential to improve the quality of patients' lives on dialysis and to ensure that more lives can be saved.
- It is possible that schemes to create incentives for people to donate their organs could be introduced, or that consent could be presumed. There is compelling evidence to suggest that presuming patients' consent to organ donation would increase donation rates.
- Ethical issues concerning whether it is ethical to sell a kidney for money are complex. While it denies a person autonomy to decide for themselves, the law seeks to protect the vulnerable by making organ sales unlawful.
- The reality continues that there are insufficient organs to meet the demand of those patients on the organ transplantation list. Methods need to be introduced to increase the supply to help improve lives of patients on dialysis or save the lives of those patients who cannot survive without a transplant.

Further reading

Bird, S. and Harris, J (2010) 'Time to move to presumed consent for organ donation', BMJ, 340, c2188.

Downie, R. (1997) 'Xenotransplantation', *Journal of Medical Ethics* 23, pages 205–6.

Hammerman, M. (2011) 'Xenotransplantation of Embryonic Pig Kidney or Pancreas to Replace the Function of Mature Organs', *Journal of Transplantation*, Article ID 501749.

Harris, J. and Erin, C. (2002) '*An ethically defensible market in organs*', BMJ, 324, page 1541.

Kluge, E. H. (2000) 'Improving organ retrieval rates: various proposals and their ethical validity', *Health Care Anal*, 8, pages 279–95.

Lavee J., Ashenazi T., Gurman G. and, Steinberg D. (2009) 'A new law for allocation of donor organs in Israel', *The Lancet*, published online 17/12/2009 DOI; 10.1016/50140-6736 (09) 61795.

Organ Donation Taskforce (2008) *The potential impact of an opt out system for organ donation in the UK – an independent report from the Organ Donation Taskforce.*

Sheddon, P. (2009) 'Consent and the Acquisition of Organs for Transplantation', HEC Forum, 21 (1), pages 55–69.

Singer, P. (1994) *Rethinking Life and Death.* Oxford: Oxford University Press.

Summers, D. et al (2010) 'Analysis of factors that affect outcome after transplantation of kidneys donated after cardiac death in the UK; a cohort study', *The Lancet*, vol. 376, Issue 9,749, pages 1301–11.

Truog, R. D. (2007) 'Brain Death – Too flawed to endure, Too Ingrained to Abandon', *Journal of Law, Medicine and Ethics*, 35, pages 273–281.

10

End of life issues: assisted suicide

AIMS AND OBJECTIVES

After reading this chapter you should be able to:

▓ Understand the differences in the definitions of euthanasia and assisted suicide
▓ Understand the statutory provisions on physician-assisted suicide and euthanasia in other jurisdictions
▓ Appreciate statutory provisions on assisted suicide
▓ Demonstrate a thorough understanding of the current common law
▓ Demonstrate a level of critical analysis of seminal judgments
▓ Appreciate the ethical debate surrounding both assisted suicide and euthanasia
▓ Demonstrate an ability to develop an informed ethical discussion.

10.1 Introduction

Arguably, the issue of assisted suicide and euthanasia is one of the most topical but controversial subjects in current medical ethics. Destined to maintain its high media profile for many years, the debates continue to rage as to whether a person who suffers unbearably from a terminal illness should have the right to an autonomous decision in how and when to end their life. Should this right outweigh the protection of society as a whole? The legal aspects concern the crucial development of a small amount of case law in an ever-changing climate of public opinion and policy. If the law allows euthanasia and/or assisted suicide, can the law adequately protect those patients who may be abused or vulnerable, and may opt for euthanasia or assisted suicide when it is not their own clear and informed choice? In this chapter we begin by considering the definitions of euthanasia and assisted suicide, and then review the legal position in England, Wales and Scotland before we look at other jurisdictions where assisted suicide and/or euthanasia are legal. Thereafter, we will consider the ethical arguments for and against assisted suicide.

10.1.2 The distinction between euthanasia and assisted suicide

In order to achieve a clear understanding of this topic it is necessary to attempt to draw a clear distinction between euthanasia and assisted suicide, as these terms can often lead to some confusion.

▓ **Euthanasia** is described as the administering of medication to a patient at the patient's express request, which has the direct aim or intention of hastening the patient's death. It is perhaps necessary to distinguish this from the principle of double effect, where the direct aim is pain relief but death is not an unwelcome by-product.

■ **Assisted suicide,** as the words suggest, is where assistance is given to the person so that the person can end his or her own life. The motive is the same for both: in order to relieve him or her of their suffering.

10.2 What is euthanasia?

The word 'euthanasia' derives from the Greek, meaning 'good death', and refers to the practice whereby a person seeks to end their life prematurely in order to alleviate their pain and suffering. Euthanasia can be categorised into three types:

■ **Voluntary** euthanasia – where the patient requests the act which causes their death.
■ **Non-voluntary** euthanasia – where the act which causes the patient's death is conducted *without* the patient's consent.
■ **Involuntary** euthanasia – where the act which causes the death is against the wishes of the patient. Given that the act of ending the person's life is without their consent, it could be more appropriate to describe this act as murder (fulfilling as it does the *mens rea* and *actus reus* of the common law definition of murder).

A distinction also needs to be drawn between active and passive euthanasia:

■ **Active euthanasia** occurs when either a medical professional or another person performs an act intended to bring about the person's death.
■ **Passive euthanasia** occurs when a medical professional or other person omits to perform an act which is keeping the person alive.

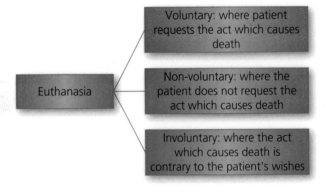

Figure 10.1 Forms of euthanasia

10.2.1 An act, or an omission to act?

Whether the distinction between an act or an omission to act is a valid legal or ethical one is hotly debated. The distinction was illustrated by Lord Goff, in *Airedale NHS Trust v Bland* [1993] AC 789, who stated:

JUDGMENT

'the law draws a crucial distinction between cases in which a doctor decides not to provide, or to continue to provide, for his patient treatment or care which could or might prolong his life, and those in which he decides, for example by administering a lethal drug, actively to bring his patient's life to an end'.

He added that, while the former situation could be lawful, the latter situation where a doctor gives a patient a drug in order to hasten his death was clearly unlawful.

10.2.2 The doctrine of double effect

In the case of *R v Cox* (1992) 12 BMLR 38 below the court explained that, where a drug has no **therapeutic** value and where it leads to a patient's death, the prescribing of the

mens rea
refers to the mental element of a criminal offence

actus reus
refers to the physical act in a criminal offence

therapeutic
where a drug has some beneficial healing power

drug is clearly unlawful. However, what is the situation where the doctor prescribes pain-relieving drugs, which at the same time results in a quicker death for the patient? This scenario is referred to as the 'doctrine of double effect'. In this situation, it appears there is no illegality. The case of *Cox*, as we shall see, does not demonstrate double effect because the potassium chloride that Cox prescribed to his patients did not have any therapeutic qualities and only hastened death.

In *Airedale NHS Trust v Bland* (1993) the court was clear in its view that the duty of care which a patient is owed is limited by whether the treatment given is in the patient's best interests. Lord Goff stated:

JUDGMENT

'... a doctor may, when caring for a patient who is, for example, dying of cancer, lawfully administer pain-killing drugs despite the fact that he knows that an incidental effect of that application will be to shorten the patient's life.'

Although the doctrine of double effect is accepted in practice, it does not sit comfortably with the criminal law. The *mens rea* or guilty element of murder is intention – the actor must have intended death (or GBH). Intention can be defined as direct intention where the result is the direct aim or purpose of the act; for example, A gives B poison in order to kill him. Oblique or indirect intention is where the consequences of the act may not be desired but may be virtually certain; for example, Dr A gives patient B a pain-relieving drug with the intention of alleviating the pain but it is virtually certain that the drug will hasten the patient's death. In these latter circumstances, the leading authority of *R v Woollin* [1999] AC 82 HL states that the jury may infer intention: the *mens rea* of murder. Thus, the difficulty is apparent and there is a fine line to distinguish between what is lawful and what is unlawful. Authorities however are unequivocal that, where a doctor prescribes a drug for a specific purpose relevant to the patient's condition, if a consequence of that drug results in hastening the patient's death, the act will not be unlawful. We consider this point in the case examples below.

CASE EXAMPLE

R v Cox (1992) 12 BMLR 38

A patient was suffering from rheumatoid arthritis. Dr Cox gave the patient a lethal amount of potassium chloride which killed the patient.

Dr Cox was convicted of attempted murder. The potassium had no therapeutic value so he could not argue that he was trying to relieve the patient's pain and suffering. Moreover, while the patient's condition was painful, it was not terminal and the drug's sole effect was to hasten the patient's death.

Ognall J confirmed that hastening death with a drug which has no therapeutic value can never be legal. He said:

JUDGMENT

'... please understand this, ladies and gentlemen, what can never be lawful is the use of drugs with the primary purpose of hastening the moment of death.'

Interestingly, Dr Cox's sentence of imprisonment was suspended (which was later reduced even further to probation), reflecting the court's recognition that his actions were borne of compassion rather than malice. However, many would argue that his actions, in determining for himself that this patient's life was not worth living, were tantamount to murder.

The GMC hearing of Dr Munro

In another more recent hearing before the General Medical Council's Fitness to Practice in 2007, consultant neonatologist Dr Munro gave lethal doses of a muscle relaxant to babies on two different occasions. The babies were close to death and on both occasions treatment had been withdrawn with their parents' consent. His actions were described as 'tantamount to euthanasia' by a GMC lawyer as he had, on each occasion, administered a drug in order to hasten each baby's death. However, the GMC concluded that, although his acts had led to a quicker death in each case, his motivation was simply to relieve the physical pain and suffering of the baby and the parents' mental suffering in watching their child die a slower and more agonising death.

In this case, the Scottish criminal justice system failed to prosecute even though on a strict interpretation he satisfied the mental element required for murder in that his acts intended to kill (or cause grievous bodily harm) (*R v Vickers* [1957] 2 QB 664). The GMC exonerated Dr Munro, stating that his fitness to practice was unaffected. Goodman observes (2010) that 'where a doctor acts compassionately in the best interests of the baby and the family, he could avoid legal and professional sanctions', and it would appear from a legal perspective that this indeed is the case.

Dr Munro's acts were undoubtedly motivated from a deep-rooted sense of compassion; indeed the deceaseds' family was grateful to him for his intervention. However, Lord Goff's dictum in *Bland* (1993) loudly resonates, and it would appear that the law lacks clarity in its distinction between active and passive euthanasia. Dr Munro administered treatment to his patients knowing it would lead to their deaths and, regardless of his motives, his acts still amounted to active euthanasia.

10.2.3 Mercy killing?

There is no criminal offence of 'mercy killing' *per se*, and the colloquial term refers to a person who kills another motivated by compassion. Nevertheless, the person who commits an act of mercy killing is likely to be charged with murder, as in criminal law the motive of the act is largely irrelevant, demonstrated in criminal cases such as *R v Steane* [1947] KB 997. If the actor's intention is to bring about death, either directly or indirectly, he or she will be charged with murder.

CASE EXAMPLE

R v Inglis (Francis) [2010] EWCA 2637

Thomas Inglis was a healthy man of 27 years of age when, in July 2007, he was being taken to hospital in an ambulance. On the way, the doors to the ambulance opened on three occasions and on the last occasion he fell out, suffering severe and irreversible brain damage. Two months later, his mother Francis Inglis attempted to kill him. He was resuscitated and remained in hospital although his condition deteriorated. A year later, despite an order restraining his mother from visiting him, she managed to gain access to the hospital and killed him by injecting him with heroin. She was convicted of murder and was sentenced to the mandatory life sentence with a minimum term of nine years' imprisonment. She appealed not against conviction but against sentence.

The Court of Appeal reduced her minimum sentence to five years. The fact that this was a mercy killing is not in doubt, and she had killed her son after a considerable amount of meticulous planning. The fact that the law pays no regard to the motive of the murderous act is shown in the words of Judge LJ in the Court of Appeal who stated,

JUDGMENT

'the law does not distinguish between murder committed for malevolent reasons and murder motivated by familiar love.'

The court rejected her plea that her son was 'already dead in all but a small physical degree' as although disabled he was very much alive. He was, however, vulnerable and the law exists to protect the vulnerable in society. No one, not even his mother, could bring his life to a premature end. It was no excuse that she ended his life through compassion, adding that 'if the defendant intentionally kills the victim in the genuine belief that it is in the victim's best interest to die, the defendant is guilty of murder'. Thus, mercy killing is murder, whether or not it is committed through compassion.

10.3 Assisted suicide: the law as it is today

Section 1, Suicide Act 1961 finally decriminalised the offence of suicide, although to date assisted suicide remains a criminal offence and therefore unlawful. Section 2(1) Suicide Act 1961 states as follows:

SECTION

'A person who aids, abets, counsels or procures the suicide of another, or an attempt by another to commit suicide, shall be liable on conviction on indictment to imprisonment for a term not exceeding fourteen years.'

The wording of the Act demonstrates that an intention is required. The terms 'aiding, abetting, counsel and procuring' may seem a little abstract and are best defined as shown in Figure 10.2. Since many of the terms are interchangeable, it is probably advisable not to compartmentalise the terms too much.

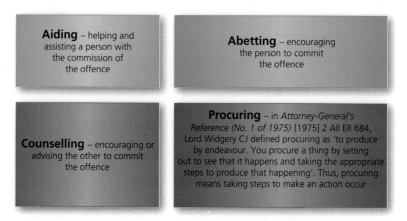

Figure 10.2 Legal definitions

By virtue of s 2(4), the consent of the Director of Public Prosecution is required before a prosecution can commence:

SECTION

'no proceedings shall be instituted for an offence under this section except by or with the consent of the Director of Public Prosecutions'.

Thus, the offence of assisted suicide distinguishes itself from many other criminal offences which begin in the more familiar mode, by way of arrest by the police and prosecution by the Crown Prosecution Service. The role of the Director of Public Prosecution has, since the case of *R (Purdy) v DPP* [2009] UKHL 45, been at the forefront of recent developments in the law relating to assisted suicide, which will be considered in greater detail shortly.

10.3.1 The Coroners and Justice Act 2009

Effective from 1 February 2010, the Coroners and Justice Act 2009 amended the Suicide Act 1961. The amendment, brought about by a concern regarding the use of websites which promoted or described ways in which to commit suicide or help others to do so, simply consolidated the law.

Prior to the Coroners and Justice 2009, the law prohibiting suicide was not only contained in the Suicide Act 1961 but also under the Criminal Attempts Act 1981, which stated under s 1(1) that it was an offence to aid, abet, counsel or procure either a suicide or an attempted suicide. In order for this offence to be satisfied, the defendant must take steps which are considered to be 'more than merely preparatory'. No physical attempt of the actual offence was in fact required.

The new offence under s 2A, Suicide Act 1961 created by s 59, Coroners and Justice Act 2009 simply consolidates the two offences.

Section 2A states as follows:

SECTION

S 2A '(1) A person ("D") commits an offence if —
   (a) D does an act capable of encouraging or assisting the suicide or attempted suicide of another person, and
   (b) D's act was intended to encourage or assist suicide or an attempt at suicide.
(1A) The person referred to in subs (1)(a) need not be a specific person (or class of persons) known to, or identified by, D.
(1B) D may commit an offence under this section whether or not a suicide, or an attempt at suicide, occurs.'

The seriousness of the offence is demonstrated by the fact that a case can only be tried in the Crown Court whereupon conviction the maximum sentence is 14 years' imprisonment.

10.3.2 What amounts to assisting a suicide?

CASE EXAMPLE

AG v Able [1984] QB 795

The Attorney-General sought a declaration to determine whether the elements of s 2 were satisfied by the publication of a book which appeared to describe various ways of committing suicide.

Woolf J at first instance stated that simply supplying the book would not satisfy the statutory provisions, and the defendant was acquitted. Thus, it would appear there has to be a nexus between the supply of the book and the acts of the victim in cases where the supply has either intended to encourage or intended to assist the victim.

10.3.3 Refusal of medical treatment

While assisted suicide remains illegal in the UK as in many countries worldwide, it is sometimes difficult to distinguish between the right of a competent patient to refuse medical treatment in circumstances where it is clear that the refusal will lead directly to their death, and the lack of a right to determine in other situations the manner in which we choose to end our own lives. Consider the following case example.

CASE EXAMPLE

Re B (Adult Refusal of Medical Treatment) [2002] All ER 449

In Chapter 2, we examined the facts of this case where a 41-year-old woman, who suffered from paralysis and was dependent on a ventilator, made her wishes clear that she wished to have the ventilator switched off. She understood that she would die as a direct result.

The court accepted that she was competent to make a decision and could refuse continuing treatment that would lead directly to her death. Butler Sloss P said:

JUDGMENT

'if ... the patient, having been given the relevant information and offered the available options chooses to refuse, that decision has to be respected by the doctors'.

The significance of this case is that a competent patient has a right to refuse medical treatment even if it will lead to the patient's death. The decision is a clear reflection of a patient's autonomy and has been embedded in English law since the decision of *Re T (Adult: Refusal of Medical Treatment)* [1992] 4 All ER 649 where the court allowed the patient to refuse medical treatment even if death was a clear possibility. Here, Ms B was afforded the comparative luxury of deciding the point at which she wanted to end her life, but only after extensive court proceedings at a point when she knew she did not want to continue living. She was well-versed in her condition and knew what to expect; she also knew what she did not want to endure. To say that her autonomy was respected is true, but only once she had overcome the hurdles of paternalism both from the doctors and from the courts.

Is the law inconsistent? On the one hand a competent patient can refuse life-saving or life-sustaining treatment; on the other hand, a competent patient such as Ms Pretty (discussed below) cannot insist on treatment to end her life even if the degree of pain or severity of their condition is similar. Ms B's life ended peacefully when her life-support machine was switched off.

Critics may determine that the doctor's final act could be interpreted as physician assisted suicide (PAS) or euthanasia, as the doctor's intentional act brought about the patient's death. The case however turns on subtleties and the courts instead referred to the withdrawal and withholding of medical treatment and, applying the dictum of Lord Goff in *Bland* (1993), considered the switching off of the ventilator as the act of withdrawing previous treatment. On the contrary, Ms Pretty was not receiving continuing treatment and could not exercise the same right to refuse medical treatment. Her case is discussed below.

10.3.4 Is there a 'right' to die?

It may seem axiomatic that a person should be endowed with the fundamental right to determine the nature and time of their death, but they are not. A person can of course take their own life, but they cannot, if they are unable to do so, lawfully end their life with the help of another.

Put more simply, the right to life does not convey a similar right to die. Article 2, ECHR states that 'Everyone's right to life shall be protected by law'. Whether a right to life also implies a right to die was explored in *R (Pretty) v DPP* [2002] 1 AC 800 – a case we consider in more detail below. However, with regards to this specific point, Lord Bingham in the House of Lords stated that:

JUDGMENT

'The right to die is not the antithesis of the right to life but the corollary of it and the state has a positive obligation to protect both.'

The significance of Art 2, ECHR is that it acts as a protection mechanism between the individual and a third party or the State. The preservation of life does not equate to the right to die in the manner of one's choosing. The House of Lords considered that this would simply stretch the interpretation of the meaning too far.

The European Court of Human Rights (2002) 35 EHRR 1 took a similar approach, stating that Article 2 could not:

JUDGMENT

'be interpreted as conferring the diametrically opposite right, namely a right to die; nor can it create a right to self-determination in the sense of conferring on an individual the entitlement to choose death rather than life'.

It is therefore fair to say that there is no relationship between the right to life and the right to die. The right to life is an 'absolute right' contained within ECHR and now entrenched in HRA 1998. The 'right to die' is an emotive (although justifiably so) and self-autonomous desire to end one's life at a time of one's choosing.

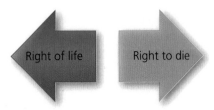

Figure 10.3 Balancing rights

In recent years, the subject of assisted suicide has dominated the media and probably remains one of the most controversial legal dilemmas and ethical issues. It is probably fair to say that the case of *Pretty* (2001) was the match to the tinderbox.

CASE EXAMPLE

R (on the application of Pretty) v DPP [2001] UKHL 61

Mrs Pretty was suffering from **motor neurone disease**, a degenerative fatal and incurable disease. She was unable to end her life without assistance. She unsuccessfully sought an assurance from the DPP that her husband would not be prosecuted if he assisted her to die. She then brought an action in judicial review claiming that the Suicide Act 1961 and the DPP's refusal to provide the assurance was incompatible with the provisions of HRA 1998.

Having already explored her argument in support of Art 2, we now focus on her reliance on Art 3 (prohibiting inhumane and degrading treatment), Art 8 (the right to respect for a private and family life), Art 9 (the right to freedom of thought, conscience and religion) and Art 14 (prohibits discrimination in respect of the convention rights).

Article 3: Diane Pretty argued that the State was imposing inhumane and degrading treatment upon her as they refused to provide her with the assurance that her husband would not be prosecuted if he were to help her die. As they failed to provide that assurance, she could not allow him to help her for fear of the repercussion of prosecution. As she could not die without assistance, her life was prolonged in a condition which she argued breached Art 3.

Article 8: she argued that refusing to allow her to die in the manner and time of her choosing breached her right to a private and family life and failed to take account of her wishes as a competent patient, making a fully informed and voluntary decision.

Having exhausted the domestic courts, she took her case to the European Court of Human Rights, who also rejected her case.

In rejecting the breach of Art 3 argument, Lord Hope said that her condition did not amount to torture, inhumane or degrading treatment and that, in any event, her condition was a direct result of the illness itself and was not a result of any infliction by the State.

motor neurone disease

is a progressive neuro-degenerative disease

The European Court of Human Rights considered the Art 8 argument carefully and did not dismiss out of hand the possibility of it being engaged. In retrospect and bearing in mind the later case of *Purdy* (2009), reliance on Art 8 was the most valuable argument. The court recognised that, as more people live longer, they should not be forced to live with mental or physical conditions that are contrary to their own wishes. However, the right to autonomy and self-determination had to be balanced against the rights of vulnerable people who could be influenced to end their life for fear of being a burden on others. The European Court of Human Rights was prepared to accept that Art 8 could be engaged but the interference of the State under Art 8(2) was justified in order to protect the vulnerable.

Article 9 was also dismissed, as was Art 14 as the latter is unable to stand alone without attaching to a convention right.

In dismissing this case, both the House of Lords and the European Court of Human Rights demonstrated their unwillingness to act in an area where only Parliament could. Mrs Pretty died shortly afterwards.

The relevance of Art 8 became apparent shortly afterwards in the case of *Purdy* (2009). Here, the courts accepted that Art 8 could, in theory, be engaged.

CASE EXAMPLE

R (Purdy) v DPP [2009] UKHL 45

Debbie Purdy, who was 45 years of age, suffers from **primary progressive multiple sclerosis**. She wanted guidance on whether, if her condition reached such a point that she considered life to be so unbearable that she wanted to end her life, her husband would be prosecuted if he helped her travel to Switzerland (where assisted suicide is lawful) to end her life. She argued that the DPP had failed to provide sufficiently clear and transparent guidance as to when a prosecution may be brought and that the failure had interfered with her rights under Art 8.

She applied by way of **judicial review** to challenge the DPP's failure to establish a specific policy which would set out the circumstances in which a person would be prosecuted for aiding, abetting, counselling or procuring a suicide contrary to s 2(1), Suicide Act 1961.

The guidance was of paramount importance as she did not want anyone 'dear to me to be made a criminal for what I see as an act of love and humanity'. If there was a risk that he would be prosecuted then she would choose to travel to Switzerland at an earlier stage, while she still could travel alone and protect him from the risk of prosecution. Lord Hope in the House of Lords described what she sought simply and accurately as 'information that she says she needs so that she can take a decision that affects her private life'.

The reality is that in recent years over 100 people have travelled from the UK to Switzerland in order to end their lives. The vast majority have had close family travelling with them. Unless they travelled alone, any help or assistance that a loved one gave them, in the organisation of the journey, during the journey or at any time before the moment of death, could be considered to be aiding and abetting and would breach the provisions of the Suicide Act 1961. While some people have been investigated by the police on their return, there have been no prosecutions to date. However, this was not a risk that Ms Purdy was ready to take. The DPP are not obliged to prosecute but have discretion to prosecute based upon an almost invisible criteria. What Ms Purdy sought was clarity and transparency in order that she could make decisions as to when she could, when the time arose, end her life. The lack of openness meant that she might be forced to travel to Switzerland and end her life at an earlier stage than she otherwise would, to alleviate the risk of her husband being prosecuted.

At first instance, the court followed *Pretty* (2001) and maintained that her rights under ECHR were not breached. Although the European Court of Human Rights had opened a window ajar for Art 8 to be accepted, this was rejected at first instance. The court held not only was Art 8 not engaged but, even if it had been, Art 8(2) would apply as the interference in this right would be proportionate and justifiable to protect the rights and freedom of others.

She was unsuccessful in the Court of Appeal but the House of Lords held in her favour. Lord Hope distinguished *Pretty* (2001) narrowly on the facts and departed from the decision stating that the right to respect for a private life in Art 8(1) was engaged. Having reached this milestone, it was still possible to derogate from that right. Article 8(2) states:

primary progressive multiple sclerosis
is a form of multiple sclerosis. A progressive auto-immune disease

judicial review
is a way of challenging the decision of public bodies in the courts

ARTICLE

'there shall be no interference … with the exercise of this right except such as in accordance with the law'.

Lord Hope stated that the 'Convention principle of legality requires the court to address itself to three distinct questions'. For our purposes the second question is of most relevance:

JUDGMENT

'whether the law or rule in question is sufficiently accessible to the individual who is affected by the restriction and sufficiently precise to enable him to understand its scope and foresee the consequences of his actions so that he can regulate his conduct without breaking the law'.

Here we have the crux of the issue; the DPP did not have a policy which was either accessible or transparent. Hence, Ms Purdy could neither understand nor foresee the consequences of her actions.

The House of Lords directed the Director of Public Prosecutions (DPP) to formulate a policy which would be accessible to the public and which would assist them in appreciating the factors that would be taken into account when deciding whether to prosecute.

The Law Lords opined that Art 8 gave a person the right to die in the manner they chose and said as follows:

JUDGMENT

'Everyone has the right to respect for their private life and the way that Ms Purdy determines to spend the closing moments of her life is part of the act of living … Ms Purdy wishes to avoid an undignified and distressing end to her life. She is entitled to ask that this too must be respected.'

The judgment makes fascinating reading but it must be put into context. Although the House of Lords stated that Art 8 was engaged, the House of Lords *did not* state that it was not an offence to assist a person to commit suicide. This is only a question for Parliament to determine. Hence, the House of Lords did not legalise assisted suicide but directed the DPP to issue appropriate guidelines to allow a person to determine the circumstances in which the DPP would be likely to prosecute in cases of assisted suicide.

KEY FACTS

Key facts on comparison between the cases of *Pretty* and *Purdy*

R (on the application of Pretty) v DPP (2001)	R (Purdy) v DPP (2009)
Suffered from motor neurone disease.	Suffers from primary progressive multiple sclerosis.
Held that Art 2 (a right to life) did not convey a right to die.	Relied on Article 8. She argued the wording of 'in accordance with the law' in Art 8(2) was relevant as the DPP guidelines were neither accessible nor transparent. Hence, she could not ascertain what was in accordance with the law.

Art 3 – her condition did not amount to torture or degrading treatment and was not inflicted by the State.	The House of Lords directed the DPP to deliver a policy which was clear and transparent and from which the reader would be able to determine when the DPP would or would not prosecute a person who may assist a suicide.
Art 8 – the derogation under Art 8(2) was relied upon as it was justified to protect the vulnerable members in society.	The House of Lords did not indicate Art 8 was engaged or legalise assisted suicide. This is a matter for Parliament.

Daniel James

In 2008, the media's attention was drawn to the plight of Daniel James, a 23-year-old man paralysed in a rugby accident in March 2007. Subsequently, he was diagnosed as **tetraplagic** and completely reliant upon his parents for even the most basic care. Not able to come to terms with the disability, he attempted suicide on three occasions and was determined to end his life, wishing to travel to Switzerland to gain the assistance he needed.

He was a fiercely independent young man, and a consultant psychiatrist had attested to his clarity of thought and his awareness and understanding of his condition. He was not influenced by his parents who had begged him not to end his life, and even booked a return flight for him in case he changed his mind. He travelled to Switzerland with his parents and, with the assistance of Dignitas, ended his life in 2008. On return, his parents were questioned by the police as they had aided, abetted, counselled or procured their son's suicide and could be charged under s 2(1), Suicide Act 1961.

In not pursuing a prosecution and in making a decision to publish reasons for this decision, Keir Starmer QC, the Director of Public Prosecutions, carefully and fully outlined which of the factors set out in the Code for Prosecutors would apply and which would not, concluding:

QUOTATION

'While there are public interest factors in favour of prosecution, not least of which is the seriousness of this offence, I have determined that these are outweighed by the public interest factors that say that a prosecution is not needed.'

This was not an act which Daniel's parents could possibly repeat and, even if the couple had been convicted, a term of imprisonment would have been extremely unlikely. The likelihood is that they would have received an absolute discharge or a fine.

In the case of *Purdy* (2009) considered above, Lord Judge LJ took the opportunity to comment on the case of Daniel James. He highlighted how the DPP had come to the conclusion it had together with the general guidance it appeared to be offering to Debbie Purdy. Of course, this did not amount to 'law' and could not be relied upon in another case, but he did however conclude his observations on the case of Daniel James by stating that 'there can be no doubt about the correctness of the decision'.

10.3.5 The DPP's response: policy for prosecutors in respect of cases of encouraging or assisting suicide

Following the case of *Purdy* (2009), the House of Lords ordered the DPP to establish a policy in order to assist the public in determining whether prosecution was a possibility in cases of assisted suicide. After a period of consultation and after issuing an interim policy, Keir Starmer QC, Director of Public Prosecutions, issued guidelines in February 2010. The focus, he explained, was on the motivation of the person suspected of aiding, abetting, counselling or procuring assisted suicide rather than the 'characteristics of the victim'.

The policy neither legalises assisted suicide nor seeks to encourage assisted suicide. Its purpose is to provide 'a clear framework' to help prosecutors decide whether to prosecute. Its publication also satisfies Ms Purdy's question: under what circumstances could her husband be prosecuted?

The DPP emphasises that each case has to be considered on its merits, and the publication of the guidelines does not reflect a relaxation in their policy of prosecution, simply a change of focus.

There are sixteen public interest factors **in favour of prosecution**. They are as follows:

- The victim was under 18 years of age.
- The victim did not have the capacity (as defined by the Mental Capacity Act 2005) to reach an informed decision to commit suicide.
- The victim had not reached a voluntary, clear, settled and informed decision to commit suicide.
- The victim had not clearly and unequivocally communicated his or her decision to commit suicide to the suspect.
- The victim did not seek the encouragement or assistance of the suspect personally or on his or her own initiative.
- The suspect was not wholly motivated by compassion; for example, the suspect was motivated by the prospect that he or she or a person closely connected to him or her stood to gain in some way from the death of the victim.
- The suspect pressured the victim to commit suicide.
- The suspect did not take reasonable steps to ensure that any other person had not pressured the victim to commit suicide.
- The suspect had a history of violence or abuse against the victim.
- The victim was physically able to undertake the act that constituted the assistance himself or herself.
- The suspect was unknown to the victim and encouraged or assisted the victim to commit or attempt to commit suicide by providing specific information via, for example, a website or publication.
- The suspect gave encouragement or assistance to more than one victim who were not known to each other.
- The suspect was paid by the victim or those close to the victim for his or her encouragement or assistance.
- The suspect was acting in his or her capacity as a medical doctor, nurse, other healthcare professional, a professional carer (whether for payment or not), or as a person in authority, such as a prison officer, and the victim was in his or her care.
- The suspect was aware that the victim intended to commit suicide in a public place where it was reasonable to think that members of the public may be present.
- The suspect was acting in his or her capacity as a person involved in the management of or as an employee (whether for payment or not) of an organisation or group, a purpose of which is to provide a physical environment (whether for payment or not) in which to allow another to commit suicide.

There are six public interest factors **against prosecution**. They are:

- The victim had reached a voluntary, clear, settled and informed decision to commit suicide.
- The suspect was wholly motivated by compassion.
- The actions of the suspect, although sufficient to come within the definition of the crime, were of only minor encouragement or assistance.
- The suspect had sought to dissuade the victim from taking the course of action which resulted in his or her suicide.
- The actions of the suspect may be characterised as reluctant encouragement or assistance in the face of a determined wish on the part of the victim to commit suicide.
- The suspect reported the victim's suicide to the police and fully assisted them in their enquiries into the circumstances of the suicide or the attempt and his or her part in providing encouragement or assistance.

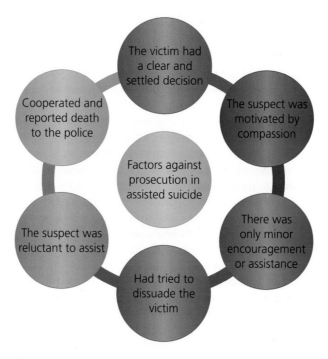

Figure 10.4 Factors against prosecution in assisted suicide

Comments on the DPP guidelines

The guidelines are a welcome step forward but the legal and ethical position of assisted dying is still fraught with uncertainty and continues to be a hugely significant public policy issue. These guidelines should rightly be seen as a triumph but they do not represent a change in the law permitting either PAS or assisted suicide.

The guidelines provide a tick-box exercise in order to assess whether the person who assists another to end their life is likely to be prosecuted. Of course, this is the intention; it is neither about the patient nor about the morality of requiring a terminally ill person to travel abroad to end their life. It is primarily about the compassion and the motive of the person who assists another to end their life. Mullock (2010) observes that this motive-based approach is surprising as the concept of compassion does not tend to be relevant at all in legal principles. Moreover, in criminal law, motive is said to be *expressly* irrelevant as the case of *R v Steane* (1947) has demonstrated. Mullock states:

QUOTATION

'By adopting a motive-centred approach, in which compassion is identified as the key determining factor, thereby confirming that it is not appropriate to seek to punish the majority of those who assist in suicide in this context, the Policy treads a sensitive path.'

The guidelines attempt to embrace the patient's autonomy, but they remain restrictive and unhelpful in other ways. For example, there is little reference to the patient's medical condition, and the issue where a patient needs physical help in taking the medication to end his or her life remains unresolved. Furthermore, the DPP have stated that the list of factors is not necessarily exhaustive, leaving elements of doubt in the mind of those patients and loved ones who wish to travel abroad to end their lives. However, the guidelines achieve their purpose. They provide a (hopefully) clear picture of whether a loved one is likely to be prosecuted if they 'aid, abet, counsel or procure'. In reality, this is what Debbie Purdy sought and the achievements are unparalleled, despite its shortcomings.

CASE EXAMPLE

The case of Kay Gilderdale

Only weeks prior to the above guidelines being published, Kay Gilderdale was acquitted of the attempted murder of her daughter. A former nurse, she had witnessed her daughter's 17-year battle with Myalgic Encephalopathy (ME), which she had contracted at the age of 14. In constant pain and with no hope of improvement, Lynn Gilderdale had pleaded with her mother to help her to die. Eventually, Kay Gilderdale succumbed to her daughter's wishes, increased her daughter's dose of morphine and gave it to her daughter to self-administer. Her mother then took further steps to ensure that her daughter's wishes were fulfilled. She had pleaded guilty to assisted suicide but the prosecution pursued a charge of attempted murder. Why did the CPS pursue this case? Although it was undoubtedly traumatic for Kay Gilderdale and her family to revisit the events that led to her daughter's death, a failure to prosecute could result in the misconceived perception that the CPS quietly condoned mercy killing.

Furthermore, there were similarities between this and the *Inglis* case (2010), not least because they were heard within days of each other. Both planned how to kill their sick children but one of the crucial differences was that Lynn Gilderdale had begged her mother to help her end her life. Nevertheless, the *Gilderdale* case contained elements that bore a hallmark not only of assisted suicide but also of mercy killing, hence the charge of attempted murder. In Daniel James's situation, his parents and his friend helped him in a number of distinct ways to travel to Dignitas to end his life. The one difference that can be drawn between the experience of James and Gilderdale is that Gilderdale also sought ways to end her daughter's life by calling 'Exit', a group which advocates suicide, in order to seek further advice. It was this act which the DPP considered crossed the threshold from a charge of assisted suicide to a charge of attempted murder.

Kay Gilderdale was acquitted of attempted murder amid a frenzy of media reports. When asked by the judge whether it was in the public interests for the case to proceed, the CPS confirmed that 'it was felt at the highest level that this was a case that should be canvassed before a jury'. Public opinion had spoken.

Daniel James	Kay Gilderdale	Francis Inglis
• Rendered tetraplegic in a rugby accident. Could not come to terms with the disability. • Was intent on ending his life. Travelled to Dignitas in Switzerland with the help of family and friends where he died. • DPP did not consider it to be in the public interest to prosecute. Referred to in the case of *Purdy* where the court indicated complete agreement with the decision not to prosecute.	• Helped to end her daughter's life at her daughter's continued request. • Daughter had suffered for many years from ME. • Mother attempted to help her end her life but had to take further advice. • Bore hallmarks of mercy killing. • Jury acquitted her of attempted murder.	• Mother had tried to end her son's life when he became brain-damaged. • Despite an injunction she managed to access the hospital and she killed her son by injecting him with heroin. • He had not asked her to help him end his life. • Convicted of murder. • The court took no account of familial love as the motive for the murder.

Figure 10.5 Key factors in cases of assisted suicide or mercy killing

ACTIVITY

Self-test questions

Ensure that your answers are supported by case law and/or statute where appropriate.

- Is suicide legal? Is assisted suicide legal?
- Distinguish between euthanasia and assisted suicide.
- What do you understand by the term 'mercy killing'?
- Does the law permit a right to die?
- Clearly explain the judgment in the case of *R (on the application of Pretty) v DPP* (2002).
- Why was Diane Pretty's case unsuccessful?
- To what extent was *R (Purdy) v DPP* (2009) successful?
- Has assisted suicide been legalised by the above judgment?
- Consider the effectiveness of the DPP guidelines.

10.4 Attempts to legislate assisted suicide in England and Wales

On no less than three occasions, Lord Joffe introduced Bills to Parliament in the hope that assisted dying for the terminally ill would be legalised in England and Wales.

In 2003, Lord Joffe introduced for the first time a Private Members' Bill to enable a competent patient to access assisted dying if that person was 'suffering unbearably', due to either a terminal or a serious and progressive physical illness.

In the second reading of the Patient (Assisted Dying) Bill June 2003, Lord Alton expressed his disapproval of the provisions of the Bill.

There was agreement from professional bodies. The British Medical Association stated 'there is consensus within the BMA that the law should not be changed to permit euthanasia or physician-assisted suicide in the UK'.

The view was echoed by the Royal College of Physicians who considered that:

QUOTATION

'key terms in the Bill are worryingly vague ... it could be extended to apply to a very large number of patients beyond those whom the sponsors had in mind when they proposed it.'

Doctors too expressed alarm at the proposals and indicated in a poll that by far the majority, some 74 per cent, would not perform assisted suicide if it was legalised.

The Bill proceeded no further, but it was only a short period of time before Lord Joffe introduced the new Assisted Dying for the Terminally Ill Bill. Its intention was not dissimilar to the previous Bill or indeed to the future Bills. While there was a lack of Parliamentary time in order for the Bill to be fully debated, the first Report of the Select Committee recommended the following:

- a clearer distinction should be drawn between PAS and euthanasia
- a definition of mental competence should take into account the need to identify patients who may suffer from either psychological or psychiatric disorder
- that the term 'unbearable' should be replaced with the term either 'unrelievable' or 'retractable'
- if assisted suicide or patient-assisted suicide is being offered as a genuine alternative to palliative care, then consideration should be given as to how patients should experience such care.

In November 2005, a new 'Assisted Dying for the Terminally Ill Bill' was introduced and, in May 2006, reached its second reading in the House of Lords. Being aimed only at those patients who had capacity, the Bill once more sought to legalise voluntary euthanasia and assisted suicide. Its 'formal' intended purpose was to

CLAUSE

'enable an adult who has capacity and who is suffering unbearably as a result of a terminal illness to receive medical assistance to die at his own considered and persistent request'.

Joffe's Bill was aimed at alleviating the suffering of those who endure unbearable pain, but the fear of the wider implications of allowing involuntary euthanasia in through the back door or exploitation of the vulnerable remained too overwhelming to allow the Bill to proceed further.

Keown (2007) contended that the provisions in the Bill 'invited both extension and abuse' and that the safeguards were simply 'illusory'. As is a common fear, if the Bill was to proceed and be subsequently enacted, the door would be opened not only for PAS that Lord Joffe was advocating, but also for non-voluntary euthanasia. It was felt that one of the major hurdles which could not be overcome was the lack of distinction between PAS and euthanasia.

Once more, Lord Joffe's Bill was rejected; on this occasion the House of Lords rejected the Bill's proposals by 148 votes to 100. What do these three failed attempts at legalising physician assisted suicide and euthanasia represent? They have in reality achieved a considerable amount as these issues are now firmly in the public domain, being debated and argued.

Probably more significantly, the cases of *Pretty* (2002) and the seminal case of *Purdy* (2009) which forced the DPP to develop a transparent policy outlining factors in favour and against prosecution have raised debate and public awareness to an even higher level. There is a sustainable view that, if there can be adequate safeguards to protect the vulnerable from abuse and a clear distinction drawn between euthanasia and PAS, assisted suicide may one day be legalised.

10.5 Attempts to legislate in favour of assisted suicide in Scotland

In January 2005, at a similar time to the introduction of Lord Joffe's third Private Members' Bill in support of assisted suicide, Jeremy Purvis MSP introduced a consultation document on his proposed *Dying with Dignity* legislation. As he only received a mere handful of signatures in favour of his proposal, he was unable to introduce it to the Scottish Parliament.

In 2010 a Private Members' Bill, the End of Life Assistance (Scotland) Bill, was introduced by independent MSP Margo MacDonald, herself a Parkinson's sufferer. The Bill proposed to remove criminal liability for assisted suicide to enable a person to die with 'dignity' and with a 'minimum of stress'. The Suicide Act 1961 is only applicable in England and Wales; thus in Scotland, where there is no specific legislation, the law on homicide applies. The End of Life Assistance (Scotland) Bill Committee was charged with reporting on the contents of the Bill. One important point for consideration was that public policy was in favour of prosecution in cases of assisted suicide. In support of this, the Holyrood Committee referred to a 2006 case where a man was convicted of culpable homicide for assisting his brother, who was suffering from Huntingdon's disease, to end his life.

Given that public policy was in favour of prosecution, it was unlikely that this Bill would have proceeded in any event, but the Committee had a number of other issues with the definitions and provisions within the Bill, and by December 2010 had failed to recommend the general principles of the Bill to Parliament.

The Bill had aimed to permit assisted suicide within strict parameters. The person seeking to end their life would have to be over the age of 16, either be diagnosed as 'terminally ill and finds life intolerable' or 'is permanently physically incapacitated to such an extent as not to be able to live independently and finds life intolerable'. Furthermore, the person would have to make a formal request on two separate occasions to a medical practitioner and a psychiatrist before he or she could proceed.

In a free vote, a majority of MSPs failed to vote in favour of the Bill's provisions. However, once more the issue of assisted suicide was examined, opened up for debate and gained greater exposure.

10.6 Legislation in other jurisdictions

10.6.1 United States of America

A number of American States have resisted the move to permit assisted suicide, and to date the States of Washington and Oregon are the only States to have legalised assisted suicide. The courts have historically viewed in a dim light challenges to the law on assisted suicide; most recently, a Connecticut Superior Court Judge in the case of *Blick v Connecticut* (2010) rejected two doctors' contention that 'aid in dying' was the same as assisted suicide.

10.6.2 Oregon

The law

Oregon introduced assisted suicide with the Death with Dignity Act 1994, although it was not enacted until 1997 because of a number of challenges. Since the date of its enactment, a total of 460 patients have died as a direct result of ingesting medication prescribed under this Act.

The Death with Dignity Act 1994 states that a terminally ill resident of Oregon can obtain from their physician a prescription for lethal medication which will end their lives. The following criteria must be fulfilled:

- The patient must be an adult (over 18 years of age) and competent.
- The diagnosis and prognosis of a terminal illness must be confirmed by two doctors. The second doctor must also confirm that the patient is acting voluntarily and is competent.
- A terminal illness is defined as having less than six months to live.
- If there is any doubt about the patient's competency, the doctor must refer the patient for evaluation.
- The patient must make two oral requests, 15 days apart and one written request. After 48 hours after the last request, the patient can then ask for the prescription to be completed.
- The patient's request must be witnessed by two people. In order to demonstrate a complete lack of influence, at least one of the witnesses must not be a relative or a potential beneficiary under a will or employed at the place where the patient is receiving treatment. Neither of the witnesses can be doctors.
- The patient must be asked to notify their next of kin, although contacting them is not obligatory.
- The prescribing doctor must report the prescription to the Oregon Department of Human Services. The pharmacist must also report the prescription.

The practice

Oregon's Department of Human Services released their Annual Report in March 2010 on statistics relating to deaths under the Death with Dignity Act 1994. The statistics make interesting reading and suggest that there is little abuse of the statutory provisions. Moreover, the statistics confirm that the fear expressed in many other US States and countries suggesting a dangerous vacuum for elderly, poor and infirmed people is largely unfounded.

Figures show that, during 2009, there were 95 prescriptions for lethal medications, an increase of just seven from the previous year. Despite the number of prescriptions, only 53 died as a result of taking their prescriptions. Nevertheless, when added to the figures of six patients who died from taking previously prescribed medications, the total figure of 59 deaths during 2009 under the statutory provisions represents 19.3 deaths through assisted suicide per 10,000 total deaths. Statistics show the majority of patients were aged 55 or over, white, middle class, well-educated and chose to end their life at home.

The greater percentage who chose to end their life suffered from cancer, although it is interesting to note that in previous years a small number of HIV/AIDS sufferers also chose to end their lives in this way.

Patients' primary motivation was a combination of a concern over loss of autonomy, a loss of dignity and being unable to do things which had previously made their lives enjoyable. These are personal considerations about the quality of a person's life, and the statistics suggest that feeling a burden to family, friends and care-givers was not an important consideration.

Even less important were concerns about the lack of pain relief and palliative care, as Oregon rates well in the provision of palliative care when compared with other US States; over 90 per cent of patients were enrolled in a hospice during the relevant period. These statistics do not suggest that patients seek PAS as the only option to a lack of palliative care.

Moreover, the figures also confirm that financial considerations were hardly relevant, and the argument that patients would seek PAS because they could not afford medical insurance or healthcare does not seem to be borne out.

Real and serious concerns about protecting people who are poor, vulnerable, female, poorly educated or elderly are simply not borne out by these statistics. Consistently, year-on-year men represent the greater percentage of patients than women, although the margin between the two sexes is never greater than seven per cent difference. Women do not therefore feel more vulnerable than men. The greatest age range is between 65–74, suggesting that elderly people who are aged 85 and over are not disproportionately more vulnerable than another age range and do not feel that they should end their lives to cease being a burden on others.

Ninety-eight per of all patients are married and educated. This too fails to support the argument that poor and uneducated people would be a vulnerable section of the population and feel bound by the black hole of PAS. Instead these statistics reflect that decisions to end a person's life are taken by those who appear to be the least vulnerable in society. They suggest that these decisions are simply a clear expression of a person's autonomy of how to end their lives when their condition is such that it renders their life, from their perspective, one that lacks the quality they desire.

10.6.3 Washington

The law

In 2008, the State of Washington introduced the Death with Dignity Act, legalising PAS for the first time after being previously rejected in 1991. A person must be able to fulfil statutory criteria which are remarkably similar to that in Oregon's Death with Dignity Act 1994. The patient must be over 18, be terminally ill, competent and a resident of the State of Washington. The doctor must ensure that the patient is making an informed decision by explaining the patient's diagnosis and prognosis to the patient, the risks associated with taking the medication (the probable result) and the available alternatives, such as palliative care. The doctor must refer the patient to a second doctor for confirmation of the diagnosis and that the patient is competent and acting voluntarily. The doctor will recommend notifying the next of kin. The patient must make an oral request followed by a written request, and then a further request at least 15 days after the initial request, which can be rescinded thereafter.

The practice

The Washington State Department of Health reported the numbers of deaths between March and December 2009 where medication with the intention of hastening death had been prescribed. There were 63 related prescriptions, although only 36 patients died after ingesting the medication. Seven died from causes unrelated to the medication, presumably the patient's underlying medical condition, and it is not known whether the four remaining patients ingested the prescribed medication. Over three-quarters of the patients concerned were suffering from cancer; 89 per cent had private medical insurance; the vast majority were white; and 61 per cent were well educated. As other statistics suggest, women were no more likely to opt for PAS than men, and the age range where patients are most likely to request euthanasia is 65–74. The older the patient is, the less likely they are to request euthanasia.

As evidenced in Oregon, by far the majority of patients chose euthanasia for concern over not being able to carry out activities that made their life enjoyable; 82 per cent thought their loss of dignity was a motivating factor; but for all patients, loss of autonomy was the most important factor. There is little to suggest that a lack of palliative care was a factor in a patient's decision as nearly three-quarters of patients were enrolled in hospice care when taking the medication, and concerns about lack of pain control was not a relevant factor. Concerns about financial obligations and being a burden to others also failed to feature significantly in the survey.

The results for both studies are remarkably similar. Neither reflects the popular view of patients opting for euthanasia for fear of being a burden on their families or motivation by financial concerns of the lack of palliative care. By far the majority of patients are well-informed and educated whose primary concerns are loss of autonomy, dignity and the ability to do things which gave them pleasure. Those who voice concern that euthanasia will be a conduit for more vulnerable patients certainly have a valuable opinion but the results of the studies in the United States simply do not support this view.

10.6.4 Montana

In January 2010 a Supreme Court of 4:3 in Montana held that PAS was not banned by State law.

CASE EXAMPLE

Baxter v Montana [2010] 09-0051, Supreme Court of Montana (Helena)

A number of patients who were terminally ill brought the action together with their doctors and the support of an American organization supporting the legalisation of PAS. Baxter was terminally ill with leukaemia and he sought medication in order to end his life. His doctor sought to challenge whether he could be prosecuted if he helped competent and terminally ill patients to die.

In late 2009, a majority judgment of the Supreme Court indicated that PAS did not appear to be contrary to public policy and that it:

JUDGMENT

'[it] ... *reflects legislative respect for the wishes of a patient facing incurable illness.* [It] also indicates legislative regards and protection for a physician who honors his legal obligation to the patient.'

The judgment means that the State's criminal law does not condemn the practice of PAS, but the Supreme Court did not rule on whether Montana's State Constitution conveys a positive right to PAS. The Montana Death with Dignity Act is currently making its way through the legislature in Montana, in line with Oregon's Death with Dignity Act.

10.6.5 The Netherlands

The law

The Netherlands has a unique approach to euthanasia and assisted suicide which reflects a society which is significantly more open and transparent. While the impression is given that euthanasia and assisted suicide are legal in the Netherlands, this is not an accurate reflection of Dutch law.

The Netherlands Penal Code distinctly provides the following:

- **Article 293** makes it an offence to end a person's life at their express consent. The offence carries a maximum sentence of 12 years, not dissimilar to the provisions of the Suicide Act 1961 in England and Wales.
- **Article 294** prohibits assisting suicide. Where a person is found to be assisting, counselling or procuring the victim's death, the offence carries a maximum sentence of 3 years or a fine.

However, the Articles above were amended by The Termination of Life on Request and Assisted Suicide (Review Procedure) Act 2001 which came into force in 2002. It states as follows:

SECTION

'A person who terminates the life of another at that other person's express and earnest request is liable to a term of imprisonment of not more than twelve years or a fine ... The offence referred to in the first paragraph shall not be punishable if it has been committed by a physician who has met the requirement of due care ... and who informs the municipal autopist of this.'

While both euthanasia and assisted suicide remain criminal offences, Art 20 provides that a doctor who ends a life following express consent or a person who assists with a suicide fulfils the 'due care' criteria which is set out in s 2, The Termination of Life on Request and Assisted Suicide (Review Procedure) Act 2001. The doctor must also report the cause of death to the coroner.

In order to be exempt from criminal liability, two conditions must be met:

■ the 'due care' criteria must be fulfilled
■ the cause of death must be reported to the coroner.

It is worth noting that the statutory provisions specifically refer to a doctor; accordingly, since a literal interpretation is applied, any other person who assists with the termination of life or assisted suicide would be guilty under the Act.

There is no statutory provision that patients have a right to insist on either ending life or assistance with the suicide and there is no obligation that the doctor must comply with the request.

The 'due care' criteria

Article 2(1) provides as follows:

■ The patient must make a voluntary and well-considered request.
■ There is no hope of improvement in the patient's condition and the patient's suffering is unbearable.
■ The patient has been informed about his or her situation and prognosis.
■ Both the doctor and the patient, in the relationship they have, appreciate that there is no other reasonable avenue to pursue in view of the patient's condition.
■ The patient must have consulted at least one other independent doctor who must have seen the patient and provided a written opinion on the due care criteria set out above.
■ The patient's life has ended or assistance with suicide has been provided with due care.

In any event, the above criteria had been practised for a number of years preceding the Act. Since late 1990 a doctor would not have been prosecuted under Arts 293 and 294 if he had complied with 'rules of careful practice', which were worded similarly to the provisions above. Not only was it considered not to be in the interests of justice to prosecute a breach of the provisions but, provided the doctor complied with the 'rules of careful practice', it was both accepted and approved of.

While the Act represents a truly bold move in a highly emotive area fraught with ethical dilemmas, in reality the Act simply reflects the common law position that had been adopted by the Dutch courts for the previous 30 years. The following case examples are cited in Jackson (2009).

CASE EXAMPLE

The *Postma* Case (1973) *Nederlandse Jurisprudentie* No. 183 District Court Leeuwarden

Dr Postma was a Dutch general practitioner who was prosecuted for ending her mother's life by administering a fatal dose of morphine. Sheldon (2007) comments that husband and wife were both popular GPs in a quiet rural village and Dr Postma (male) had expressed his opinion that a person should be entitled to a 'good and conscious death' in an article in 1965. Dr Postma's mother was severely ill; she was paralysed as a result of a brain haemorrhage, and found it difficult to speak or hear, but she had repeatedly expressed her wish to die. The daughter injected her mother with a lethal dose of morphine which ended her life. Drs Postma then reported the matter to the nursing home and Dr Postma (female) was subsequently charged under Art 293 which carries a maximum sentence of 12 years' imprisonment.

Dr Postma was sentenced to one week's suspended sentence and 12 months' probation. While she was convicted, the leniency of the sentence reflects not only the empathy of the courts, but the existence of four crucial factors:

- There was no hope of recovery.
- Her pain was unbearable.
- She had repeatedly asked for her life to be terminated.
- It was performed by her doctor, having consulted with him or her.

Although the Postmas were never intending this case to be a landmark case and were not at that time advocating a change in the law, they were committed to the principle that a person whose pain and life is unbearable should be able to end it at the time of their choosing. Within a few weeks of Dr Postma's conviction, the Dutch Voluntary Euthanasia Society was established.

CASE EXAMPLE

The *Alkmaar* Case (1984) *Nederlandse Jurisprudentie* 1982 No. 106 Supreme Court, The Netherlands

A 95-year-old woman was seriously ill. There was no chance that her condition would improve. Her condition deteriorated; she was unable to eat or drink and lost consciousness. When she regained awareness, she begged the doctor to end her life. She had also previously signed an advance declaration requesting euthanasia if her condition worsened. Dr Schoonheim finally succumbed to her request.

Although he was initially convicted, the case was subsequently referred to the court of The Hague which quashed his conviction. Dr Schoonheim relied upon the defence of necessity. As Sjef Gevers explains:

QUOTATION

'a doctor will not be convicted if he or she has carefully balanced the conflicting duties and made a decision that can objectively be justified, taking into account the special circumstances of the case'.

In other words, where there is a conflict of duty between the doctor's duty to preserve life and as Jackson describes 'his duty to relieve unbearable suffering' (2009), he can balance the scales by relieving the unbearable suffering of the patient, provided that he can objectively justify his decision-making process. This is referred to as the defence of necessity.

In the same year as the judgment, the Royal Dutch Medical Association confirmed that there could be circumstances in which euthanasia was acceptable. The purpose was to provide some much needed guidance to the profession. The criteria reflected the court's decisions at common law and also the due care criteria above.

With no specific mention of the patient having to be terminally ill, the following case concerned the euthanasia of a mentally ill patient.

CASE EXAMPLE

The *Chabot* case (1994) *Nederlandse Jurisprudentie* 1994 No. 65 Supreme Court, The Netherlands

A Dutch psychiatrist helped an acutely unhappy patient to commit suicide. She had been unhappily married and both of her sons had died. She said that she wanted to die and would not accept any help for her depression. Since she had not been diagnosed with any mental condition, she had capacity to make the decision.

Chabot was convicted of assisted suicide despite being acquitted twice. He had assisted in the death of a woman who had no medical condition save for unbearable grief following the death of her two sons. Despite the possibility of a three year sentence, no penalty was imposed.

As a direct result of the Chabot case, the guidelines were changed to allow doctors to help patients who suffered mentally to such an extent that their lives were irreversibly unbearable to terminate their lives.

More recently and generating more public concern, a case of assisted suicide concerning a 65-year-old Alzheimer's patient was reported to the Netherland's assessment committee system. It was decided that the criteria was fulfilled and euthanasia was lawful. It now appears to be acceptable and, more importantly, lawful that Alzheimer's patients may now be able to request PAS or assisted suicide as well as those that are severely depressed. It is perhaps questionable whether this was the Dutch Parliament's intention when the 2001 Act was passed. Many critics would consider this to be a significant step towards the slippery slope (see below).

The practice

Although there was initial concern that some assisted suicides were unreported, since 1990 it has been necessary for the doctor to inform the authorities of a death and they then refer it to the prosecutor's office. Only once the prosecutor is satisfied that all the criteria have been satisfied can the deceased be released for burial. Once this procedure was introduced, the number of reported cases increased significantly to 40.7 per cent in 1995 (Van Der Wal *et al* (1996)). More recently, cases are reviewed by a regional review committee who will not refer the case to the prosecutor until they are satisfied that the criteria have been complied with.

The *Remmelink Report* in 2001 considered statistics from 1990, 1995 and 2001 with a view to ascertaining whether there was a marked increase over the years. The figures show that the number of deaths of both assisted suicide and PAS between 1995 and 2001 was relatively constant. However, recent statistics reported in the Dutch press suggest that the number or deaths from euthanasia in 2010 has increased significantly and possibly disproportionately by 13 per cent to 2,636, compared with 10 per cent the previous year. At the time of writing, the reasons for this increase are unclear although it is possible that the increase is due to the stigma of euthanasia being slowly eroded. In any event, the Health Ministry is currently investigating the recorded increase.

Statistical analysis provided by the Netherlands is crucial to the continuing debate and, while the numbers of deaths related to end of life decisions may seem alarmingly high, they are compatible overall with data provided from Oregon.

In 2005, only 1.7 per cent of total recorded deaths were as a result of euthanasia and a mere 0.1 per cent were the result of PAS. Rather than a year-on-year increase as might be expected, the number of deaths from euthanasia was considerably lower than in 2001 when the recorded percentages were 2.6 per cent and 0.2 per cent respectively ('End of Life Practices in the Netherlands Under the Euthanasia Act 2007', *New England Journal of Medicine*, 2007, 356, pages 1957–65.)

In the years of the study (1990, 1995, 2001 and 2005), euthanasia was more common than assisted suicide, ranging between 1.7–2.6 per cent of all reported deaths, while assisted suicide represented no more than a relative constant of 0.2 per cent of deaths. In line with Oregon, cancer was the most common cause of decisions leading either to PAS or assisted suicide which were most frequently carried out by the patient's GP in their own home and within one week of their estimated end of life.

10.6.6 Belgium

In 2002, the Belgium Euthanasia Act was passed which legalised euthanasia subject to satisfying the criteria. Assisted suicide has not been included in the Act.

A doctor will not commit an offence if euthanasia is committed and the following criteria are met:

- The patient must be over the age of 18 and competent or an 'emancipated minor'.
- The request for euthanasia must be voluntary, well considered and repeated.
- The patient must not be subjected to any undue influence.
- The patient must be suffering from an incurable physical or mental condition that causes unbearable pain or distress.
- The doctor must discuss the patient's condition with him or her, together with the repeated requests and the offer of palliative care and come to the decision together that there is no viable alternative.
- The doctor must consult another doctor about the patient's condition and advise the patient of the discussion. The second doctor must examine the patient's file and be certain that the patient's physical conditions are constant and unbearable, and in the case of a mental condition be satisfied that the mental condition cannot be alleviated.
- The request must be in writing and can be withdrawn at any time.
- An advance directive can be made in the case of a competent patient.
- Doctors are not obliged to comply with a request but must inform the patient accordingly.

Smets T *et al* conducted a survey in 2010 into the frequency of end-of-life decisions from a sample of death certificates in Flanders within a five-month period in 2007. The number of deaths estimated to be related to euthanasia was 1,040 which represents about 1.9 per cent of all deaths. Only about half of the deaths related to euthanasia were reported to the Federal Control and Evaluation Committee, although the survey explained this by stating that doctors who considered their cases to be euthanasia were extremely likely to report it, and doctors who failed to report the death were generally not of the opinion that it was euthanasia, given the proximity of actual death to the estimated life expectancy.

Similar to euthanasia data provided by other jurisdictions, patients were more likely to be under 80 years of age, suffering from cancer, and preferred to die at home.

10.6.7 Switzerland

The law

Article 114 of the Swiss Penal Code which is referred to as euthanasia or murder on request states that a person who kills another on the basis of his or her serious and insistent request can be convicted and sentenced to a term of imprisonment. In Switzerland, intentional killing is not automatically considered to be murder, unlike the law in England and Wales, although the charge can be increased to murder. Article 115 states that inciting or assisting a person to commit suicide is a criminal offence if the motive is considered to be 'selfish'. If the motive is altruistic and compassionate, it would appear that no criminal offence is committed.

The practice

Dignitas is one of three organisations in Switzerland who assist those who wish to end their life. Dignitas is the only body who will accept foreigners. Exit, which does not accept non-Swiss residents, had over 50,000 members in 2008.

Between 1998 and 2010, statistics released by Dignitas show that a total of 1,138 patients chose to end their life there. There were a total of 30 different nationalities with Germans representing 62 per cent of all patients. Between 1998 and 2009, 160 British patients ended their lives at Dignitas – 17 per cent of all patients.

KEY FACTS

Key facts on relevant jurisdictions where some form of assisted dying is permitted

Jurisdiction	What the legislation permits	Legal provision
Belgium	PAS	Belgian Euthanasia Act 2002
Netherlands	PAS and assisted suicide	The Termination of Life on Request and Assisted Suicide (Review Procedure) Act 2001
Oregon (USA)	PAS	Death with Dignity Act 1994
Montana (USA)	PAS	There is no legislative provision but, in 2009, the Supreme Court indicated that there is 'nothing in Montana Supreme Court precedent of Montana statutes indicating that physician aid in dying is against public policy'.
Washington State (USA)	PAS	Death with Dignity Act 2008
Switzerland	Assisted suicide	Swiss Penal Code 1942

10.7 Is there any prospect of legislation in the UK?

A Commission on Assisted Dying was set up in November 2010 to independently investigate whether the UK law is in need of reform, or whether the DPP guidelines are sufficiently adequate to represent the law in the twenty-first century.

The Commission's stated aim is to:

- investigate the circumstances under which it should be possible for people to be assisted to die
- recommend the type of system that could be established in order to allow people to be helped to die
- identify the type of person who should be entitled to assistance with dying, and
- consider adequate protection for vulnerable people to prevent them from feeling pressurised to opt for an assisted death.

While the Commission is independent, it has been criticised from its inception as being pro assisted suicide and euthanasia, given its membership and funding. Arguably, the time for statutory reform has never been more appropriate; the DPP guidelines, while of significant benefit, do not address the question of whether a person has a fundamental right to an autonomous decision on how and when to end their life.

The cynic may observe that, given three unsuccessful Private Members' Bills, an equally unsuccessful Private Members' Bill in Scotland and failed amendments to the recent Coroners and Justice Act 2009, any outcome of the Commission on Assisted Dying is doomed to failure. However, media awareness has probably never been greater and public opinion appears to be quietly in favour. Moreover, the DPP guidelines are only intended to be guidelines and are probably not fit for long-term use. It is not for the courts to legislate and, while prosecutions are likely to be very few and far between, if the Commission does report favourably, it may now be time for a forward-looking government to consider legislation.

The most obvious form legislation could take is to embody the DPP guidelines, setting them out as exceptions to s 2(1) of the Suicide Act 1961 of aiding, abetting, counselling or procuring a suicide. As already discussed, the guidelines are not without their own critics, being largely about the person assisting rather than the victim.

In addition or as an alternative, Mason and Mulligan (1996) propose an amendment to the wording of s 2(1) which would retain the offence of assisted suicide but permit a form of PAS. The wording suggested would be as follows:

QUOTATION

'The provisions of s 2(1) shall not apply to a registered medical practitioner who is providing assistance to a patient who is suffering from a terminal illness or from a progressive and irremediable condition, and who is prevented, or will be prevented, by physical disability from ending his or her life without assistance, and who acts with the patient's consent or, if this is not available, in the patient's best interests.'

They propose a stage-by-stage approach in order to gauge legislative response. Arguably, any amendment to s 2(1) should not include reference to the incompetent patient. This area should still be reserved for the courts as in *Bland* (1993); alternatively separate provisions should apply specifically to the incompetent patient.

If the law is to move forward then legislation cannot be piecemeal or coy. Legislation must provide for the future. If the Commission on Assisted Dying reports positively and it moves forward, any proposed legislation should provide not only for assisted suicide but also for PAS, failing which there may be circumstances in which a patient may not actually be able to end their life even though it may be lawful to do so. It seems illogical that a person can end their life if they can swallow tablets that will lead to death, but cannot obtain a doctor's help if they cannot.

10.8 Ethical issues and assisted suicide

10.8.1 Autonomy

One of the most significant ethical arguments in favour of euthanasia is the principle of autonomy. Previously we have seen in *Re T (adult: refusal of medical treatment)* (1992) that a competent adult patient may refuse life-sustaining treatment even if it will lead to certain death.

Lord Donaldson explained that the appeal concerned a person's autonomous decision about the right to decide how to live their life, even if their decision made death more likely:

JUDGMENT

'This appeal ... is not in truth about "the right to die". There is no suggestion that Miss T wants to die ... This appeal is about the "right to choose how to live".'

We have also seen that the converse does not apply. In most jurisdictions, a competent patient may not insist that a doctor ends his life and cannot enlist the help of family or friends to help him end his own life. Here, in the UK, it is a crime. Why should the criminal law impose sanctions? We will address each of the arguments in turn but firstly we will consider the principle of autonomy.

Autonomy means that a person has the right to decide how to live their lives without State intervention. I am free to pursue dangerous pursuits and hobbies even if they carry inherent risks. I can pursue a potentially dangerous career such as fire-fighting or belong to the military even though both may carry a risk of death. I can even decide to commit suicide which is not unlawful since the Suicide Act 1961. However, the act I cannot pursue is that which is probably most desperately desired – the act of requesting a doctor or family or friends to end my life or to help me end my life if the medical condition I suffer from is so beyond measure that death is the preferred and only option. Hence, it could be argued that the autonomy which is afforded to me throughout my life, including the choice to make wrong or dangerous decisions, is denied to me at death.

Harris observes (1995):

QUOTATION

'Euthanasia should be permitted, not because everyone should accept it is right … but … to deny a person control of what … must be one of the most important decisions of life, is a form of tyranny, which like all forms of tyranny, is an ultimate denial of respect for persons.'

The theme of tyrannical oppression is echoed by philosopher Ronald Dworkin:

QUOTATION

'Making someone die in a way that others approve, but he believes a horrifying contradiction of his life, is a devastating, odious form of tyranny.'

In *Reeves v Commissioner of Police for the Metropolis* [2000] 1 AC 360, Lord Hobhouse gave an impassioned dissenting speech in favour of autonomy:

JUDGMENT

'Personal autonomy includes the right to choose conduct which will cause that person's death and the right to refuse to allow others to obstruct that choice.'

If a person has a terminal condition and is in unbearable pain despite the availability of palliative care, being alive can be tantamount to being enslaved. It may be tempting to try and argue as in *Pretty v UK* (2002) that such an act is contrary to Art 3, ECHR (the prohibition of inhumane and degrading treatment). However, we have already seen from the judgment of the European Court of Human Rights that Art 3 was not breached as there was 'no … act or "treatment" on the part of the United Kingdom'. The State had not caused her condition; her illness had.

The argument against autonomy

In medical law there is considerable reference to the value of autonomy in positive terms, and modern medicine prides itself in moving from paternalism towards patient autonomy. Arguably, in this respect, although we may view the terminally ill patient's autonomous decision of when to die as desirable, we can lose sight of the wider picture.

Keown (2002) explores the idea of autonomy with this approach: if I choose to murder A, this is an expression of my autonomy but it is clearly not only undesirable, it breaches fundamental values. If we choose to exercise our autonomy then we can do so, but this must be within a guided framework. Just because a decision is an autonomous one, does not mean it is acceptable. He asks 'Is there a right to choose … paedophilia?' This is undesirable because it will have a negative impact on others and because it is contrary to the moral framework in which we live. He explains that we live in a community, not isolated from others, and therefore the choices we make impact upon other people's lives.

If patient B is suffering unbearably from a terminal condition and exercises the autonomous decision to end his life, this affects his loved ones, although some would argue his family would prefer to watch him die in this way than witness a slow and painful death. But, if we look at this again and patient B is permitted to choose to end his life with the assistance of another, his autonomous decision can have a negative effect on society as a whole.

The reality is that 'the interests of the individual cannot be separated from the interests of society as a whole' (House of Lords Select Committee 1993). While we applaud autonomy, the fundamental problem in this context is that the exercise of one person's autonomy is another person's burden.

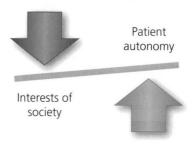

Patient autonomy

Interests of society

Figure 10.6 The interests of the individual vs the interests of society

10.8.2 Dying with dignity

The freedom to be able to die with dignity is the direct result of the exercise of a person's self-determination and autonomous wish to end their life. It is therefore no coincidence that patients cite a loss of dignity as one of the primary reasons for choosing PAS or euthanasia. Death with dignity has become a phrase synonymous with a person's desire for the right to die. Indeed it is no coincidence that the leading campaigners in the UK are named Dying in Dignity; legislation in the US is called the Death with Dignity Acts; and the clinic in Switzerland is named Dignitas – Latin for worthiness and nobility.

Macklin (2003) argues with some force that 'dignity is a useless concept in medical ethics and can be eliminated without any loss of content'. Admittedly, it is difficult to define what amounts to dignity in this context, but often it is associated with a person's attributes. Allmark (2008) observes that health professionals cannot ensure that a person dies with dignity but can ensure that a person has a death without indignity. In order to do this, Allmark explains that barriers to dignity have to be removed such as unbearable pain, as far as is possible, and a person's autonomy respected.

In the case of *Pretty* (2002), she unsuccessfully argued that Art 3, ECHR conferred upon her the right to die with dignity, but in *Purdy* (2009) her pleas for clarification for when her husband may be prosecuted if he assisted her to die stemmed from the need to die with dignity. The underlying desire was that they both wanted to be able to die with dignity when they deemed the time was right for them. While Pretty was unable to achieve this, Ms B (*Re B* (2002)) was granted her wish.

10.8.3 Pressure to seek euthanasia or PAS

While we acknowledge that autonomy is one of the fundamental and respected principles, there is a concern that elderly or vulnerable people might feel compelled or duty-bound to request euthanasia or PAS if it was legalised. There is a plausible argument that elderly people would consider that they had had a 'fair innings' and that it would not be a tragedy for them to die aged 70-plus. They may fear being a physical or emotional burden on their family and friends. Indeed, there are those who argue that, if a person is a burden on others, then it is their positive duty to end their lives. Baroness Warnock was recently quoted in the magazine *Church of Scotland, Life and Work*, as saying:

QUOTATION

'I'm absolutely, fully in agreement with the argument that if pain is insufferable, then someone should be given help to die, but I feel there's a wider argument that if somebody absolutely, desperately wants to die because they're a burden to their family, or the state, then I think they too should be allowed to die.'

Of course, being *allowed* to die does not have the same implication as being *duty-bound* to die, but elderly people may feel compelled to act.

More protectively, Lord Alton in the second reading of the Patient (Assisted Dying) Bill in June 2003 expressed concern over the proposed legislation (which subsequently failed) as he referred to the subjective duty that elderly people might feel to die. He commented that the introduction of assisted suicide in the UK would:

QUOTATION

'create a subjective duty to die for the old, create a stigma for disabled people and hinder progress in the palliative care that represents the real hope and comfort for the terminally ill and disabled'.

George (2007) observes that a woman is more likely to choose PAS or assisted suicide rather than a man as they may wish to avoid becoming dependent. If one accepts a woman's role is traditionally more caring than a man's, it may be difficult for some women to accept some form of role reversal in later life. George quotes Carol Gilligan who states as follows:

QUOTATION

'... while society might affirm publicly the woman's right to choose for herself, the exercise of such choice brings her privately into conflict with the conventions of femininity, particularly the moral equation of goodness with self-sacrifice. Although independent assertion in judgment and action is considered to be the hallmark of adulthood, it is rather in their care and concern for others that women have both judged themselves and been judged.'

Women may be more likely to choose assisted suicide as an unintended product of their stereotypical role, reflecting the idea of being selfless and being unwilling to accept the potential of role reversal of care.

People with disabilities may also feel vulnerable. There is a common misconception that disabled lives are of less value and may not be worth living. Although *Pretty* (2002) sought a right to die with dignity, this should not be read as suggesting that a disabled person should be under a duty to die or, in the alternative, they would lack dignity. The essence of vulnerability is conveyed in the following quote; Baroness Campbell from the Equality and Human Rights Commission and a sufferer from spinal muscular atrophy herself, said:

QUOTATION

'Disabled people's lives are invariably seen as less worthwhile than those of non-disabled people. Descriptions such as tragic, burdensome and even desperate are routinely used without objection. Unless one is extraordinarily strong, this negativity impacts on the individual disabled person. If suicide were a legally and socially acceptable option, too many would succumb to this fate, believing being "put out of misery" to be expected of them...'

Ironically, if assisted suicide was legal, it may actually prolong life rather than shorten it. Dr Anne Turner suffered from incurable and progressive, degenerative supra nuclear palsy. Having previously failed to take her own life, she decided to travel to Switzerland to end her life before her condition deteriorated further. However, Dr Turner chose to end her life at a time when she could still manage to travel herself. Debbie Purdy's concern was that, if she did not know whether it was likely that her husband would be prosecuted if he assisted her in travelling, she might have to travel to Switzerland alone at an earlier time, while she still could. The effect of legalising assisted suicide may be that some patients will not feel the need to end their lives earlier to protect their loved ones from prosecution.

10.8.4 The effect on the doctor–patient relationship

One of the basic tenets of medicine comes from the Latin phrase *Primum Non Nocere*, roughly translated as 'above all do no harm'. As patients, we have an expectation that our doctor will care for us. Knowing that a doctor can end our lives could undermine the trust between doctor and patient, particularly in the more vulnerable patient, who may be concerned that PAS could be exercised without his express consent. Conversely, if PAS was legalised and a patient expressly consented to PAS, to deny that patient their death with dignity would be positively doing harm to that patient. However, the Hippocratic Oath states that 'to please no one will I prescribe a deadly drug, nor give advice that may cause his death' which suggests that one of the most fundamental principles of medical practice dating from the fourth century BC is in direct conflict with euthanasia.

10.8.5 The slippery slope argument

One of the most cogent arguments against the legalisation of assisted suicide and euthanasia is the fear of where it might lead. Imagine legislation in the UK that legalised PAS and which was drafted in similar terms to Oregon's Death with Dignity Act. Imagine now the Act sometime in the future.

While legislation would refer to a competent adult who has expressed a clear and informed request to end his life due to the unbearable illness of a terminal disease, it could now apply to situations where a patient has not made a specific request and, in time, the move to non-voluntary PAS could then invariably move to PAS of the incompetent patient.

If a competent patient made a free and informed decision as a last resort to end his life due to unbearable pain from a terminal illness, each of these elements can be open to abuse either intentionally or unintentionally. While it may be the doctor's duty to ensure that each of these factors is complied with, it is likely that their application will be subjectively applied, with the outcome of an inconsistent approach throughout the UK.

Why does the pain have to be unbearable? Why does the patient have to wait until the pain becomes unbearable before he seeks PAS? If he knows this is what will surely happen, why wait until that stage comes? Why not seek PAS just before, in order to achieve that 'good' death? We have already seen in the *Chabot* case (1994) in Holland that a patient with Alzheimer's and severe depression both sought and obtained PAS. This seems to provide the evidence to support this argument of a slippery slope, that legislation that was once intended to apply to those with terminal illness becomes diluted over time and can now apply to those suffering from non-terminal illness.

How far can the slippery slope extend?

While we speak in hypothetical terms about the extremes of involuntary euthanasia and its potential dangers, it is worth recalling the Action T4 Euthanasia Programme in Nazi Germany that officially spanned the years 1939–41, although in reality extended far beyond 1941. The programme sought to destroy or murder those whose lives were not deemed by the Nazi regime to be of value, whether they were Jewish or disabled. With an initial interpretation of 'mercy killing', it was applied to people suffering mental illness and finally became the basis of orchestrated genocide. Evidence suggests that over 275,000 people were killed in this way. One however should avoid drawing parallels between involuntary euthanasia today and Nazi Germany. The meaning which the Nazi regime gave to euthanasia is entirely different, using the term euthanasia to justify the systematic slaughter of innocent victims under the guise of medical intervention, and determining for themselves whose lives were not worth living based upon an agenda of ethnic cleansing.

Is there statistical evidence to support the slippery slope argument?

A survey conducted by Onwuteaka-Phillipsen *et al* into deaths in the Netherlands concluded that the rate of PAS had not significantly increased between the years 1990, 1995 and 2001, and that the majority of those patients who chose PAS were white, educated, between aged 65–79 and were most likely to suffer from cancer.

The data showed that in 39 per cent of all deaths in the Netherlands, the patient had made a decision that 'probably or certainly hastened death'. However, in about 1,000 cases per year, a decision was made to administer medication which would have the effect of hastening death where the patient had *not explicitly requested it*. This figure should not be taken out of proportion as it is considerably fewer than those patients who had made a specific request, but the amount is still significant. It also appears to be the case that, where PAS took place without the patient's consent, this occurred at a slightly younger age than where a patient had explicitly requested PAS. The most common age group was under 64 years of age and the most common illness was cancer, as with PAS.

In real terms, it appears that one out of every five PAS is in fact without the patient's consent which leads some critics to remark that, although superficially the PAS statistics appear to be constant and controlled, the reality is that euthanasia is out of control. Indeed Jochensen and Keown comment (1999) that 'The reality is that a clear majority of cases of euthanasia, both with and without request, go unreported and unchecked. Dutch claims of effective regulation ring hollow.'

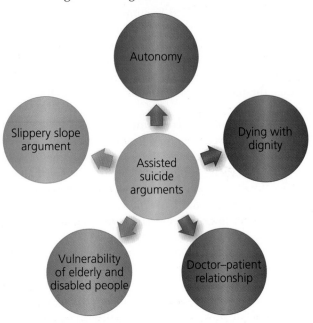

Figure 10.7 Assisted suicide arguments

In summary, while we may consider that PAS is desirable to avoid a person suffering a protracted and painful death, the patient cannot be considered in isolation. Some potential consequences are undesirable, with a negative impact on society that may be hard to control.

A step too far or practical progression?

In January 2011, a presentation was given at the Belgian Royal Medical Academy 2010 where doctors advocated organ donation after euthanasia. In patients where euthanasia is sought but their organs are of good quality, such as neuromuscular disorders, patients can be counselled to donate their organs to waiting recipients. The benefit is extremely significant as, if patients consent, organs become available to those in need and appropriate arrangements can be made for recipients. This could represent a significant increase in numbers of good quality organs available for transplantation, giving others waiting a greater opportunity of improving their quality of life, or just simply surviving.

It was argued that harvesting organs in this manner is both feasible and productive. The procedure would entail obtaining the patient's specific consent and ensuring a clear separation between the euthanasia procedure and organ procurement. Patients would undergo tests to assess the suitability of their organs and be prepared for surgery in hospital rather than being able to die at home. After completion of euthanasia, patients would be kept on a ventilator pending surgery.

Does this represent the beginning of a slippery slope? It is possible that the elderly or vulnerable may feel an increased obligation to end their lives with euthanasia, especially if they feel their lives have little value. Conversely, it may give those who are choosing to die by euthanasia a sense of wellbeing and purpose at the end of their lives, knowing that their death will benefit a significant number of other patients.

One concern is whether or not the organ donation is intended to be purely altruistic. Let us suppose for one moment that financial incentives or a form of payment for organ donation was introduced. If the donor received payment for the organs then there is a more significant concern. Vulnerable people who might feel they are a burden to their family both physically and financially may see the possibility of donating their organs at the end of their lives as both a release for their families, not only from having to care for their loved ones, but also from financial restraints. Poor and elderly patients may consider they have little left to live for, and to be able to support their families at the end of their lives by choosing euthanasia and agreeing to donate their organs may be seen as attractive. There might also be the concern that some less scrupulous families would also ply undue pressure upon their elderly relatives, for whom they care and provide, to choose an early death in order to release them from their burden. It would then be difficult to ensure that the patient's consent was free from influence and oppression.

ACTIVITY

Self-test questions

- To what extent is autonomy the overwhelming factor in favour of assisted suicide?
- What is autonomy balanced against? You might look to the judgments in *Pretty* and *Purdy* for guidance.
- What effect could legalising assisted suicide have on elderly and disabled people?
- Would euthanasia damage the doctor–patient relationship?
- Explain what is meant by the slippery slope in the context of assisted suicide and euthanasia.

SUMMARY

- Having read this chapter, it is possible that your own personal views on assisted suicide and PAS have been severely challenged.
- In the UK assisted suicide remains illegal although case law illustrates that the DPP is unlikely to prosecute.
- Since the DPP guidelines, introduced as a result of the case of *Purdy,* a patient can more easily determine whether or not there is likely to be a prosecution for aiding or abetting a suicide.
- There have been several attempts to legislate but the concern for protection of the public has on each occasion outweighed the autonomy of the individual.
- Legislation in some States in America and other European countries allows patients the self-determination to die at a time of their choosing, reflecting their desire to die with dignity; statistics do not necessarily show that elderly or vulnerable people are being abused.
- The ethics of assisted suicide and PAS largely focus on a person's autonomy to determine when to end their life, when they determine their life has become too unbearable to continue, balanced against protection of the vulnerable, for society fears they may be influenced or abused to end their lives prematurely. However, in countries where PAS is legal there is little evidence of this.

■ Despite ever-increasing public awareness and growing public opinion in support of assisted suicide in the UK there is, at present, little prospect for decriminalising assisted suicide or permitting PAS. Nevertheless, the prospects of prosecution for assisted suicide are limited, providing it can be clearly established that the person who aided and abetted acted entirely out of compassion and the guidelines set down by the DPP are stringently met.

SAMPLE ESSAY QUESTION

Kay suffers from a progressive degenerative condition, the effect of which will render her entirely dependent upon her partner Mark within a short period of time. She has decided after lengthy discussions with Mark that she wishes to end her life before she reaches the stage when she is no longer able to enjoy the quality of life she has previously experienced. However, there is likely to be a stage where she will need his assistance. Mark is willing to help her but she is concerned that assisted suicide remains illegal in the UK and he may be prosecuted if he helps her travel to Switzerland where she can legally end her life with assistance.

Advise Kay on her specific concerns. Not only is she concerned about the legal implications, but she would like to be more fully informed about the ethical issues that arise when considering assisted suicide.

- It would be appropriate in an introduction to this problem question to set out the relevant law.
- Although the Suicide Act 1961 decriminalised the offence of suicide, assisted suicide remains a criminal offence and therefore unlawful.
- Section 2(1) states that a person who aids, abets, counsel or procures the suicide of another can on conviction be sentenced to a maximum of 14 years. The DPP's consent is necessary under s 2(4) for a prosecution to proceed.
- Applying statute to this problem question, it is apparent that Mark can be criminally liable if he helps Kay to end her life by travelling to Switzerland where assisted suicide is legal.

- It is now necessary to turn to common law and consider the approach of the courts over recent years to the issue of assisted suicide. It would be appropriate to start with the case of *Pretty* (2002). She sought an assurance from the DPP that her husband would not be protected if he assisted her in her plea to end her life. Take care to refer to Arts 2, 3 and 8 as these are the grounds that Diane Pretty relied on. Ensure that you are able to explain that Art 8 could not be engaged as the interference under Art 8 (2) was justified.
- Ensure that you understand why *Pretty* is relevant. While it is relevant in its own right, the case of *Pretty* lays the groundwork for the case of *Purdy* (2009). These two cases must be dealt with in detail.
- Purdy wanted guidance on whether her husband would be prosecuted if he helped her travel to Switzerland to end her life. Her argument, which it is important to express, was that the DPP had produced insufficiently clear guidelines as to when and in what circumstances a prosecution may be brought. She argued that it was this failure that interfered with her Art 8 rights.

- When discussing *Pretty* and *Purdy*, firstly ensure that you have read the case and can demonstrate some depth of knowledge. Note the words of Lord Hope; either quote them or be able to express the judgment very clearly in your own words. The guidelines were insufficiently precise for Ms Purdy to understand the scope of the restrictions or to be able to appreciate the consequences. It was for this reason that the DPP were required to produce a new accessible policy.

- When you discuss case law, apply the case to the question. These cases are fundamentally important to the law on assisted suicide and no answer would be complete without them.
- It may be also prudent to mention the case of Daniel James, as the case was referred to in *Purdy* as an appropriate example of where the DPP did not prosecute. Most cases where parties have travelled to Switzerland to end their lives have not prosecuted.

- Next, discuss the DPP's response. From the guidelines one can determine that having considered the six public interest facts against prosecution, it is unlikely that Mark will be prosecuted. The reasons for this are that Kay has made a clear and informed decision to commit suicide. Mark is motivated by compassion. Apply the other factors, but if Kay is determined to end her life and Mark is motivated by no other reason apart from compassion, it is most unlikely that Mark will be prosecuted.

- Next, turn to the ethical advice. Although these comments appear briefer to the reader, an equal amount of time should be spent on the law and the ethics.
- Autonomy: consider this argument as a justification for permitting assisted suicide. Kay should be able to determine how she wants to live her life. See Lord Donaldson's comments in *Re T* (1992). If we deny Kay her autonomy, it suggests a lack of respect for her as a person. However, if we are to permit her autonomy, we also need to consider the impact on society as a whole.
- If Kay is allowed to end her life at a time she desires, it allows her to die with dignity. Although it is difficult to define precisely what is meant by the term 'dignity', and some academics refuse to acknowledge such a concept exists at all, it is still of value to Kay who may decide that her life lacks dignity when she requires help for all her personal tasks.
- Arguments against assisted suicide include the concern that elderly and disabled people would feel duty-bound to end their lives for fear of being a burden on others. Is this relevant to Kay? Does she feel duty-bound to end her life because of her disability? Should the State interfere and restrain her from being able to do so?

- Explore as many ethical arguments as you can. It is impressive if you are able to support your discussion with academic commentary. Apply the arguments to Kay throughout.

- In your conclusion, it will be the case that Mark is unlikely to be prosecuted. Your discussion of case law should reflect depth of knowledge and application of the law to the question.
- When discussing ethics, ensure that your arguments are coherent. Kay wishes to be advised. Therefore, your discussion should be informed and succinct.

Further reading

Allmark, P. (2008) 'Death with Dignity', *Journal of Medical Ethics*, 28, pages 255–7.

George, K. (2007) 'A woman's choice? The gendered risk of voluntary euthanasia and physician assisted suicide', *Medical Law Review*, 15 (1) (1–3).

Goodman, J. (2010) 'The case of Dr Munro: Are there lessons to be learnt?' *Medical Law Review*, 18 (4) pages 564–77.

Harris, J. (1995) 'Euthanasia and the Value of Life' in Keown (ed) *Euthanasia examined.* Cambridge: Cambridge University Press.

Jackson, E. (2009) *Medical law: Text, Cases and Materials*, second edition. Oxford: Oxford University Press.

Jochemsen, H. and Keown, J. (1999) 'Voluntary euthanasia under control? Further empirical evidence from the Netherlands' *Journal of Medical Ethics*, 25, pages 16–21.

Keown, J. (2002) *Euthanasia, ethics and public policy.* Cambridge: Cambridge University Press.

Keown, J. (2007) 'Physican-Assisted Suicide, Lord Joffe's Slippery Bill', *Medical Law Review*, 15 (1) pages 126–135.

Macklin, R. (2003) 'Dignity is a useless concept', *BMJ*, 327, pages 1419–20.

Mason, J. K. and Mulligan, D. (1996) 'Euthanasia by stages', *The Lancet*, 347, page 810.

Mullock, A. (2010) 'Overlooking the criminally compassionate: what are the implications of prosecutorial policy on encouraging or assisting suicide?' *Medical Law Review*, 18(4), pages 442–70.

Onwuteaka-Phillipsen, B., Van der Heide, A., Koper, D. *et al* (2003) 'Euthanasia and other end of life decisions in the Netherlands in 1990, 1995 and 2001', *The Lancet,* vol. 362, Issue 9381, pages 395–9.

Sheldon, T. (2007) Obituary to Andries Postma, *BMJ*, 334: 320.

Sjef Gevers (1996) 'Euthanasia: law and practice in The Netherlands', *British Medical Bulletin*, 52 (No. 2) pages 326–33.

Smets, T., Bilsen, J., Cohen, J. *et al* (2010) 'Reporting of euthanasia in medical practice in Flanders, Belgium: cross sectional analysis of reported and unreported cases', *BMJ*, c5174.

Van Der Wal, G., Van Der Maas, P. J., Bosma, J. M. *et al* (1996) 'Evaluation of the notification procedure for physician assisted suicide in the Netherlands', *New England Journal of Medicine*, 335, pages 1706–11.

Wilkinson, D. and Savulescu, J. (2011) 'Should we allow organ donation euthanasia? Alternatives for maximizing the number and quality of organs for transplantation', *Bioethics*, doi: 10.1111/j.1467-8519.2010.01811.

11

End-of-life decisions

By the end of this chapter you should be able to:

■ Demonstrate an understanding of the 'best interests' principle when applied to the issue of withholding or withdrawing treatment from a patient in a persistent vegetative state
■ Understand the effect of the Human Rights Act 1998 on common law in cases of this nature
■ Appreciate the legal and ethical complexities concerning withdrawal of treatment from adults and the minor child.

permanent vegetative state
a long term condition where where the patient is in a coma like state with no periods of wakefulness or has no cognitive function

Previously we have seen that where a patient lacks competence, medical professionals will act in the patient's best interests. Here, we explore what amounts to 'best interests' in circumstances where the patient lacks competence and had not contemplated how he or she would wish to be treated if the situation arose.

11.1 Withholding and withdrawing medical treatment

The seminal case of *Bland* (1993) below illustrates the difficult choices to be made, where a patient lacks competence due to a **permanent vegetative state** (PVS). How are decisions to treat such a patient made? Can treatment be withdrawn, and if so, when?

CASE EXAMPLE

Artificial ventilation
where the patient is dependent upon artificial ventilation to help them breathe.

nutrition and hydration
where the patient receives any form of nutrition of food and fluid via a tube

Airedale NHS Trust v Bland [1993] AC 789

Anthony Bland was a young man aged 17 years when he suffered appalling crush injuries at the Hillsborough football ground disaster in 1989. He was left in a permanent vegetative state. Patients suffering from such a condition can on occasions appear to be awake, and can respond to some stimuli but have no cognitive function. Three-and-a-half years later, it was apparent to the medical professionals caring for him that he was not going to improve. Together with his family, the Trust sought a declaration from the courts that:

1) **Artificial ventilation,** and artificial **nutrition and hydration** (ANH) and all forms of life-sustaining treatment be discontinued.
2) Once discontinued, life sustaining treatment be withheld.

The consequences of withdrawing life-sustaining treatment and then withholding treatment (switching off the life support machine) would have the effect of allowing Anthony Bland to die peacefully and without pain or distress.

The issues (1)

The doctors were seeking to withdraw and withhold life-sustaining treatment from Anthony Bland in order to cause his death. Would this not satisfy the physical element (*actus reus*) and mental element (*mens rea*) for murder?

In a majority decision, the court held that withdrawing and withholding life-sustaining treatment and switching off the life support machine could fulfil the definition of murder, which Lord Browne Wilkinson defined as 'causing the death of another with intent to do so'. Thus, it appears straightforward that a murder charge would in theory follow if the medical professional switched off a patient's life support machine. As far as the *mens rea* is concerned, the mental element of murder would be satisfied as there would be an intention to cause the patient's death. But what about the *actus reus*?

How was this problem overcome? The court distinguished between a *positive* act which causes the death of a person and an *omission* to act to prevent death. In these circumstances, the withdrawal of treatment would amount to an *omission* rather than a *positive act*. The reasoning for this was that, by withdrawing life-sustaining treatment, the patient was simply being returned back into the position that he was in when he first sustained the injury. Lord Browne Wilkinson expressed this reasoning:

JUDGMENT

'The positive act of removing the nasogastric tube presents more difficulty. It is undoubtedly a positive act, similar to switching off a ventilator in the case of a patient whose life is being sustained by artificial ventilation. But in my judgment in neither case should the act be classified as positive, since to do so would be to introduce intolerably fine distinctions.'

Lord Goff explained as follows:

JUDGMENT

'... discontinuation of life support is, for present purposes, no different from not initiating life support in the first place. In each case, the doctor is simply allowing his patient to die in the sense that he desisting from taking a step which might, in certain circumstances, prevent his patient from dying as a result of his pre-existing condition; and as a matter of general principle an omission such as this will not be unlawful unless it constitutes a breach of duty to the patient.'

Hence, since withdrawal and withholding of life-sustaining treatment could be described as an omission, the medical professionals could not be liable for murder.

The issues (2)

Could ANH be considered as basic care or treatment?

As ANH was considered to be treatment rather than basic care (such as washing), the treatment could be legitimately withdrawn. This is a controversial decision in itself, as inserting the tube in which the patient is fed is clearly treatment, but critics argue that the feeding of the patient with the use of the tube amounts to basic care.

The issues (3)

Does an omission as Lord Goff explained above amount to a breach of duty of care?

The duty of a medical professional only extends as far as acting in the patient's best interests. In this case, Anthony Bland's best interests were difficult to define as, due to his condition, life-sustaining treatment was no longer in his best interests. While this may sound callous, it is entirely accurate. As Lord Mustill said:

JUDGMENT

'... although the termination of his life is not in the best interests of Anthony Bland, his best interests in being kept alive have also disappeared'.

The court concluded that it was not in the best interests of Anthony Bland to continue to receive life-sustaining treatment, not because it was preferable he should die rather than to be living, but that continuing treatment would no longer benefit him. It was not therefore in his best interests that it should continue.

The issues (4)

How can a medical professional withdraw and withhold a patient's treatment when such an act would violate the most sacrosanct of principles – the sanctity of life? Such a violation goes against the understanding of every medical professional's vocational commitment endorsed in the Hippocratic Oath.

Lord Keith addressed this very point, pointing out that the principle of sanctity of life:

JUDGMENT

'... is not an absolute one ... In my judgment it does no violence to the principle to hold that it is lawful to cease to give medical treatment and care to a PVS patient who has been in the state for over three years, considering that to do so involves invasive manipulation of the patient's body to which he has not consented and which confers no benefit upon him'.

Similarly, in cases where an adult competent patient refuses to be treated:

JUDGMENT

'the principle of the sanctity of human life must yield to the principle of self-determination ... On this basis, it has been held that a patient of sound mind may, if properly informed, require that life should be discontinued'.

Hence, a competent patient's autonomy outweighs the sanctity of life.

One further point worthy of consideration is the effect of withdrawing and withholding medical treatment of a PVS patient. Put simply, once life-sustaining treatment is withdrawn, the patient will die. If a patient is assisted in his breathing by artificial ventilation then the act of withdrawing ventilation leads to a speedy death. If the patient is only reliant on ANH, which is then withdrawn, the patient will not endure a quick death but will 'die slowly, though painlessly, over a period of weeks from lack of food'. It is worth contemplating the difference between this act and passive active euthanasia; how far apart are the two acts? In the case of *Bland* the court conveniently described the withdrawal of treatment as an omission, rather than an act, so it becomes more difficult to draw any parallel between the omissions and euthanasia. Once ANH has been withdrawn, it is challenging to be able to morally justify allowing the person to die from thirst or hunger. While painless for the patient, it is far from painless for the family who, knowing their loved one is dying, has to endure the emotional agony of watching the patient fade away. Moreover, how does allowing someone to die from thirst and hunger suggest compatibility with the principle of sanctity of life? Lord Browne-Wilkinson commented:

JUDGMENT

'How can it be lawful to allow a patient to die slowly, though painlessly, over a period of weeks from lack of food but unlawful to produce his immediate death by a lethal injection, thereby saving his family from yet another ordeal to add to the tragedy that has already struck them? I find it difficult to find a moral answer to that question. But that is undoubtedly the law'.

The future

Finally on the case of *Bland*, the court indicated that it would be necessary for future cases to apply to the courts for a declaration that treatment could be withdrawn and withheld in order for a body of practice decisions to be established. Thus, every PVS case would be dealt with on its merits, which would ensure that the patient was adequately protected and the public could have confidence in the decisions of the court and the medical profession. It would also serve as protection for the doctor, in order to avoid damage to the patient–doctor relationship.

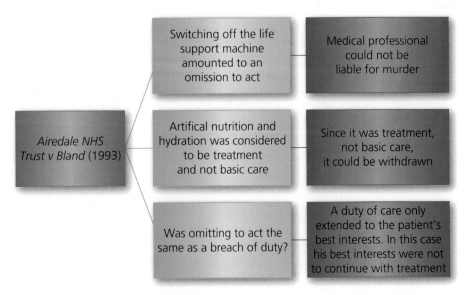

Figure 11.1 The judgment of *Bland* (1993)

11.2 Post *Bland* (1993)

After *Bland* (1993), a number of cases involving patients in PVS came before the courts. One of the first cases to deal with facts similar to *Bland* is discussed below.

CASE EXAMPLE

nasogastric tube
is used for feeding
artificially

Frenchay Healthcare Trust v S [1994] 2 All ER 403

Following a drug overdose, the patient sustained severe brain damage. He had been receiving nutrition and hydration by way of a **nasogastric tube** but this had ceased to be possible and a tube had been surgically inserted into his stomach instead. The tube had become displaced and an operation was needed in order to replace it. Without the operation, he would not be able to carry on living. The Trust sought an emergency declaration not to replace the tube as the treating doctors were of the opinion that it was not in S's best interests to undergo surgery.

The medical evidence was not as conclusive as in *Bland* (1993). There was evidence that S may have had some very limited awareness and might be able to, on some level, suffer pain. Nevertheless, the court accepted the opinion of those treating S that his condition was permanent and had little hope of recovery. The court allowed the emergency declaration.

Here, the court indicated that while, as a general rule, the Trust should seek a declaration and thereafter allow the court an opportunity to investigate the facts in detail, there are situations where there may be insufficient time for detailed reflection in the manner recommended by the House of Lords in *Bland* (1993). If the court is under pressure from emergency applications, it does not have the benefit of weighing up detailed expert advice, and perhaps has insufficient time to give due consideration to the most crucial of decisions. The effect of this decision is to relax the restrictions that *Bland* (1993) sought to impose, as this case demonstrates there was even some question as to whether S was in a PVS at all.

We can see in the case examples below that the courts have not automatically adopted the same approach as in *Bland*.

CASE EXAMPLE

NHS v J [2006] All ER 73

The patient, a 53-year-old woman, had suffered a brain **haemorrhage** and had been in a PVS for a period of three years. The Trust, medical experts and the family were of the view that medical treatment should cease. When the case reached court, evidence was put before the judge that made him question the possibility of an alternative treatment which might stimulate the patient. The family did not wish her to be treated, believing she would suffer as a result. The court refused to allow the declaration and instead authorised a short course of alternative treatment. Subsequently, following treatment which did not benefit the patient, the parties returned to court and withdrawal of treatment was authorised as it was, after a trial of the alternative treatment, considered in her best interests.

---

haemorrhage
a considerable level of bleeding from ruptured blood vessels

Professional guidance

The BMA issued guidelines in 2007 entitled *Withholding and Withdrawing Life Prolonging Medical Treatment: Guidance for Decision Making* (third edition) which endorses the common law approach in *Bland* (1993). In further guidance on end-of-life decisions in 2009, the BMS stated with specific reference to patients in PVS that:

QUOTATION

'When medical treatment ceases to provide a net benefit to the patient, this primary goal of medicine cannot be realised and the justification for intervening is gone. Unless some other justification can be demonstrated, most people would accept that treatment should not be prolonged. The BMA does not believe that it is appropriate to prolong life at all costs, with no regard to its quality or the burdens of the intervention.'

Thus, the guidance explains that the primary purpose for intervention in a patient's medical condition is to provide a benefit and, once that ceases to be a possibility, the justification for intervention ceases to exist. The guidance continues as follows

QUOTATION

'Patients with progressive, degenerative conditions can have their lives prolonged considerably but this will not necessarily reverse a patient's disease. Other patients, for example those with very severe brain damage, may remain stable for many years if life-prolonging treatment is provided, but this may be with no hope of recovering more than very minimal levels of awareness of their surroundings. They may lack the ability to interact with others or the capacity for self-directed action. In such severely damaged patients, treatment or intervention to prolong life by artificial means may fail to provide sufficient benefit to justify the intervention and the proper course of action may be to withhold or withdraw further treatment.'

It is apparent from the above that withdrawal of life-prolonging treatment is not necessarily confined to situations where the patient is in a PVS. The case below illustrates precisely that point.

CASE EXAMPLE

Re D (Adult: Medical Treatment) [1998] 1 FLR 411

D had suffered serious brain damage as a result of a road traffic accident. The Trust sought a declaration that it would be lawful to withdraw ANH. Although she was described as being in a PVS and had no awareness, it was felt this was not a conclusive diagnosis as the Royal College of Physicians guidelines 1993 had not been precisely met.

Despite the fact the criteria were not fulfilled, Sir Stephen Brown was of the view that the patient experienced 'no evidence of any meaningful life whatsoever' and was suffering a 'living death'. He concluded that it was not in the 'patient's best interests artificially to keep her body alive'. The declaration was granted.

The case shows considerable departure from the scale of illness indicated in *Bland* (1993) as, although the patient was severely disabled and had limited awareness, she was not, according to the Royal College of Physicians, in a PVS as such.

CASE EXAMPLE

Re R (Adult: Medical Treatment) [1996] 2 FLR

R suffered from serious learning difficulties and cerebral palsy. He had a serious brain condition and it was likely he was both deaf and blind. He lived in a residential home but had been admitted to hospital on a number of occasions. R's psychiatrist was of the opinion that the next time he was admitted to hospital with a life-threatening condition, he should not be resuscitated. Members of staff were sufficiently concerned about the Do Not Resuscitate order that they sought judicial review of the decision.

In deciding whether the Do Not Resuscitate order was lawful, the court reasoned it was important to act in the patient's best interest, even if that meant not taking every step to prolong life. In these circumstances, Sir Stephen Brown said 'it would not be in the best interests of R to subject him to cardio-pulmonary resuscitation in the event of his suffering a cardiac arrest', and that it was a question for medical professionals whether to withhold future medical treatment 'in the light of prevailing circumstances'.

Whereas in *Bland* (1993) the court indicated that all PVS cases should seek a declaration from the courts, the same does not necessarily apply to non-PVS patients. Since the court considered it to be in R's best interests not to resuscitate him in the future, the case demonstrates the apparent ease with which it can be determined to be in the patient's best interests for treatment to be withdrawn. Arguably, if the patient is not in pain, best interests should be to continue treatment. However, the courts maintain that, where the quality of the patient's life is such that continuing treatment would render the patient's life intolerable, treatment could be withheld.

KEY FACTS

Key facts on post-*Bland* cases

Case	Principle
Frenchay Healthcare Trust v S (1994)	Allowed the emergency declaration not to replace the feeding tube even though the patient was not in exactly the same PVS as Anthony Bland.
Re R (Adult: Medical Treatment) (1996)	Patient was not in a PVS but had a number of complex difficulties. Court accepted that it would not be in his best interests to resuscitate in the event of a life-threatening episode.
Re D (Adult: Medical Treatment) (1998)	The patient was not in a PVS but there was no evidence of meaningful life. A declaration to withdraw ANH was granted.
NHS v J (2006)	The court ordered a short course of alternative treatment first as there was a view that it may be of some benefit. Once this proved to be unsuccessful, the declaration sought was allowed.

11.3 The impact of the Human Rights Act 1998 on *Bland* (1993)

The case below was one of the earliest to rely on the provisions of the HRA 1998 after it came into force in 2000. From the judgment it is apparent that human rights legislation has had little direct effect and the courts instead relied on the common law principle of 'best interests' by applying the judgment in *Airedale NHS Trust v Bland* (1993).

CASE EXAMPLE

NHS Trust A v M, MHS Trust B v H [2001] Fam 348

The case concerns two patients, M and H, who had both been in a PVS for periods of three years and nine months respectively. The medical teams of both patients had decided that it was not in their best interests to continue ANH, the withdrawal of which would cause neither of the patients any suffering. Both Trusts, supported by the patient's families in each case, sought a declaration from the courts that it was lawful to discontinue ANH in respect of both patients, bearing in mind Sched 1, HRA 1998 which states that:

SECTION

'Everyone's right to life shall be protected by law. No one shall be deprived of his life intentionally save in the execution of a sentence of a court following his conviction of a crime for which this penalty is provided by law.'

Although it was obvious that the withdrawal of ANH from patients who were in a PVS would bring about their death, the court concluded (as in *Bland* (1993)) that where the decision to withdraw treatment was made by a team of medical professionals who had come to a decision that treatment was no longer in the patient's best interests, the withdrawal of treatment was an *omission* to act rather than an intentional act which deprives the patient of his life. The term 'deprivation of life' was said to confer a positive act by someone who was acting on behalf of the State rather than an omission to act. In these particular circumstances, Art 2 was not violated as the circumstances were not such that a positive obligation on the State to prolong life was imposed. Art 3 did not apply in cases where patients were in a PVS since they had no appreciation of any treatment they were receiving or that may be withdrawn.

CASE EXAMPLE

A Hospital v W [2007] EWHC 425

Following a cycling accident, W was left profoundly brain-damaged and had been in a PVS for at least a year. The hospital, with the family's support, sought a declaration that it was no longer in her best interests to receive life-sustaining medical treatment and thus, treatment could be lawfully withdrawn.

The court applied *Bland*, confirming that W was in a PVS and life-sustaining treatment could not be of any benefit to her as there was no prospect of recovery. The court then confirmed that, in these circumstances, the withdrawal of artificial hydration and nutrition did not violate Art 3, ECHR.

Professional guidance

The most recent advice from the GMC entitled *Treatment and care towards the end of life* came into force in July 2010. The advice builds upon common law decisions, ethical principles, the Mental Capacity Act 2005 and the Incapacity (Scotland) Act 2000 together with the requirements of the Human Rights Act 2000. At the time of writing, this guidance represents the most up-to-date guidance in relation to end-of-life decisions. The guidance states that a medical professional 'must not be motivated by a desire to bring about the patient's death, and must start from a presumption in favour of prolonging life'. Therefore, all reasonable steps must be taken to 'prolong a patient's life but there is no absolute obligation to prolong life irrespective of the consequences of the patient's views, if they are known or can be found out'. The guidance continues by explaining that the doctors must decide whether it is in the patient's best interests to continue treatment and must consult with the patient's relatives if appropriate (paragraphs 15-16) and other members of the patient's healthcare team.

11.4 Patients in a minimally conscious state

Some 18 years have passed since the judgment in *Bland* and the recent case of *W (by her litigation friend, B) v M (by her litigation friend, the Official Solicitor) and S and A NHS Primary Care Trust* 2011 EWHC 2443 discussed below. This period of time is hugely significant in terms of medical development as a clear distinction can be drawn between patients in a persistent vegetative state, now referred to as VS, and those in a minimally conscious state (MCS). With the benefit of new assessment methods a patient's true condition can be determined and expert evidence heard in the case below suggests that patients originally diagnosed as VS could now be diagnosed as MCS.

The term coined by an American research team in 2002 distinguishes MCS from VS in a number of crucial ways and is defined as a

'... condition of severely altered consciousness in which minimal but definite behaviour evidence of self or environmental awareness is demonstrated' Neurology Feb. 12, 2002 Vol. 58, No. 3 349–363)

The implication of the distinction for legal purposes cannot be underestimated since a patient in VS is likely to be permitted a declaration for life-sustaining treatment to be withdrawn and withheld, following the judgment in *Bland*, but for those patients who in the future are declared to be in a MCS the courts must closely consider the medical evidence in order that the patient's best interests are carefully weighed and life-sustaining treatment is not unethically withdrawn.

CASE EXAMPLE

W (by her litigation friend, B) v M (by her litigation friend, the Official Solicitor) and S and A NHS Primary Care Trust [2011] EWHC 2443 (Fam)

M was a 43-year-old active woman when she suffered from viral encephalitis which left her with extensive brain damage. Since 2003 she has been entirely dependent on others for her care and has been fed artificially. Initially she was in a coma from which she emerged. She was then diagnosed as being in a PVS or VS state. In 2007 the family together with the Trust's support sought a declaration that life-sustaining treatment including artificial nutrition and hydration be withdrawn. Although evidence from the family was that M would not wish to live in this condition, and she had indicated as much prior to the onset of encephalitis, she had not made an Advance Directive. Had she done so, and it was valid and applicable, it would have been unlawful for the Trust to continue to treat her.

The medical evidence

In preparation for the application, M underwent a number of tests which determined she was not in a VS but a MCS. M is able to demonstrate levels of consciousness, albeit inconsistently, and can on occasions respond to commands. These occasions are not reflex actions and, thus, on some level there is an element of functioning to M's life. She can, according to the evidence, experience emotions and pleasure from either music or from interaction with people caring for her.

The issue

This was the first time a court had to determine whether a patient who was in a MCS could have life-sustaining treatment withdrawn. The issue for the court to determine was whether it was in M's best interest for life-sustaining treatment including artificial nutrition and hydration to be withdrawn. M's best interests were defined by application of section 4 of the Mental Capacity Act 2005 and by case law, primarily *Airedale NHS Trust v Bland*. Accordingly, with the MCA in mind the views and wishes of the family would be taken into account and could bear great weight in the court's judgment.

In situations where patients are in a MCS, the court can adopt a 'balance sheet' approach having consideration of all the facts and the evidence, which in each case will be unique to the next, in order to determine whether to err on the side of the fundamental principle of preservation of the patient's life (which in itself is not absolute, according to Lord Goff in *Bland*) or permit a patient to 'die in dignity' and, in M's case, adhere to the family's wishes.

The Official Solicitor argued if it was accepted M was in a stable MCS, it would be inappropriate to adopt the balance sheet argument as it would be unlawful to withhold and withdraw life-sustaining treatment from her. Baker J rejected this approach maintaining it was necessary to compare the advantages of withdrawing treatment as against the advantages of continuing treatment.

The judgment

Having set out the advantages and disadvantages based upon the evidence and facts of this particular case, Baker J held in favour of the preservation of life, and in doing so the application for a declaration permitting withdrawal and withholding of life-sustaining treatment was unsuccessful. Although Baker J took the family's wishes into account together with their evidence that M would not wish to live in this condition, he concluded that the evidence would not carry great weight. The court also rejected expert evidence that her life was largely surrounded by negative experiences, choosing instead to focus of the more positive aspects of her life. The 'Do Not Resuscitate' order remained in place as it was accepted that it would not be in M's best interests in her condition to receive cardio-pulmonary resuscitation.

The future

In setting down guidelines for the future, Baker J stated as follows:

- Cases involving application for declarations concerning patients in MCS should be made to the Court of Protection.
- Cases will be allocated to one High Court Judge who will be responsible for time management and will hear the final hearing.
- Patients should be clearly diagnosed as early as possible with accuracy in order that the correct diagnosis as to the patient's condition is made.

Baker J also stated that it was 'alarming' that legal funding had not been available for the family to apply for the declaration and that it was 'intolerable' that they had to rely on the goodwill of the solicitors to represent them pro bono. Non-means-tested funding should be available for cases of this nature, failing which, it was certainly possible that Article 6 of ECHR could be infringed.

The significance of the judgment cannot be over estimated. The onus is upon the medical professionals to ensure that patients are adequately tested so that a condition that may have been diagnosed as VS is not a much higher degree of awareness such as MCS. One dare not contemplate whether previous patients have had treatment withdrawn and withheld when modern assessment tools would diagnose a MCS rather than a VS state but with medical advances comes increased responsibility that such a case cannot occur in the future.

While we have every sympathy with M and her family, if the law was to permit life-sustaining treatment to be withheld in M's case, what we are really saying as able bodied people is that those patients, who due to a variety of conditions whether minimally responsive or not, have lives less valuable than ours and those lives are not worth living. If M has some pleasure in life and any pain and suffering she may experience can be appropriately managed, it must be unethical to determine that she has a life that has no value. It is indeed a weighing scale between advantages and disadvantages but, if there are advantages and pleasures to her life, albeit limited, then it is ethically unacceptable to determine that treatment can be withdrawn and withheld.

Such is the future for patients in a minimally conscious state and clearly each case must be judged on its merits but this case is also likely to pave the way for patients in other conditions of awareness. Perhaps one would agree that it is likely to only be a matter of months or years before a patient with 'locked in syndrome' applies to the court in a similar vain.

ACTIVITY

Self-test questions

Ensure that your answers are supported by case law where appropriate.

- Ensure that you understand what is meant by a PVS.
- Carefully explain how treatment could be legally withheld and withdrawn from Anthony Bland.
- How have cases subsequent to the seminal case of *Airedale NHS Trust v Bland* (1993) been decided?
- How has the above judgment been applied to cases which do not fit the criteria of PVS exactly?
- What effect has HRA 1998 had on this area of the law?

11.5 The Human Rights Act 1998 and end-of-life decisions

In Chapter 10 we examined the cases of *R (Pretty) v DPP* (2002) and *R (Purdy) v DPP* (2009) in which both applicants' arguments were based upon provisions in the Human Rights Act 1998. In *R (Purdy) v DPP* (2009), the House of Lords accepted in principle that her desire to end her life through the means of assisted suicide fell within the scope of Art 8. This was a significant development from *R (Pretty) v DPP* (2002) where the House of Lords had rejected Ms Pretty's argument based on Art 8, and she was forced to take her case to the European Court of Human Rights. In *Pretty v UK* (2002) the Court accepted that Art 8 was engaged, as she had a right to determine for herself the way in which she should end her life. The court however then derogated under Art 8(2) saying that it was both necessary and proportionate to prohibit assisted suicide in order to protect the vulnerable members of society.

In *R (Purdy) v DPP* (2009), the House of Lords accepted that she had a right under Art 8 to determine how to end her life, even if this entailed assisted suicide. The court then (as in *Pretty*) argued that the derogation under Art 8(2) could be justified but that the derogation had to be justified in law. In order for the derogation to be justifiable, the law had to be sufficiently clear in order that people who were contemplating assisted suicide knew and understood the potential impact of the law. The law was not clear and it was this point that led to the court directing the DPP to produce appropriate guidelines.

From these cases, we get a flavour of the impact of human rights legislation. Despite the apparent success of Debbie Purdy, this is not a complete human rights success story. The value of HRA 1998 in this respect was to identify the lack of clarity in the law and it was the court who sought to rectify this element. The court was not permitting assisted suicide; indeed the court was adamant that the derogation from Art 8 was justified in order to protect vulnerable elements of society; the value of the human rights should not therefore be overplayed in these seminal cases.

It should also be remembered that, as far as Art 2 is concerned, the European Court of Human Rights in *Pretty v UK* (2002) unequivocally stated that:

JUDGMENT

'Article 2 cannot, without a distortion of language, be interpreted as conferring the diametrically opposite right, namely a right to die; nor can it create a right to self-determination in the sense of conferring on an individual the entitlement to choose death rather than life.'

It is in this direction we now turn our focus. The case below illustrates the use of Arts 2, 3 and 8 in a case where the patient wished clarification that ANH would *not* be withdrawn if he became incompetent. We have already explored the law in *Re C (Adult: Refusal of Medical Treatment)* (1994) where it was established that a competent patient has every right to refuse medical treatment even where it will lead to his or her death. The question we now ask is whether a patient can with the use of HRA 1998 *insist* on medical treatment.

CASE EXAMPLE

R v (Burke) v GMC [2005] 3 FCR 169

Leslie Burke suffers from a progressive degenerative disease and, at some point in the future, he will require ANH in order to keep him alive. If ANH was withdrawn or withheld, he would die of starvation (nutrition) or thirst (hydration). He was concerned that the GMC guidelines on the withholding and withdrawing of ANH were incompatible with the law and would in any event be contrary to his wishes to *continue* to receive ANH, without which if he was incompetent, he would simply die. He brought proceedings for judicial review and sought to rely on the provisions of HRA 1998 to enforce his argument that he had a right to receive continuing treatment.

His argument is seen in Figure 11.2.

Article 2: right to life	Article 3: right not to be subjected to inhuman and degrading treatment	Article 8: right to a private and family life
• Withdrawing or withholding ANH against his express wishes competently made would violate Art 2. • Refusing an incompetent patient ANH could amount to a violation of Art 2.	• Withdrawing or withholding ANH against his express wishes would violate Art 3.	• Withdrawing or withholding ANH against his express wishes violates Art 8.

Figure 11.2 Leslie Burke's arguments to receive continuing treatment

The Court of Appeal overturned the court of first instance, where Munby J had upheld Mr Burke's arguments deciding that the GMC guidelines did breach his Convention rights. Crucially, the court recognised that while the patient's autonomy was paramount, it did not follow that there was a right to insist on specific treatment.

Lord Phillips explained as follows:

JUDGMENT

'Autonomy and the right to self-determination do not entitle the patient to insist on receiving a particular medical treatment regardless of the nature of the treatment. Insofar as a doctor has a legal obligation to provide treatment this cannot be founded simply upon the fact that the patient demands it.'

Thus, the principle we derive from this case is that a patient cannot insist on medical treatment without reservation. However the court continued by explaining:

JUDGMENT

'where life depends upon the continued provision of ANH there can be no question of the supply of ANH not being clinically indicated unless a clinical decision has been taken that the life in question should come to an end. This is not a question that can lawfully be taken in the case of a competent patient who expresses the wish to remain alive.'

The court explained that where ANH was clinically indicated then it would be provided. Here, the focus was on 'duty' rather than 'rights'. The court put is as follows:

JUDGMENT

'So far as ANH is concerned, there is no need to look far for the duty to provide this. Once a patient is accepted into a hospital, the medical staff come under a positive duty at common law to care for the patient ... A fundamental aspect of this positive duty of care is a duty to take such steps as are reasonable to keep the patient alive. Where ANH is necessary to keep the patient alive, the duty of care will normally require the doctors to supply ANH.'

But where clinical indications are that ANH is not in the patient's best interest, it will not be given and can be withdrawn. Hence, even though the competent patient may express his wishes to life-prolonging treatment, if he loses competency and the circumstances are such that it is not in the patient's best interests to receive ANH, this withdrawal or withholding will not violate Art 2.
The court expressed this as follows:

JUDGMENT

'where life involves an extreme amount of pain, discomfort or indignity to a patient, who is sentient but not competent and who has manifested no wish to be kept alive, these circumstances may absolve the doctors of the positive duty to keep the patient alive. Equally the courts have recognised that there may be no duty to keep alive a patient who is in a persistent vegetative state.'

The judgment of the court despite its potential complexities is surprisingly straightforward. The GMC guidelines were entirely acceptable. If a medical professional withdraws life-prolonging treatment from a *competent patient* who has not refused medical treatment, it follows that the patient's right to life will be violated and it is likely that any act by the medical professional will be tantamount to murder. However, where the medical professional considers ANH not to be in the *incompetent* patient's best interests, ANH could be withdrawn or withheld, despite any advance directive being made while the patient was competent.

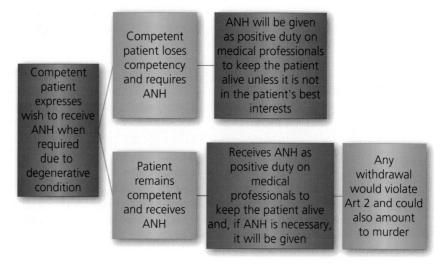

Figure 11.3 The judgments in this case

Mr Burke took his case to the European Court of Human Rights *(Burke v UK Application 19807/06* (2006)). The court rejected any suggestion that his rights were breached. In concluding that his application had been 'manifestly unfounded' they repeated the principle that patients could not demand treatment unless the treatment was clinically indicated and, furthermore, there was no legal obligation on the medical profession to seek prior authorisation before withdrawing ANH.

11.6 The minor child

Issues such as withdrawing and withholding medical treatment from the minor child are invariably distressing, primarily for the bereaved families. One must also regard the bigger picture–the distress caused to the treating medical professionals, the dilemmas faced by the courts, and also the student of such a topic who has to cast aside their own feelings and focus on the principles of the case. The judgments illustrate that, regardless of the severity of the condition or the parent's wishes as regards their child's treatment, the courts' approach is to act in the best interests of the child.

CASE EXAMPLE

Re B (A Minor) (Wardship: Medical Treatment) [1990] 3 All ER 927

B suffered from Down's syndrome and had an intestinal blockage. She required an operation to relieve her condition, without which she could die. Her health was such that she had a life expectancy of 20–30 years. Her parents refused to consent to the operation, being of the view that it was more compassionate to allow her to die than to live with learning difficulties. The local authority made her a ward of court and sought an order from the courts that the operation should be carried out.

At first instance the judge respected the parents' view and refused to make the order. On appeal, the focus altered. It was not the parents' wishes that were the overriding consideration but what was in the best interests of the child.

The crucial point for consideration was indicated by Templeman J, who stated:

JUDGMENT

'at the end of the day it devolves on this court in this particular instance to decide whether the life of this child is demonstrably going to be so awful that in effect the child must be condemned to die, or whether the life of this child is still so imponderable that it would be wrong for her to be condemned to die'.

In a similar sentiment, Dunn LJ referred to a life that would be 'intolerable' and so full of 'pain and suffering' that it would not be in the child's best interests to undergo the operation.

In this case, the reality was whether to permit an operation to proceed which would give this patient a further life expectancy of 20–30 years or whether to end the life of the patient who suffered from learning difficulties just because she also had an intestinal complaint.

The court allowed the appeal on the basis that the child could survive another 20–30 years with the operation, albeit with disability. Hence, the court weighed up her condition and, determined that her life would be neither 'intolerable' nor 'awful' if she carried on living and given her life expectancy, considered that the operation should proceed. Given that there are approximately 60,000 people suffering from Down's Syndrome in the UK, any other decision by the court would have the effect of condemning those who suffer from Down's Syndrome as having lives that are not worth living.

CASE EXAMPLE

Re C (A Minor) (Medical Treatment) [1998] 1 FCR 1

A young girl suffered from **spinal muscular atrophy** – a fatal condition for which on occasions she required assistance with ventilation. She had been on ventilation in intensive care for several weeks, and it was the doctor's view that her condition was so severe that ventilation as a form of life-sustaining treatment was of no benefit to her. Continuing ventilation was in their opinion simply continuing her distress and suffering without providing her with any clear benefit. A clinical decision was made that, in the event of a further respiratory arrest, ventilation would not be carried out. Her parents as Orthodox Jews believed a person should not stand aside and watch another die where steps can be taken to avoid it. Such steps were, in this case, ventilation. The doctors sought an order from the courts that non-ventilation would be a lawful course of action.

In a heart-rending judgment, Sir Stephen Brown referred to the term 'no chance' situation. This phrase is defined in the Royal College of Paediatrics and Child Health's (1997) publication entitled *Withholding or Withdrawing Lifesaving Treatment in Children, a Framework for Practice*. The guidance defines 'no chance' situations as:

spinal muscular atrophy
a condition which causes progressive muscular degeneration

QUOTATION

'where the child has such severe disease that life-sustaining treatment simply delays death without significant alleviation of suffering. Medical treatment in this situation may thus be deemed inappropriate …'

Bearing the guidance in mind, Brown continued that C's condition is:

JUDGMENT

'so grave that it is not in her best interests that she should be further ventilated, and if, when ventilation is withdrawn, it should not be reinstituted in the event of a further respiratory arrest. The doctor's view is that such treatment would be futile, it would not improve her quality of life and would subject her to further suffering without conferring any benefit.'

The parents wished to continue treatment, but their preferred course of action was one which the doctors could not clinically support. In these circumstances, the courts could not act in the child's best interests by disregarding the medical evidence before them. Accordingly the court granted an order in the terms sought by the doctors.

The judgment in *Re C* illustrates the challenges faced by the courts when parents of a minor child cannot through religious observance or complex emotions accept clinical advice as to the best interests for the child. The real difficulty lies not with the courts but with the relationship between the medical professional and the child's parents when the course of action cannot be agreed between them. The court referred to the judgment in *Re J (a minor) (medical treatment)* [1992] 2 FCR 753 (which we consider in more detail shortly) and in particular the judgment of Lord Donaldson, where he stated:

JUDGMENT

'No one can dictate the treatment to be given to the child – neither court, parents nor doctors. There are checks and balances. The doctors can recommend treatment A in preference to treatment B. They can also refuse to adopt treatment C on the grounds that it is medically contra-indicated or for some other reason is a treatment which they could not conscientiously administer. The court or parents for their part can refuse to consent to treatment A or B or both, but cannot insist on treatment C. The inevitable and desirable result is that choice of treatment is in some measure a joint decision of the doctors and the court or parents.'

And, in the absence of parental consent, the court must act in the best interests of the child.

The leading case of withdrawing and withholding medical treatment from a child is discussed below.

CASE EXAMPLE

Re J (a minor) (Wardship: medical treatment) [1991] Fam 33

J had been born prematurely. He had suffered brain damage and required artificial ventilation. An episode in which he had stopped breathing left him reliant on artificial ventilation. The doctors treating him were of the opinion that he was likely to become a serious spastic quadriplegic with a shortened life expectancy. The only real sensation he would be able to experience would be pain. The local authority whose care he was in sought an order that in the event of further convulsions, he should not be resuscitated by means of artificial ventilation unless it seemed to be right to do so.

Taylor LJ identified three important issues:

1) Firstly, the best interests of the child must be the court's 'prime and paramount' consideration. In order to achieve that goal, although the views of the parents should be taken into account, they cannot override the court's view of the child's best interests. This principle was clearly relevant in *Re C (A Minor) (Medical Treatment)* (1998) where the parents could not accept the clinicians' judgment that their child should not be artificially ventilated should the need arise.

2) The court explained that the sanctity of life was so important that it 'imposes a strong presumption in favour of taking all steps capable of preserving it, save in exceptional circumstances'. However, as the court observed, the difficulty is to define what the exceptional circumstances are.

3) Given that the court is only concerned with prolonging life, the court took great care in emphasising that 'the court never sanctions steps to terminate life. That would be unlawful. There is no question of approving, even in a case of the most horrendous disability, a course aimed at terminating life or accelerating death.'

Having emphasised these crucial principles, the court now had to consider the plight of a seriously ill child and the quality of life he would enjoy if life-sustaining treatment was given.

The approach of the court was to 'judge the quality of life the child would have to endure if given the treatment and decide whether in all the circumstances such a life would be so afflicted as to be intolerable to that child'. The emphasis is on the quality of life to the *child*, not to the medical professional making that decision.

Thus the test should be 'whether the child in question, if capable of exercising sound judgment, would consider the life intolerable'.

Having set down the principles by which cases of this nature should be approached, the court concluded that if J was to be artificially ventilated, the act itself would result in deterioration in his condition, and the consequent treatment would lead to further distress and suffering. These factors combined led the court to conclude that the quality of life would be so poor as to justify the medical professionals' view.

This case contrasts to *Re B* (1990) above as B's Down's Syndrome was not 'demonstrably ... so awful' or so 'intolerable' as to justify the court sanctioning the end of B's life. In J, sadly, the condition was considerably different. J was profoundly brain-damaged with severe associated disabilities. In these circumstances, the court approved the withholding of life-sustaining treatment. Perhaps these two cases are relatively easy to distinguish, as J's disability is most apparent, whereas B's Down's Syndrome still enabled her to live a lengthy and content life. The difficulty for the courts may be in determining a case which on the facts falls in the middle of severe intolerable disability and disability that is not so profound as to be judged either 'intolerable' or 'awful'.

CASE EXAMPLE

An NHS Trust v B [2006] EWHC 507 (Fam)

An 18-month-old boy suffered from severe and degenerative spinal muscular atrophy. His life expectancy was limited. The Trust sought a declaration that it would be lawful to withdraw ventilation from him as the burden of permanent ventilation combined with unknown cognitive function was so great that it outweighed any potential benefits. It would therefore be in his best interests that it would be withdrawn. His parents did not agree with the Trust's position and sought a declaration that a procedure be performed in order that he could receive long-term ventilation.

In an unusual judgment that effectively sided with the parents, Holman J recognised that the welfare of the child was their paramount consideration and, with that point in mind, the court rejected the doctors' medical evidence supporting withdrawal of medical treatment. The child was aware of his family and experienced other pleasures despite the fact that he had never left hospital and his experiences were very limited. Even though he suffered from some pain and suffering, these burdens did not outweigh the obvious benefits and accordingly ventilation would continue, although it would not be in his best interests for any further invasive procedures to be carried out as these could impose additional pain.

The case below, heard soon after, illustrates a painful contrast.

CASE EXAMPLE

Re K (a minor) (2006) EWHC 1007 (Fam)

The Trust treating the child K sought a declaration to remove the feeding tube from her abdomen, allowing her to die peacefully. She had been born prematurely with an inherited severe condition which caused muscle weakness. She had to be fed via a line into her abdomen and, aged five-and-a-half months, her condition was so poor that it was not a question of if she would die but when she would die. All parties, including her parents, agreed with the medical professional opinion that life-prolonging treatment should cease.

Sir Mark Potter granted the declaration, describing her life as one filled with 'regular pain, distress and discomfort and unrelieved by the pleasures of eating'. In contrast to Baby B above, she had no pleasurable experiences and, given that her life expectancy was less than a year, she was unlikely to have any in her short existence. As there could be no improvement in her condition, the court concluded it would be in her best interests to remove the tube, ensure she was pain-free and allow her to die in the care of those who loved her.

Key facts on the minor child

Case	Judgment
Re B (A Minor) (Wardship: Medical Treatment) (1990)	The best interests of the child rather than the parents' views were the paramount consideration. The child's life would not be so intolerable or full of pain and suffering to justify supporting the parental opinion.
Re C (A Minor) (Medical Treatment) (1998)	Life-sustaining treatment would simply delay death and thus it would not be in her best interests to continue treatment.
Re J (a minor) (Wardship: medical treatment) (1991)	The paramount consideration of the courts was the child's best interests and, while the sanctity of life is fundamental, it could be overridden by the child's best interests. This was not the same as ending life or quickening the pace of death as this would be unlawful.
An NHS Trust v B (2006)	The child had some level of awareness and the benefits of treatment would outweigh the burden as the child's suffering was controlled and, at the time of the judgment, containable.
Re K (a minor) (2006)	In contrast to the above case, the baby had no discernable pleasure and suffered pain. It was in her best interests that treatment should cease.

The case below is a very unusual case where there was a very poor relationship between the child and the treating doctors, to the extent that the parents took the case to the European Court of Human Rights.

CASE EXAMPLE

Glass v UK (2004) 39 EHRR 15

The first applicant was a child who had severe mental and physical disabilities and required 24-hour care. He suffered from recurrent respiratory tract infections and the second applicant, his mother, was concerned that he would be given drugs to hasten his death when she had been told that he was suffering from terminal lung disease. A **'Do Not Resuscitate' order** had been placed upon her son's medical records. The relationship between the treating staff and the mother broke down with the police attending to avoid the mother taking the child home. She did not agree with the doctors' view that her son was dying. They applied to the European Court of Human Rights, maintaining that the right to respect for their private lives had been breached in that the dispute between the treating medical professionals and the staff should have been referred to the courts in the first instance, and that they erred in believing their son's condition was an emergency which required them to act as a matter of necessity.

The decision to impose treatment on the child in light of his mother's objections interfered with his right to respect for his private life and his right to physical integrity. Once the parties were clearly in dispute, the Trust should have applied to the court in order to diffuse the situation and to determine what course of action would be taken in a future emergency. As the Trust had overridden the parent's wishes and had no authorisation of the court, Art 8 had been violated.

While this case is a very unusual one, it is easy to lose sight of the importance of the relationship between the treating medical staff and the parents of the child. Clearly, the Trust

'Do not resuscitate' order

An order which permits a doctor not to resuscitate a patient if they stop breathing in order to alleviate further suffering for the patient should have applied to the courts once they felt that it was in the child's best interests not to continue to ventilate the child if a further episode required treatment. To place a 'Do Not Resuscitate' order on the child's notes against the parents' wishes and without a court order will only alienate loved ones.

Earlier in Chapter 2 on Consent, we considered the case of *Re A (Children) (Conjoined Twins: Surgical Separation)* (2001).

CASE EXAMPLE

Re A (Children) (Conjoined Twins: Surgical Separation) [2001] 1 FLR 267

Here, in a highly unusual case, conjoined twin girls were born. Mary was the weaker twin, being parasitic upon the other for her blood supply pumped by the other twin, Jodie's heart. It was apparent that if the twins were not separated, either both would die or Mary would die which would require separation from Jodie in any event. The parents refused consent for the operation to proceed and the Trust applied for a declaration that the operation could proceed without parental consent on the basis that it was in the child's best interests. This case, however, presented novel difficulties:

- What was in the best interests of the twins?
- What was in Mary's best interests?

Given Mary's physical condition, this was a particularly difficult decision. Mary was largely dependent on Jodie for her blood supply, and her heart and lungs had failed. She had a greatly reduced brain capacity and was possibly blind as well. The operation would not be in Mary's best interests as it would undoubtedly cause her death. Ward LJ referred to Lord Brandon in *F v West Berkshire Health Authority* (1990) where he stated that:

JUDGMENT

'The operation will only be in her best interests if, but only if, it is carried out in order either to save her life or to ensure improvement or prevent deterioration in her physical or mental health.'

Clearly the surgery could not be said to be in Mary's best interests as it would lead to her death.

- What was in Jodie's best interests?
- The separation would be in Jodie's best interests as the operation would save her life and without her twin who 'sucks the lifeblood of Jodie' (*per* Ward LJ) she would have every chance of living a full and normal life.
- Given the lack of synergy of the interests of each twin, how can one balance these interests?

In order to reach this decision it was wrong to consider which life had greater value as every life has equal value regardless of disability. Therefore, one could not approach this dilemma by weighing up which twin would have a more useful life. The twins both had the same right to life and the court had the welfare of both twins to consider. On balance the opportunity of giving Jodie a chance of a normal life by performing the operation outweighed the inevitable death that would be caused to Mary. This course of action was the least damaging; although one twin would surely die, the other could lead a normal and full life.

As surgery was deemed by the court to be the best course of action, the next question must surely be as follows:

- Was it a criminal offence to separate the twins?

As the operation would surely kill Mary, the act of separating the twins could amount to murder. The *mens rea* of murder is defined in the cases of *R v Nedrick* (1986) 8 Cr App R (S) 179 and *R v Woollin* (1996). These cases state that the offence of murder will be committed where death (or grievous bodily harm) is a virtual certainty of the defendant's acts and the defendant appreciates as much. Operating on the twins would satisfy both elements and so, by operating on the twins, the surgical team were potentially committing murder. Of course this would not be an issue if the medical team could avail themselves of a valid defence.

The defence of necessity had previously received a sceptical reception in criminal law following the case of *R v Dudley and Stephens* (1884) 14 QBD 273 DC. Here, some castaways killed and ate the cabin boy who was the smallest and weakest of their number, arguing that, had they not, they would have surely died themselves. The argument was rejected by the court and the same principle was repeated many years later in the case of *R v Howe* [1987] AC 417 that one life should never be chosen over the other: one should never appoint another to die in order to protect oneself.

How could the defence of necessity be applied in the current case? Brooke LJ considered the three requirements for the defence of necessity, namely that:

1. the act is needed to avoid inevitable and irreparable evil
2. no more should be done than is reasonably necessary for the purpose to be achieved
3. the evil inflicted must not be disproportionate to the evil avoided.

Given the circumstances the court could reach the decision that 'the interests of Jodie must be preferred to the conflicting interests of Mary' and held that the requirements for necessity were satisfied.

Without doubt, this is an unusual and tragic case where the court felt their way through complex legal and ethical territory. Although it was almost unique on its facts, this case does at least provide us with an indication of how the courts approach the task of determining what decision would be in the child's 'best interests'.

Having considered a number of cases concerning severely ill children, it has become apparent that the courts are guided by the weight of the medical evidence. One might even describe the courts' approach as entirely deferential to medical opinion. Perhaps no case has been as complex or has been before the courts on so many occasions as the case involving Charlotte Wyatt – a case which attracted considerable media attention.

CASE EXAMPLE

Re Wyatt (No. 3) (A child) (Medical treatment; Continuation of Order) [2005] EWHC 693 (Fam)

Charlotte Wyatt was born prematurely at 26 weeks' gestation in 2003 and had suffered considerable and complex medical difficulties since her birth. Due to her prematurity she suffered from acute lung disease. She never left hospital after her birth. As there were disputes and disagreements between the treating medical professionals and Charlotte's parents, the Trust invoked the inherent jurisdiction of the court in order to determine what was in the best interests of Charlotte.

In 2004 Hedley J made a number of declarations in relation to Charlotte's best interests. These provided authority to the medical professionals treating Charlotte that it would be lawful not to ventilate her if she suffered an infection which was resistant to antibiotics and which led or might lead to a collapsed lung. The declarations were not limited in time and were thus continuously in place.

Charlotte continued to defy all medical expectations and survived the winter of 2004. Charlotte's parents again applied to the court seeking to set aside the declarations. One of their areas of complaint was that the courts were determining what treatment would be appropriate in circumstances that had not arisen and, quite possibly, which might not occur in the future. Hedley J refused to discharge the declarations, stating that medical evidence still supported non-ventilation in the event of a respiratory collapse.

The decision above was subject to appeal *(Re Wyatt (A Child) (Medical Treatment: Continuation of Order)* [2005] EWCA Civ 1181). Here, the court took pains to emphasise the nature of the case. It was not itself concerned with whether treatment should be withdrawn from Charlotte in order to allow her to die; the primary issue for the court was what would happen if she required ventilation in order to be kept alive. Medical opinion in 2004 and 2005 was accepted by the court. This said it was not in Charlotte's best interests to be resuscitated as, firstly, it was possible that ventilation might actually kill her; secondly, that it would be painful; finally, because it would not improve her underlying condition. In a lengthy judgment Wall LJ explained there were a number of factors to be taken into account. Although the welfare of the child is paramount and there is a rebuttable presumption in favour of prolonging life, it is also necessary to consider the patient's perspective and conclude, taking all factors into account. Thus, when considering the best interests of a child when determining withholding of medical treatment, best interests included medical, emotional and welfare issues, not just whether the child's life would be intolerable. The declarations remained in place and would be kept under clinical review with the clinicians discussing Charlotte's condition with the parents before any steps are taken.

The last judgment was given in 2006. Here, Hedley J gave his fifth judgment as Charlotte's condition had improved slightly and indeed she had left hospital on a couple of occasions. However, there had also been a serious deterioration. Sadly, communication with the family had been more difficult as the parents had separated. She had contracted a severe infection and had a cough which she could not shake off. Her parents felt that if she was ventilated she would recover. The court maintained its position, having close regard to the medical evidence that ventilation and intubation were not in her best interests. However, it is important to note that the declarations of the court simply provide that it is lawful for the treating staff not to ventilate in the event of a respiratory collapse; it does not restrain them from doing so. At the time of writing, it would appear that Charlotte Wyatt still remains in foster care.

The above litigation was referred to in another case, *T and another v An NHS Trust and another* [2009] EWCA Civ 409 which also attracted considerable media attention.

CASE EXAMPLE

T and another v An NHS Trust and another [2009] EWCA Civ 409

The case concerned an acutely ill nine-month-old boy who was suffering from a genetic mitochondrial condition. The lower court had granted orders and declarations allowing ventilation to be withdrawn and palliative care offered to the child so that he could die peacefully with the least distress. His parents could not support the decision and the Trust applied for an emergency declaration that it would be lawful to withdraw ventilation, and that it was not under a further duty to provide invasive treatment.

The court accepted that further treatment was futile and would only increase the child's suffering. It was also argued on behalf of the child that there had been a breach of Art 8 as the application should not be brought as an emergency. In referring to the cases of *Portsmouth NHS Trust v Wyatt* (2005) and *Glass v UK* (2004) the court rejected that the emergency application was a breach of Art 8, ECHR. Moreover, with reference to Art 2, while the right to life was absolute and life-sustaining treatment must be given, it did not follow that there would be a breach of Art 2 if life-sustaining treatment that was futile according to medical opinion was not given. The case of *R (on the application of Burke) v GMC* (2005) was applied with the effect that there could not be a breach of either Arts 2 or 8 if life-sustaining treatment was no longer in the patient's best interests.

Self-test questions

Ensure that your answers are supported by case law where appropriate.

* Can a patient insist on life-sustaining treatment or will the medical professional always act in the best clinical interests of the patient?
* What approach have the courts taken in relation to life-sustaining treatment and the minor child? What is the predominant view?
* How did the courts wrestle with the best interests dilemma in *Re A (Children) (Surgical Separation)* (2001)?

SUMMARY

■ In an area fraught with medical complexities and ethical dilemmas, common law illustrates that, for patients who in a PVS, medical treatment can be withdrawn and withheld if it is considered to be in the best interests of the patient.

■ This does not mean that it is in the patient's best interests to die, but that there are no best interests in keeping the patient alive. In other words, treatment has become futile.

■ The judgment in *Bland* (1993) has been followed in a number of cases and has survived the provisions of HRA 1998.

■ We have seen from the case of *Burke* (2005) that the 'best interests' principle prevails and that there is no right to insist on medical treatment unless it is supported by clinical indications.

■ Treatment of the minor child is, as expected, fraught with emotion but the courts uphold the principle that the welfare of the child is of paramount importance and this will override parental wishes.

■ The best interests of the patient are the primary consideration of the courts. The case of *Re A (Children) (Conjoined Twins: Surgical Separation)* (2001) probably demonstrates, more than any other case, the profound ethical and legal dilemmas faced by the medical professionals and the courts. Often, there is no happy ending.

Further reading

Herring, J. (2010) *Medical Law and Ethics*, third edition, Chapter 9. Oxford: Oxford University Press.

Jackson, E. (2010) *Medical Law; Text, Cases and Materials*, second edition, Chapter 17. Oxford: Oxford University Press.

Pattinson, S. (2009) *Medical Law and Ethics*, second edition, Chapters 15 and 16. London: Sweet and Maxwell.

Glossary of terms

actus reus
    refers to the physical act in a criminal offence

admixed embryo
    an early stage embryo which combines both human and non-human material

artificial nutrition and hydration
    where the patient receives any form of nutrition of food and fluid via a tube

artificial ventilation
    where the patient is dependent upon artificial ventilation to help them breathe

beneficence
    doing good for one's patients

blastocyst
    the cluster of cells after fertilisation of egg and sperm which must then move from the fallopian tube to the uterus

breach
    the infringement of a legal obligation

cardio-respiratory/cardiopulmonary
    relating to the heart and lungs

claimant
    the aggrieved patient himself/herself, or a person claiming on their behalf

conjoined
    twins fused by one embryo failing to divide into two

CTG
    cardiotocography is the technology which records the foetal heartbeat

defendant
    the person against whom the claim is brought

dialysis
    a way of cleaning the blood by passing it through a machine to replace the normal function of a kidney

'Do not resuscitate' order
    an order which permits a doctor not to resuscitate a patient if they stop breathing in order to alleviate further suffering for the patient

fecundity
    the ability to produce further pleasures

gametes
    are reproductive cells, either eggs (or ova) or sperm

gender dysphoria
    a condition where a person feels a lack of certainty about his or her birth gender

genotype
    the genetic make up of an individual

haemorrhage
    a considerable level of bleeding from ruptured blood vessels

human somatic nuclei
    the nucleus of a human biological cell

ICU
    intensive care unit – a specialised hospital unit providing intensive care treatment

in-vitro fertilisation (IVF)
    a form of assisted reproduction where eggs or ova are removed from a woman's ovary. In laboratory conditions, the eggs are then fertilised with male sperm and return to the woman's uterus

judicial review
    a way of challenging the decision of public bodies in the courts

loco parentis
    Latin term for where a person or an organisation acts 'in place of a parent'

mastectomy
    a surgical procedure for the removal of one or both of a woman's breasts

mens rea
    refers to the mental element of a criminal offence

motor neurone disease
    neuro-degenerative disease

neo-gastric tube
    can be used as a method of feeding by inserting a plastic tube through the nose, down the throat and into the stomach

non-malfeasance
    not harming one's patients

permanent vegetative state
    a long term condition where the patient is in a coma like state with no periods of wakefulness or has no cognitive function

pluripotent cells
    cells which cannot develop into a complete organism

primary progressive multiple sclerosis
    a form of multiple sclerosis. A progressive auto-immune disease

primitive streak
    a faint white area on the end region of the embryonic disc along which the embryo will develop

propinquity
    close or proximate

retrolental fibroplasia
    an eye disease detected in babies born prematurely

spinal muscular atrophy
a condition which causes progressive muscular degeneation

tetraplagic
the term given to describe a person who has lost control of arms and legs by illness or injury

therapeutic
where a drug has some beneficial healing powers

totipotent cells
cells which are capable of forming entire organisms

transsexualism
where a person of one gender strongly identifies him or herself as a member of the opposite sex

vasectomy
a surgical procedure for male sterilisation

Index